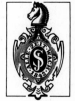

H. Schmidt-Gayk · F. P. Armbruster
R. Bouillon (Eds.)

Calcium Regulating Hormones, Vitamin D Metabolites, and Cyclic AMP

Assays and Their Clinical Application

With 142 figures and 58 tables

Springer-Verlag Berlin Heidelberg New York
London Paris Tokyo Hong Kong Barcelona

Professor Dr. med. Heinrich Schmidt-Gayk
Im Breitspiel 15, D-6900 Heidelberg

Franz Paul Armbruster, Dipl.Ing. (chem.)
Immundiagnostik GmbH
Wilhelmstraße 7
D-6140 Bensheim

Professor Dr. Roger Bouillon
Katholieke Universiteit Leuven
Laboratorium voor Experimentele Geneeskunde
en Endocrinologie (LEGENDO),
Gasthuisberg,
B-3000 Leuven

ISBN 3-540-52229-8 Springer-Verlag Berlin Heidelberg New York
ISBN 3-387-52229-8 Springer-Verlag New York Berlin Heidelberg

Library of Congress Cataloging-in-Publication Data
Calcium regulating hormones, vitamin D metabolites, and cyclic
AMP assays and their clinical application / H. Schmidt-Gayk,
F.P. Armbruster, R. Bouillon (eds.). p. cm.
Includes bibliographical references. Includes index.
ISBN 3-540-52229-8 (alk, paper) ISBN 0-387-52229-8 (alk. paper)
1. Parathyroid hormone--Analysis. 2. Calcitonin--Analysis.
3. Vitamin D--Analysis. 4. Cyclic adenylic acid--Analysis.
I. Schmidt-Gayk, H. (Heinrich), 1944. II. Armbruster,
F. P. (Franz Paul), 1957 . III. Bouillon, R.
[DNLM: 1. Biological Assay--methods. 2. Calcitonin--analysis.
3. Calcium--analysis. 4. Parathyroid Hormone--analysis.
5. Radioimmunoassay--methods. 6. Vitamin D--metabolism.
QV 276 C1442] QP572.P3C35 1990 616.07'56--dc20 DNLM/DLC
for Library of Congress 90-10022

© Springer-Verlag Berlin Heidelberg 1990
Printed in Germany

The use of registered names, trademarks, etc. in this publication does not imply, even in the absence of a specific statement, that names are exempt from the relevant protective laws and regulations and therefore free for general use.

Product liability: The publisher can give no guarantee for information about drug dosage and application thereof contained in this book, in every individual case the respective user must check its accuracy by consulting other pharmaceutical literature.

Typesetting: Macmillan India Ltd., Bangalore, India
Printing: Color-Druck Dorfi, Berlin; Bookbinding: Lüderitz & Bauer, Berlin
2127/3020-543210 – Printed on acid-free paper.

List of Contributors

Aker, I., Clinical Laboratory, Department of Surgery, University of Heidelberg, D-6900 Heidelberg, F.R.G.*

Armbruster, F. P., Immundiagnostik GmbH, Wilhelmstr. 7, D-6140 Bensheim

Bellet, D., Unité d'Immunochimie, Institut Gustave-Roussy, and Faculté des Sciences Pharmaceutiques et Biologiques, Paris, France

Birringer, H., Clinical Laboratory, Department of Surgery, University of Heidelberg, D-6900 Heidelberg, F.R.G.*

Blind, E., Department of Endocrinology, University of Heidelberg, D-6900 Heidelberg, F.R.G.

Böhler. U., Clinical Laboratory, Department of Surgery, University of Heidelberg, D-6900 Heidelberg, F.R.G.*

Bohuon, C., Department of Clinical Biology, Institut Gustave-Roussy and Faculté des Sciences Pharmaceutiques et Biologiques, Chatenay Malabry, France

Bothe, V., Clinical Laboratory, Department of Surgery, University of Heidelberg, D-6900 Heidelberg, F.R.G.*

Bouillon, R., Katholieke Universiteit Leuven, Laboratorium voor Experimentele Geneeskunde en Endocrinologie, Onderwijs en Navorsing, Gasthuisberg, B-3000 Leuven, Belgium

Fischer, S., Department of Surgery, Abt. 2.1.1, University of Heidelberg, D-6900 Heidelberg, F.R.G.

Flentje, D., Department of Surgery, Abt. 2.1.1, University of Heidelberg, D-6900 Heidelberg, F.R.G.

Ghillani, P., Uniteé d'Immunochimie, Institut Gustave-Roussy, F-94805 Villejuif Cedex, France

Grauer, A., Department of Endocrinology, University of Heidelberg, D-6900 Heidelberg, F.R.G.

Herfarth, K., Department of Surgery, Abt. 2.1.1, University of Heidelberg, D-6900 Heidelberg, F.R.G.

Hitzler, W., Clinical Laboratory, Department of Surgery, University of Heidelberg, D-6900 Heidelberg, F.R.G.

Horst, R. L., National Animal Disease Center, U.S. Department of Agriculture, Agricultural Research Service, P.O. Box 70, Ames, IA 50010, USA

Kunst, G., Clinical Laboratory, Department of Surgery, University of Heidelberg, D-6900 Heidelberg, F.R.G.*

Limbach, H. J., Im Breitspiel 15, D-6900 Heidelberg, F.R.G.

Mayer, E., Lindenstraße 17, D-5450 Neuwied 22, F.R.G.

Motté, Ph., Institut Mérieux, 1541 avenue Marcel Mérieux, F-69280 Marcy l'Etoile, France

Ratcliffe, J. G., Wolfson Research Laboratories, Department of Clinical Chemistry, Queen Elizabeth Medical Centre, Birmingham B15 2TH, United Kingdom

Ratcliffe, W. A., Wolfson Research Laboratories, Department of Clinical Chemistry, Queen Elizabeth Medical Centre, Birmingham B15 2TH, United Kingdom

Raue, F., Department of Endocrinology, University of Heidelberg, D-6900 Heidelberg, F.R.G.

Reichel, H., Department of Nephrology, University of Heidelberg, D-6900 Heidelberg, F.R.G.

Reinhardt, T. A., National Animal Disease Center, U.S. Department of Agriculture, Agricultural Research Service, P.O. Box 70, Ames, IA 50010, USA

Scharfenstein, H., Clinical Laboratory, Department of Surgery, University of Heidelberg, D-6900 Heidelberg, F.R.G.*

Scharla, S., Department of Endocrinology, University of Heidelberg, D-6900 Heidelberg, F.R.G.

Schmidt-Gayk, H., Im Breitspiel 15, D-6900 Heidelberg, F.R.G.

Schneider. H.-G., Department of Endocrinology, University of Heidelberg, D-6900 Heidelberg, F.R.G.

Stadler, A., Clinical Laboratory, Department of Surgery, University of Heidelberg, D-6900 Heidelberg, F.R.G.*

Troalen, F., Unité d'Immunochimie, Institut Gustave-Roussy, F-94805 Villejuif Cedex, France

Vogel, G., Clinical Laboratory, Department of Surgery, University of Heidelberg, D-6900 Heidelberg, F.R.G.*

Walch, S., Im Breitspiel 15, D-6900 Heidelberg, F.R.G.

Zillikens, D., Clinical Laboratory, Department of Surgery, University of Heidelberg, D-6900 Heidelberg, F.R.G.*

* address all correspondense to the first editor.

Preface

There are very few books available containing details on the assay of calcium regulating hormones. The volume Assay of Calcium Regulating Hormones, edited by D. D. Bickle, was published in 1983, but since then rapid progress has been made in our understanding of calcium matabolism and in the assays of calcium regulating hormones. To mention just a few:

A revised structure of parathyroid hormone (PTH) has been confirmed by cDNA techniques. The peptides with the correct structure are commercially available, and assays for intact PTH have been developed that exhibit extreme sensitivity and specificity.

Parathyroid hormone-related protein (PTH-rP) is a substance that has been recently discovered. Assays for PTH-rP have been developed, but many questions remain to be answered about the clinical usefulness of the assay of PTH-rP.

The clinical significance of vitamin D metabolites in serum has become much clearer, and more direct measurements of 25-hydroxyvitamin D and 1,25-dihydroxyvitamin D allow an easier diagnosis and more appropriate therapeutic intervention.

The diagnostic value of new peptides from the calcitonin gene has been investigated. Highly sensitive immunoradiometric assays for the measurement of calcitonin in serum or plasma have recently been introduced, facilitating the diagnosis of early familiar medullary thyroid carcinoma. It is hoped that the physiology and pathophysiology of calcitonin may be clarified by these new assays.

We have felt the lack of a recent review on calcium regulating hormones and related topics and have consequently attempted to provide a collection of clinical reviews and detailed assay protocols. The first chapters deal with clinical information relevant to calcium regulating hormones. These chapters are followed by a description of methods for the assay of calcium regulating hormones, many of which have already been described in other publications. As they are all updated, these second-generation assays replace older methods. Because some assays have been in clinical use for years, it is now possible to evaluate their clinical utility. We hope that the book will be welcomed by physicians and chemists working in laboratories and clinics involved with calcium-related diseases and that it will be useful for years to come.

We are pleased to have been able to cooperate with experts in endocrinology, who have provided up-to-date constributions from their particular areas of expertise. We also thank Springer-Verlag for its valuable assistance in preparing the book.

Heidelberg, July 1990   H. Schmidt-Gayk

Contents

3   Parathyroid Hormone-Related Protein

4   Cyclic AMP

5   Vitamin D: Assays of 25-Hydroxyvitamin D (Calcidiol) and 1,25-Dihydroxyvitamin D (Calcitriol)

1 Introduction

Calcium metabolism is regulated by three specific hormones: parathyroid hormone (PTH), calcitriol, and calcitonin. Other factors may also contribute to the regulation, among them parathyroid hormone-related protein (PTH-rP). The activity of PTH and PTH-rP is in part reflected by the concentration of cyclic AMP in urine.

Methods for the quantitative measurement of calcium regulating hormones, vitamin D metabolites, and cyclic AMP are necessary for the reliable diagnosis of disorders affecting calcium metabolism. Clinically, a reliable assay for the quantitation of parathyroid gland activity is most often requested. To assess parathyroid function, many assays for PTH are available. Until recently, PTH was measured mainly by assays detecting the mid-regional or the carboxyl-terminal part of the hormone. Since 1987 the assay of intact PTH has gained wider acceptance.

At the beginning of this century vitamin D was still considered a single substance produced in one tissue (the skin) and acting on one system (calcium-bone homeostasis). We now realize that it is part of a complex system in which many tissues or cells contribute to the formation of vitamin D metabolites and bear receptors for calcitriol. Measurement of the main vitamin D metabolites has been improved markedly by the advent of more direct measurements of 25-hydroxyvitamin D (calcidiol) and 1,25-dihydroxyvitamin D (calcitriol).

Calcitonin (CT) was discovered in the 1960s by Copp and colleagues, who first recognized the calcium-lowering effect of this hormone which is produced and secreted by the thyroid C-cells. The physiological function of CT remains uncertain, but its diagnostic role as a marker of medullary thyroid carcinoma, a tumor of the C-cells, is indisputable. This diagnostic tool might be extended to include the peptides encoded by the calcitonin gene, i.e., calcitonin gene-related peptide and katacalcin. Highly sensitive immunoradiometric assays for the measurement of CT have recently been introduced, and they may help to elucidate the physiological function of CT.

Chapter 1.1

Clinical Application of Intact Parathyroid Hormone Determination*

E. Blind, D. Flentje, and S. Fischer

Introduction

The concentration of calcium ions in blood is, along with calcitriol and calcitonin, mainly regulated by parathyroid hormone (Parathyrin, PTH). In patients with disorders of calcium metabolism, measurement of serum PTH plays an important role, specifically to differentiate hypercalcemia due to primary hyperparathyroidism from other hypercalcemic disorders, in which a high serum calcium tends to suppress the secretion of PTH [30]. Conversely, in the differential diagnosis of hypocalcemia, serum PTH measurements may be useful to distinguish hypoparathyroidism from other causes [21]. In secondary hyperparathyroidism, commonly caused by chronic renal failure, PTH can be measured to assess parathyroid overactivity.

Measurement of serum PTH concentrations is complicated by the fact that there are several fragments of the hormone in the circulation, as a result of the metabolism of PTH either peripherally or within the parathyroid glands [22]. The biologically active intact hormone represents only a small portion of the total PTH immunoreactivity, and it is, in fact, present in the circulation in very low amounts (10^{-11}–10^{-12} mol/liter) [11]. PTH is an 84-amino acid peptide, the sequence of which is shown in Fig. 1. Intact PTH is cleaved, mainly by the liver, between the amino acid residues 34–37 into fragments which include the N-terminal or the C-terminal sequence of the hormone. The N-terminal fragments contain the biologically active sequence of PTH and are cleared quickly from the circulation. In contrast, biologically inactive midregion and C-terminal fragments disappear less rapidly from the circulation and thus are present in higher concentrations.

The immunoheterogeneity of PTH in serum has led to the development of several different PTH radioimmunoassays (RIAs). Many of them detect a specific part of the hormone ("fragment assays") and their usefulness is often restricted to certain questions. The most widely used PTH RIAs are directed against the midregion or C-terminal part of the hormone. Although these assays

---

* This work was supported by Deutsche Forschungsgemeinschaft (Schm/7-1). Parts of this chapter have been published in *Journal of Clinical Endocrinology and Metabolism*.

```
              1  2  3  4  5  6  7   8  9 10 11 12 13 14 15 16
Human-PTH:  NH₂-SerValSerGluIleGlnLeuMetHisAsnLeuGlyLysHisLeuAsn
Bovine-PTH:     Ala. . . . . . . . Phe. . . . . . . . . . . . . . . . Ser
Pig-PTH:        . . . . . . . . . . Phe. . . . . . . . . . . . . . . . Ser
Rat-PTH:        Ala. . . . . . . . . . . . . . . . . . . . . . . . . . Ala
```

```
            17 18  19 20 21 22 23 24 25 26 27 28 29 30 31 32 33
            SerMetGluArgValGluTrpLeuArgLysLysLeuGlnAspValHisAsn
            . . . . . . . . . . . . . . . . . . . . . . . . . . . . . . . .
            . . .Leu. . . . . . . . . . . . . . . . . . . . . . . . . .
            . . .Val. . . . . .MetGln. . . . . . . . . . . . . . . . .
```

```
            34 35 36 37 38 39 40 41 42 43 44 45 46 47 48 49 50
            PheValAlaLeuGlyAlaProLeuAlaProArgAspAlaGlySerGlnArg
            . . . . . . . . . . . . .SerIle. . . Tyr. . . . .GlySer. . . . . . .
            . . . . . . . . . . . . .SerIleVal. His. . . . .Gly. . . . . . .
            . . . . . Ser. . . . .ValGlnMet. . .Ala. . .GluGlySerTyr. . . . .
```

```
            51 52 53 54 55 56 57 58 59 60 61 62 63 64 65 66 67
            ProArgLysLysGluAspAsnValLeuValGluSerHisGluLysSerLeu
            . . . . . . . . . . . . . . . . . . . . . . . . . . . .Gln. . . . . . .
            . . . . . . . . . . . . . . . . . . . . . . . . . . . .Gln. . . . . .
            . . .Thr. . . . . . . . . . . . . . .AspGlyAsnSer. . . . . .
```

```
            68 69 70 71 72 73 74 75 76 77 78 79 80 81 82 83 84
            GlyGluAlaAspLysAlaAspValAsnValLeuThrLysAlaLysSerGln -COOH
            . . . . . . . . . . . . . . . .Asp. . . . .Ile. . . . . . . Pro. . . .
            . . . . . . . . . . . . .Ala. . .Asp. . . . .Ile. . . . . . . Pro. . . .
            . . . . .Gly. . . . . . . . . . Asp. . . . .Val. . . . . . . . . . . .
```

Fig. 1. Amino acid sequence of human, bovine, porcine and rat PTH [13, 15]. The human sequence is shown as determined by Keutmann et al. [15] except for position 76, which was found to be asparagine (instead of aspartic acid) by nucleotide sequencing of cloned cDNA encoding human PTH messenger RNA [14]. The revised amino acid sequence was supported by immunological data of native human PTH [10]

detect mainly biologically inactive fragments of PTH, many of them can clearly discriminate patients with primary hyperparathyroidism from normal persons [20, 32]. In renal dysfunction, however, the elevated results obtained by these assays must be interpreted with caution, because midregion and C-terminal fragments are removed from the circulation mainly by glomerular filtration [9, 22]. In the differential diagnosis of hypercalcemia these assays are less useful [30], for reasons which are discussed in this chapter. In those patients, N-terminal assays, which do detect both intact PTH and biologically active N-terminal fragments, are more reliable but, on the other hand, do not always detect primary hyperparathyroidism. Furthermore, many PTH RIAs are not sufficiently sensitive to distinguish normal from subnormal PTH values [21]. Recently, Armitage has reviewed the clinical utility of different PTH assays and the role that PTH metabolism has played in their development [2].

The best way to study the secretory activity of the parathyroid glands directly may be to measure the biologically active intact hPTH(1-84) molecule. PTH RIAs, however, have proved to be either not sufficiently sensitive for reliably detecting the small amounts of intact hormone in normal subjects or not sufficiently specific to avoid detection of circulating PTH fragments [2, 17, 19]. Chapter 2.8 deals further with the problems of measuring intact PTH and summarizes the methods and characteristics of intact PTH assays which have been published to date. The two-site immunoradiometric assay (IRMA) technique is now available to measure intact PTH [4, 6, 27]. This method overcomes the limitations of older assays as it is both sensitive enough to detect the low amounts of intact hormone in normal subjects and specific enough to prevent nonspecific serum effects and cross-reaction with inactive fragments. The usefulness of our assay (Chap. 2.8) in the investigation of patients with various disorders of calcium metabolism is shown in this chapter. The results are compared with those obtained using a well-established serum midregion PTH assay.

Methods and Subjects

Two-Site Assay of Intact PTH

The development and characteristics of the assay are described in Chap. 2.8 in detail and were reported previously [4]. An N-terminal PTH antiserum (code G774) was raised in a goat immunized with extracts from human adenomatous glands, while a C-terminal antiserum (code R82) was raised in a rabbit immunized with synthetic hPTH(53-84). A solid-phase system was established by covalently linking the N-terminal antiserum to cellulose particles. These particles were used to separate intact PTH and N-terminal fragments from plasma samples (analyzed in duplicate), thus avoiding any interference from other plasma proteins, including biologically inactive midregion and C-terminal fragments in the subsequent steps of the assay. In the second step, the C-terminal antiserum was added and finally labeled at the second free binding site of this antibody with $[^{125}I]$ Tyr^{52}-hPTH(53-84). The radioactivity bound was proportional to the content of intact PTH in the tubes, since the peptide acted as a link between the solid-phase bound N-terminal antibody and the indirectly labeled C-terminal antibody. The assay was sufficiently sensitive to allow detection of intact PTH in all normal subjects. The assay did not cross-react with several synthetic PTH fragments (Table 1). In addition, there was no interference with large amounts of the biologically inactive fragment hPTH(39-84). Further characteristics of this assay are shown in Table 1.

Table 1. Characteristics of the immunoradiometric two-site assay for intact hPTH(1-84) and the RIA of midregion hPTH(44-68)

	Intact PTH	Midregion PTH
Assay standard[a]	hPTH(1-84)	hPTH(44-68)
Detection limit (pmol/liter)	0.6	15
Normal range (pmol/liter)[b]	2.0–6.3	< 15–40
Sample volume/tube (µl)	200	100
Overall incubation time (h)	65	50
Cross-reactivity[c]		
hPTH(1-34), hPTH(28-48)	0.0	0.0
hPTH(1-44), hPTH(39-84)	0.0	
hPTH(64-84)		0.0
hPTH(44-68), hPTH(53-84)	0.0	1.0
hPTH(1-84)	1.0	0.4[d]
Reference	Blind et al. [4]	Schmidt-Gayk et al. [32]

[a] Synthetic peptides. Mol wts: hPTH(1-84), 9425; hPTH(44-68), 2838

[b] The reference limits are those reported in the initial clinical validation of the methods and are based on results from 58 normal subjects for the intact [4] and on 124 normal subjects for the midregion assay [32]

[c] Relative reactivity of synthetic peptides expressed on a molar basis. The reactivity with the assay standard was considered 1.0. Zero cross-reactivity was confirmed with concentrations up to 2000 pmol/liter for the midregion RIA and up to 6400 pmol/liter for the intact PTH assay

[d] 440 pmol/liter hPTH(1-84) was equipotent to 180 pmol/liter hPTH(44-68) at a 50% bound-to-free ratio

Radioimmunoassay of Midregion PTH

The midregion PTH assay was performed as described previously [32], except that determinations were carried out in duplicate. A version of this assay, which has been further developed, is described in Chap. 2.4. The antiserum (code MS6) was raised in a guinea pig immunized with extracts from human adenomatous glands. Purified ^{125}I-labeled Tyr^{43}-hPTH(44-68) was used as tracer to perform an equilibrium assay. Bound from free labeled PTH was separated by the second antibody method. The PTH recognition site of the antibody in this RIA was between amino acid residues 53 and 63. Table 1 shows some further assay characteristics.

Samples and Measurement

Clinical chemistry reports were reviewed to determine the patient's total serum calcium on the date the specimens were obtained for PTH measurement. If no such calcium values were available, total serum calcium was determined by flame photometry in the same specimen in which PTH was determined. When multiple preoperative serum PTH and calcium values were available in patients with primary hyperparathyroidism, the mean value was calculated.

We accepted both serum and plasma samples for measurement of intact PTH if the specimens were assayed soon after the plasma or serum had been separated from blood or stored at $-30\,°C$ until assay; the results are hereafter referred to as serum results. The PTH measurements were performed in several different assays over a period of 11 months. Serum intact PTH was measured in all patients (see below), whereas midregion PTH was determined in fewer patients because serum had not been available from some patients. PTH was measured by an immunochemiluminometric assay of intact PTH (Chap. 2.9) in 30 of the 100 patients with primary hyperparathyroidism.

Study Subjects

We studied the following groups of subjects:

1. Fifty-two ostensibly healthy blood donors and members of the laboratory staff (20 women and 32 men; age range 21–58 years).
2. One hundred patients (76 women and 24 men) with primary hyperparathyroidism (in 84 primary hyperparathyroidism was confirmed surgically, in the other 16 patients primary hyperparathyroidism was presumed but operation was either not performed or was unsuccessful) with serum total calcium concentrations ranging from 2.56 to 3.80 mmol/liter [mean 2.97 (SD 0.28), median 2.91 mmol/liter].
3. Two patients with parathyroid carcinoma and elevated serum total calcium concentrations (2.90 and 3.05 mmol/liter) at the time of PTH measurement.
4. Twenty-five patients (21 women and 4 men) with either idiopathic or surgical hypoparathyroidism, treated with calciferol, who had serum total calcium values ranging from 1.52 to 2.26 mmol/liter [mean 1.95 (SD 0.24)].
5. Two patients with pseudohypoparathyroidism.
6. Forty patients (24 women and 16 men) with severe malignancy-associated hypercalcemia [18 patients with breast carcinoma, 10 with carcinoma of the bronchus, 4 with hypernephroma, and 8 with malignancy of other sites (mediastinum, pancreas, cervix, prostate, melanoma)], with serum total calcium values ranging from 2.42 to 4.22 mmol/liter [mean 3.17 (SD 0.46)]; some of these patients had compromised renal function.
7. Twenty-seven patients (14 women and 13 men) with chronic renal failure (17 treated by hemodialysis).
8. Twenty patients with end-stage renal failure who had received a renal graft within the previous 4 years.

Results

Normal Subjects

In the 52 normal subjects, serum intact PTH concentrations ranged from 1.5 to 6.8 pmol/liter [mean 3.9 (SD 1.3)], but there was no significant correlation between serum total calcium and intact PTH values. The serum midregion PTH concentrations, measured in 36 of these subjects, ranged from undetectable (< 15) to 57 pmol/liter.

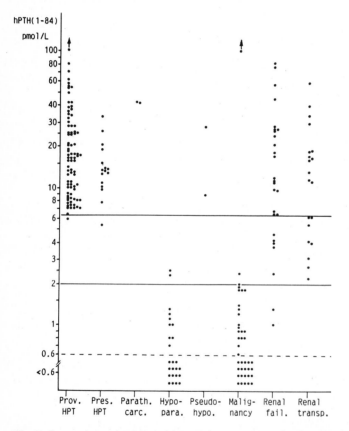

Fig. 2. Serum intact hPTH(1–84) concentrations in 100 patients with presumed (*Pres. HPT*; n = 16) or proven (*Prov. HPT*; n = 84) primary hyperparathyroidism, 2 patients with parathyroid carcinoma (*Parath. carc.*), 25 patients with hypoparathyroidism (*Hypopara.*), 2 patients with pseudohypoparathyroidism (*Pseudohypo.*), 40 patients with malignancy-associated hypercalcemia (*Malignancy*), 27 patients with chronic renal failure (*Renal fail.*; among them 17 patients receiving hemodialysis), and 20 patients after renal transplantation (*Renal transp.*). *Solid lines* indicate the limits of the normal range, the *dotted line* marks the detection limit, and the *arrows* indicate values beyond the scale

Results in Patients with Primary Hyperparathyroidism

Of 100 patients with primary hyperparathyroidism, 98 had serum intact PTH concentrations above the upper limit of the normal range (Fig. 2), whereas the sensitivity of the midregion assay was less (Fig. 3, Table 2). The percentages of patients with only slightly elevated serum PTH values were similar, however (Table 2). The mean serum intact PTH concentration (21.1 pmol/liter) was 3.3-fold higher than the upper limit of normal compared with 4.6-fold for the serum midregion PTH concentration (184 pmol/liter).

The relationship between serum total calcium, intact PTH (Fig. 6), and midregion PTH was studied in patients with primary hyperparathyroidism.

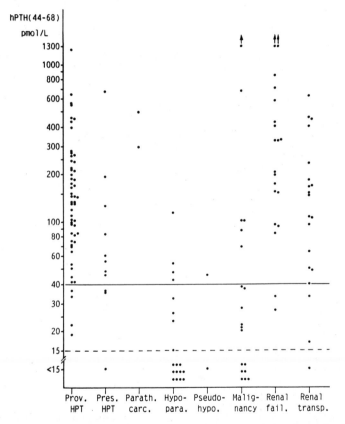

Fig. 3. Serum midregion hPTH(44-68) concentrations, determined in most of the patients shown in Fig. 2: presumed primary hyperparathyroidism ($n = 11$), proven primary hyperparathyroidism ($n = 55$), parathyroid carcinoma ($n = 2$), hypoparathyroidism ($n = 19$), pseudohypoparathyroidism ($n = 2$), malignancy-associated hypercalcemia ($n = 19$), chronic renal failure ($n = 20$), and renal transplantation ($n = 20$). The *solid line* indicates the upper limit of the normal range, the *dotted line* marks the detection limit, and the *arrows* indicate values beyond the scale

Table 2. Serum PTH values in hypercalcemic patients with malignancy and in patients with primary hyperparathyroidism, as determined by serum hPTH(1-84) and midregion hPTH(44-68) assays

	Intact PTH	Midregion PTH
Primary hyperparathyroidism[a]		
Within normal range	1/66 (2%) (2/100)	7/66 (11%)
Elevated above ULN[b]	65/66 (98%) (98/100)	59/66 (89%)
1.2-fold above ULN	58/66 (88%) (89/100)	54/66 (82%)
1.4-fold above ULN	49/66 (74%) (79/100)	51/66 (77%)
Malignancy		
Below normal range	37/40 (93%)	—
Within normal range	2/40 (5%)	13/19 (68%)
Elevated above ULN	1/40 (3%)[c]	6/19 (32%)[c]

[a] In the patients with primary hyperparathyroidism intact PTH was measured in 100 patients (results in parentheses), whereas midregion PTH and intact PTH, as determined by IRMA, were measured in 66 specimens
[b] ULN, Upper limit of the corresponding normal range (6.3 pmol/liter for the intact IRMA and 40 pmol/liter for the midregion RIA)
[c] One patient in this group had ectopic PTH production

Table 3. Relationship between intact hPTH(1-84), midregion hPTH(44-68), and serum total calcium values in 49 patients with primary hyperparathyroidism

Intact PTH	$= 12.8 + 0.038 \times$ midregion PTH	$r = 0.57$
Intact PTH	$= -69.7 + 30.1 \times$ calcium	$r = 0.54$
Midregion PTH	$= -1181 + 456 \times$ calcium	$r = 0.58$

Intact PTH and midregion PTH in pmol/liter; calcium in millimoles per liter; r = coefficient of correlation

Linear regression analysis revealed only a moderate correlation between all three parameters (Table 3).

Parathyroid Hormone in Primary Hyperparathyroidism During Parathyroid Surgery

In ten patients with a solitary parathyroid adenoma the clearance of intact PTH was studied during parathyroid surgery (Fig. 4). The mean basal value before removal of the adenoma was 18.2 pmol/liter (SD 10.1) and fell to 3.8 pmol/liter (SD 1.3) within 15 min after clamping of the adenoma. The average concentration of intact PTH in the peripheral circulation fell by 44%

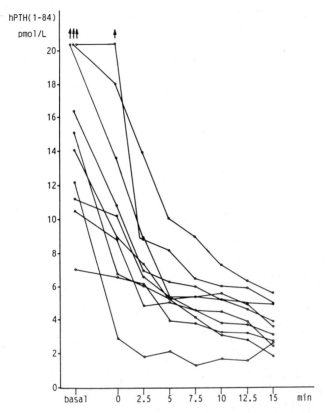

Fig. 4. Serum intact PTH concentrations in ten patients with a solitary parathyroid adenoma during parathyroid surgery, determined before, during (= 0 min), and after clamping of the adenoma. The *arrows* indicate values beyond the scale

(SD 16) within 5 min after clamping of the individual adenoma. In the subsequent 10 min, however, the concentration fell less quickly by 33.1% (SD 21.5).

In one patient intact PTH values were compared with the midregion PTH immunoreactivity during parathyroid surgery (Fig. 5). The serum intact PTH concentration was elevated approximately fourfold and fell by 45%, from 23.3 to 12.9 pmol/liter, within 5 min after clamping of the parathyroid adenoma, whereas the serum midregion PTH concentration fell much more slowly (by 11%, from 110 to 98 pmol/liter) within the same time.

Parathyroid Hormone in Hypoparathyroid and Pseudohypoparathyroid Patients

In the 25 hypoparathyroid patients serum intact PTH was undetectable ($n = 15$) or below the normal range ($n = 8$) in 92%. Two patients had values in the low normal range. With the midregion assay we were not able to distinguish these

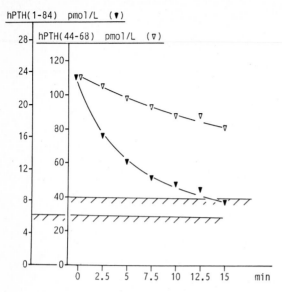

Fig. 5. Serum intact PTH (▼) and midregion PTH (▽) concentrations in a patient during parathyroid surgery, determined after clamping of a parathyroid adenoma. The *solid lines* indicate the upper limits of normal

patients from normal subjects, because midregion PTH was not detectable in all normal subjects by this method. Four patients had slightly elevated serum midregion PTH values. The two patients with pseudohypoparathyroidism had elevated serum intact PTH levels.

Results in Malignancy-Associated Hypercalcemia

The patients with malignancy-associated hypercalcemia usually had low serum intact PTH levels (Fig. 2, Table 2). Hence, these patients could be easily distinguished from the patients with primary hyperparathyroidism, even when their serum total calcium concentrations were only slightly elevated (Fig. 6). The separation of these groups by the midregion assay was less good; six patients had elevated values (Fig. 3, Table 2).

One patient with a bronchial carcinoid had evidence of the very rare condition of true pseudohyperparathyroidism i.e., ectopic PTH secretion. This patient had extremely high serum intact (253 pmol/liter) and midregion (3970 pmol/liter) PTH concentrations which became normal together with serum calcium after removal of the tumor.

Two patients had normal serum total calcium levels on the day the PTH sample was obtained (Fig. 6), although they had previously been hypercalcemic.

To lower the serum calcium level, 13 of these patients were treated with a diphosphonate. In parallel to the normalization of the calcium levels, intact

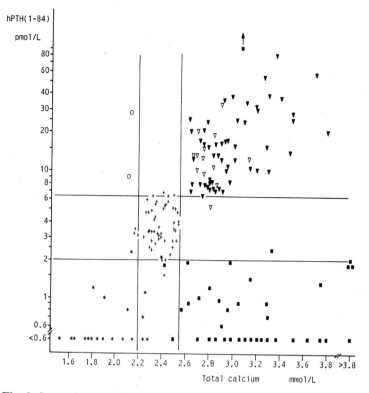

Fig. 6. Serum intact PTH concentrations in normal subjects and patients with disorders of calcium metabolism, plotted against simultaneously measured serum total calcium values: 52 normal subjects (+), 67 patients with proven (▼) or presumed (▽) primary hyperparathyroidism, 19 patients with hypoparathyroidism (∗), 2 patients with pseudo-hypoparathyroidism (○), and 38 patients with malignancy-associated hypercalcemia (■). The *solid lines* mark the limits of the normal ranges, and the *arrow* indicates a PTH value beyond the scale

PTH rose significantly from a subnormal mean value of 0.7 pmol/liter to a mean value of 5.2 pmol/liter. Figure 7 shows the nonlinear inverse correlation between both parameters.

Parathyroid Hormone in Chronic Renal Failure and After Renal Transplantation

In 20 of the 27 patients with chronic renal failure serum PTH was determined simultaneously in both assays. Two patients with high serum intact (27 and 78 pmol/liter) and midregion (1340 and 3900 pmol/liter) PTH values had elevated serum total calcium values and therefore presumably tertiary hyperparathyroidism. In the other 18 patients serum total calcium values were either within (n = 10) or below (n = 8) the normal range. Serum intact PTH

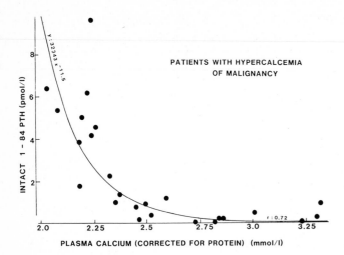

Fig. 7. Relationship between calcium levels (corrected for protein) and intact hPTH(1-84). In 13 patients with malignancy-associated hypercalcemia PTH levels were suppressed during hypercalcemia; after lowering the calcium levels the release of PTH increased substantially [31]

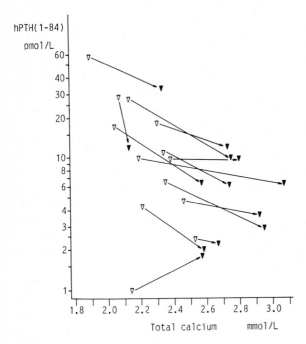

Fig. 8. Relationship between serum total calcium and intact hPTH(1-84) in 13 renal dialysis patients, showing that intact PTH concentrations are lower after (▼) than before (▽) dialysis as serum calcium levels rise

Table 4. Serum intact hPTH(1-84), midregion hPTH(44-68), and total calcium values in 13 patients with chronic renal failure before and after dialysis

Parameters (normal range)	Before dialysis	After dialysis	% Change[a]
Total calcium (2.20–2.55 mmol/liter)			
Mean (± SD)	2.23 ± 0.18	2.68 ± 0.25	+ 20.2
Median	2.21	2.73	+ 23.5
Range	1.89–2.53	2.13–3.07	
Intact PTH (2.0–6.3 pmol/liter)			
Mean (± SD)	15.2 ± 15.6	8.3 ± 8.3	− 45.4
Median	9.8	6.3	− 35.7
Range	1.0–58	1.8–33	
Midregion PTH (< 15–40 pmol/liter)			
Mean[b] (± SD)	252 ± 238	234 ± 207	− 7.0
Median	198	180	− 9.9
Range[b]	27–850	35–795	

[a] The percentage changes are calculated as the average of the percentage change in each individual patient

[b] These values were calculated after exclusion of one patient's midregion PTH value of 705 pmol/liter before and 1700 pmol/liter after dialysis. With this patient included, the corresponding mean serum midregion PTH values before and after dialysis were 286 and 347 pmol/liter, respectively

was less often elevated (15 of 20 patients) than serum midregion PTH (18 of 20 patients). These 20 patients had mean serum intact PTH values of 20.3 pmol/liter (3.2-fold elevated above the upper limit of normal) and midregion PTH values of 521 pmol/liter (13-fold elevated).

Similarly, the serum PTH values of 20 renal graft patients were more often normal (8 of 20 patients) in the intact assay than in the midregion assay (4 of 20). The mean values were 16.0 pmol/liter intact PTH and 178 pmol/liter midregion PTH.

The relationship between total serum calcium and PTH concentrations was studied in 13 renal dialysis patients immediately before and after dialysis. Lower serum calcium values before dialysis were correlated with higher serum intact PTH concentrations (Fig. 8). The increase in serum total calcium during dialysis resulted in a decrease in intact PTH concentrations in all but one patient (Fig. 8, Table 4). The change in midregion PTH was less distinct (mean − 7%) than that in intact PTH (mean − 45%).

Venous Gradients of PTH

In 12 patients selective venous catheterization was performed, in most instances because of suspected primary hyperparathyroidism and previously unsuccessful neck surgery. The intact PTH assay discriminated more clearly between peak concentrations near an adenoma and peripheral concentrations than did the midregion assay. Figure 9 shows as an example the patient with the highest peak to peripheral values: serum intact PTH was 25-fold higher in the peak sample than peripherally (470 vs. 19 pmol/liter), whereas midregion PTH was only 5.3-fold higher (980 vs. 185 pmol/liter). Individual serum intact PTH concentrations in the renal veins and the hepatic vein of each patient are shown in Fig. 10. The concentration in the inferior vena cava below the junction of the renal veins shown in the figure may be considered the peripheral value. Serum intact PTH values lower than the inferior vena cava (peripheral) concentration were constantly found in both the hepatic and renal veins. On average, the concentration was 17% below the peripheral value in the renal veins and 38% below the peripheral value in the hepatic vein. In two patients serum midregion PTH was also determined; no significant differences among the values in the renal, hepatic, and peripheral veins were detected. In one patient who had received a parathyroid allograft after total parathyroidectomy, serum PTH was determined in the veins of both the normal arm and the graft site. The serum intact

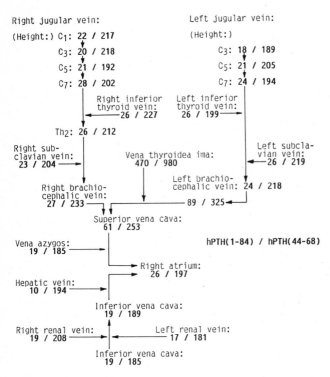

Fig. 9. Serum PTH concentrations in samples obtained by selective venous catheterization of a patient with a retrosternal parathyroid adenoma. Both serum intact PTH (*left-hand values*) and midregion PTH (*right-hand values*) were determined in all samples (pmol/liter)

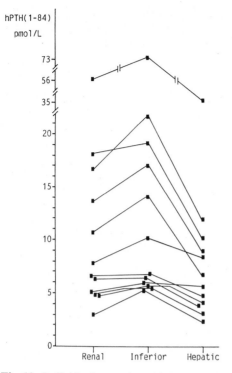

Fig. 10. Individual serum intact hPTH(1-84) values in 12 patients in the hepatic vein, the inferior vena cava below the renal veins, and the renal veins (average of both sides, except for 1 patient). The specimens were obtained by venous catheterization

PTH near the graft site was high (48 pmol/liter) compared to the value in the other arm (2.7 pmol/liter). The midregion PTH values were less different (135 and 17 pmol/liter, respectively).

Discussion

Intact PTH in Primary Hyperparathyroidism

Intact PTH was measured with this assay in 100 patients with primary hyperparathyroidism. The assay identified nearly all of these patients, although the values were only slightly elevated in some patients. The simultaneously performed midregion assay was less sensitive in this respect. Furthermore, discrimination of borderline cases was hampered by the higher between-run variation of the midregion assay (21%) for concentrations in the upper normal range. In small numbers of patients with primary hyperparathyroidism, several investigators have found midregion assays to be more [26] or less [16, 25] sensitive than the intact method used in each study.

Malignancy-Associated Hypercalcemia and Differential Diagnosis

Hyperparathyroid patients were excellently distinguished from patients with malignancy-associated hypercalcemia, except for one patient of the latter group with elevated serum PTH levels in whom ectopic PTH secretion was found. The lowest value in the primary hyperparathyroid group was still more than twice as high as the highest value in the malignancy group. This difference seems to be a feature of most assays detecting intact PTH [4, 6, 12, 25, 27]; the assay for intact PTH described by Hackeng et al. [12], based on an extraction step and subsequent region-specific RIA, distinguished both patients with primary hyperparathyroidism and those with nonparathyroid hypercalcemia only incompletely from normal subjects but was, nevertheless, able to discriminate between both patient groups.

Such discrimination is often not achieved with RIAs of PTH fragments [20, 25, 30]. The midregion assay we used gave elevated values in one-third of the patients in the malignancy group. Ashby and Thakkar [3] found a similar proportion of patients with slightly elevated results whereas Mallette et al. [20] with their very sensitive midregion assay found only 5% elevated values in patients with normal serum creatinine. The latter assay, however, yielded only slightly lowered average values in this group.

Because PTH production by nonparathyroid tumors is very rare [24], elevated midregion PTH results in these patients must be ascribed either to reduced renal clearance of these fragments or to nonspecific effects in the assay. Impaired renal function is common in these patients, and hypercalcemia itself can cause a decrease in the glomerular filtration rate, followed by an increase in midregion PTH. There is still some controversy about the serum factors that may cause elevated results in such assays. Occasionally, some factor(s), probably an immunoglobulin, interacts with anti-PTH-antibodies and thus inhibits tracer binding [18]. Recently, Suva et al. [34] isolated a tumor factor (PTH-related protein or PTH-related peptide; PTHrP), which showed an amino acid sequence homology with PTH in the first 13 amino acid residues. This peptide is a potent stimulator of some bioassays for PTH and may contribute to both hypercalcemia in malignancy and apparently elevated PTH results in some conventional N-terminal RIAs [23].

In contrast, a positive signal in the two-site assay for intact PTH requires the recognition of the PTH molecule at two distinct sites by two different antibodies. The increased specificity of the intact assay, therefore, prevents false-positive results.

Parathyroid Hormone in Renal Diseases

In patients with chronic renal failure, serum midregion PTH was much more elevated than was serum intact PTH compared to the group with primary hyperparathyroidism. In the former patients, both increased PTH release and decreased filtration of these fragments by the kidneys could contribute to the elevated serum midregion and C-terminal PTH results to an individually varying degree [9]. The presence of secondary hyperparathyroidism, in a clinical sense, may therefore be overestimated by midregion assays. In the intact assay twice as many patients had serum PTH values in the normal range than in the midregion assay. It is likely that the intact PTH assay reflects the secretory activity of the parathyroid glands more closely. Similarly, Hackeng et al. [12], using the extraction assay of intact PTH mentioned above, found normal values in more than half of 502 hemodialysis patients. Andress et al. [1] found that an assay cross-reacting exclusively with N-terminal fragments and the intact hormone may be a better predictor of bone disease in hemodialysis patients than a midregion assay. In the renal transplantation group the results were likewise more frequently in the normal range when measured in the intact PTH assay than in the midregion RIA. Elevated midregion PTH results in the presence of normal intact PTH values may simply reflect a less adequate function of the kidney transplant.

Parathyroid Hormone Levels in Hypoparathyroidism

Apart from borderline situations and the rare condition of pseudohypoparathyroidism, it is usually possible to establish the diagnosis of hypoparathyroidism by using other diagnostic procedures, but serum PTH results in these patients, compared to those in normal subjects, are a good indicator of whether a PTH assay can reliably detect low PTH concentrations. In hypoparathyroidism, serum intact PTH values were below the normal range in 92%. Hence, measurement of intact PTH based on the two-site immunoradiometric or immunoluminometric technique [4, 6, 27] permits detection of hypoparathyroidism, whereas no data for these patients are obtainable from assays of intact PTH based on other methods [12, 16]. Very few conventional RIAs or IRMAs of the one-site type were sensitive enough to show a comparable discrimination (Chap. 2.2).

Metabolism and Secretion of PTH

The assay specifically detects intact or mainly intact PTH with a short half-life. The half-life in patients who underwent removal of a single parathyroid adenoma was approximately 5 min initially whereas the disappearance rate was less rapid 5–15 min after removal. This is in agreement with the results of Hackeng et al. [12] and Curley et al. [8], who reported a similar half-life of 5 min for their assays of intact PTH. Brasier et al. [5] found a half-life of 21 min in eight patients but could not exclude a rapid initial component of less than 5 min. An even shorter half-life of approximately 2.5 min for an N-terminal specific assay has been reported [29].

   An initial half-life of roughly 5 min was also found in experiments in which calcium was injected intravenously to suppress PTH secretion (results not shown).

In dialysis patients, rising serum calcium levels resulted in a more marked decrease in intact PTH concentrations than in midregion PTH, due to the fact that changes in midregion PTH have to be detected against a high background of circulating fragments. For the same reason, the intact assay was superior to the midregion assay in detecting the site of an adenoma by selective venous catheterization. In nonparathyroid hypercalcemia, serum calcium values corrected for protein concentration and intact PTH, as determined by this assay, were inversely correlated [31]. In addition, the intact assay is sensitive enough to detect PTH levels well below the lower limit of the normal range and also small changes within the normal range. This is especially useful for investigating calcium metabolism in healthy persons. Sokoll et al. [33] were able to demonstrate a significant negative correlation between intact PTH and both total and ionized calcium in serum of postmenopausal women. This was not the case between midregion PTH and calcium. In our study there was no significant correlation between intact PTH and total calcium, which might have been caused in part by the more heterogeneous group of normal persons.

Serum midregion PTH concentrations were higher than the intact PTH concentrations in veins draining a parathyroid adenoma in one patient and a parathyroid allograft in another patient. The parathyroid tissue, therefore, secreted a substantial amount of PTH fragments which contained the amino acid sequence 53-68 but did not cross-react in the intact assay. The lower intact PTH concentrations in the hepatic and renal veins emphasize the role that these organs play in the peripheral metabolism of the intact hormone [7, 22, 28]. The liver appears to be the major organ responsible for the degradation of intact PTH since the levels in the venous effluent were 38% lower, in contrast to a decrease of only 17% in the renal veins.

Two-Site Assays of Intact PTH

The results obtained by different two-site assays of intact PTH may be better comparable than those obtained with different RIAs, because detection is restricted to a relatively homogeneous group of circulating peptides, i.e. the intact or mainly intact hormone. In addition, there is a tendency to use consistently synthetic hPTH(1-84) as standard and, despite several differences of assay design, two-site assays of intact PTH yielded similar values in normal subjects ([4, 6, 27]; see Table 2, Chap. 2.8).

Conclusion

The new generation of assays for intact PTH based on the two-site technique has overcome several limitations of many conventional RIAs. The high sensitivity of these assays makes PTH detectable in all normal subjects, which is necessary for recognizing conditions with lowered PTH levels and for detecting

PTH changes within the physiological range. The assays reflect the secretory activity of the glands very closely and are less influenced by biologically inactive PTH fragments and nonspecific effects because of their high specificity. Levels of intact PTH are increased in nearly all patients with primary hyperparathyroidism and are widely separated from the low levels in patients with malignancy-associated hypercalcemia, as strikingly demonstrated in this study. Additionally, in chronic renal failure intact PTH assays probably do reflect the secretory activity of the parathyroid gland more closely than older assays. We conclude that this new two-site assay of intact PTH is superior to the midregion RIA and meets the needs for assessing parathyroid function under various clinical conditions.

References

1. Andress DL, Endres DB, Maloney NA, Kopp JB, Coburn JW, Sherrard DJ (1986) Comparison of parathyroid hormone assays with bone histomorphometry in renal osteodystrophy. J Clin Endocrinol Metab 63:1163–1169
2. Armitage EK (1986) Parathyrin (parathyroid hormone): metabolism and methods for assay. Clin Chem 32:418–424
3. Ashby JP, Thakkar H (1988) Diagnostic limitations of region-specific parathyroid hormone assays in the investigation of hypercalcaemia. Ann Clin Biochem 25:275–279
4. Blind E, Schmidt-Gayk H, Armbruster FP, Stadler A (1987) Measurement of intact human parathyrin by an extracting two-site immunoradiometric assay. Clin Chem 33:1376–1381
5. Brasier AR, Wang CA, Nussbaum SR (1988) Recovery of parathyroid hormone secretion after parathyroid adenomectomy. J Clin Endocrinol Metab 66:495–500
6. Brown RC, Aston JP, Weeks I, Woodhead JS (1987) Circulating intact parathyroid hormone measured by a two-site immunochemiluminometric assay. J Clin Endocrinol Metab 65:407–414
7. Corvilain J, Manderlier T, Struyven J, Fuss M, Bergans A, Nijs N, Brauman H (1977) Metabolism of human PTH by the kidney and the liver. Horm Metab Res 9:239–242
8. Curley IR, Wheeler MH, Aston JP, Brown RC, Weeks I, Woodhead JS (1987) Studies in patients with hyperparathyroidism using a new two-site immunochemiluminometric assay for circulating intact (1-84) parathyroid hormone. Surgery 102:926–931
9. Freitag J, Martin KJ, Hruska KA, Anderson C, Conrades M, Ladenson J, Klahr S, Slatopolsky E (1978) Impaired parathyroid hormone metabolism in patients with chronic renal failure. N Engl J Med 298:29–32
10. Gleed JH, Hendy GN, Kimura T, Sakakibara S, O'Riordan JLH (1987) Immunological properties of synthetic human parathyroid hormone: effect of deamidation at position 76. Bone Mineral 2:375–382
11. Goltzman D, Henderson B, Loveridge N (1980) Cytochemical bioassay of parathyroid hormone. Characteristics of the assay and analysis of circulating hormonal forms. J Clin Invest 65:1309–1317
12. Hackeng WHL, Lips P, Netelenbos JC, Lips CJM (1986) Clinical implications of

estimation of intact parathyroid hormone (PTH) versus total immunoreactive PTH in normal subjects and hyperparathyroid patients. J Clin Endocrinol Metab 63:447–453

13. Heinrich G, Kronenberg HM, Potts JT Jr, Habener JF (1984) Gene encoding parathyroid hormone. Nucleotide sequence of the rat gene and deduced amino acid sequence of rat preproparathyroid hormone. J Biol Chem 259:3320–3329

14. Hendy GN, Kronenberg HM, Potts JT Jr, Rich A (1981) Nucleotide sequence of cloned cDNAs encoding human preproparathyroid hormone. Proc Natl Acad Sci USA 78:7365–7369

15. Keutmann HT, Sauer MM, Hendy GN, O'Riordan JLH, Potts JT Jr (1978) Complete amino acid sequence of human parathyroid hormone. Biochemistry 17:5723–5729

16. Lindall AW, Elting J, Ells J, Roos BA (1983) Estimation of biologically active intact parathyroid hormone in normal and hyperparathyroid sera by sequential N-terminal immunoextraction and midregion radioimmunoassay. J Clin Endocrinol Metab 57:1007–1014

17. Mallette LE (1983) Immunoreactivity of human parathyroid hormone (28-48): attempt to develop an assay for intact human parathyroid hormone. Metab Bone Dis Rel Res 4:329–332

18. Mallette LE, Nammour H (1987) False-positive elevations of midregion parathyroid hormone: inhibition of radioligand binding by a heterophilic antibody in patient serum. In: Cohn DV, Martin TJ, Meunier PJ (eds) Calcium regulation and bone metabolism, basic and clinical aspects. Excerpta Medica, Amsterdam, p 550 (Proceedings of the 9th International Conference on Calcium Regulating Hormones and Bone Metabolism, vol 9)

19. Mallette LE, Renfro M, Lemoncelli J, Rosenblatt M (1981) Radioimmunoassays for the 28-48 region of parathyroid hormone detect intact PTH but not hormone fragments. Calcif Tissue Int 33:375–380

20. Mallette LE, Tuma SN, Berger RE, Kirkland JL (1982) Radioimmunoassay for the middle region of human parathyroid hormone using an homologous antiserum with a carboxy-terminal fragment of bovine parathyroid hormone as radioligand. J Clin Endocrinol Metab 54:1017–1023

21. Mallette LE, Wilson DP, Kirkland JL (1983) Evaluation of hypocalcemia with a highly sensitive, homologous radioimmunoassay for the midregion of parathyroid hormone. Pediatrics 71:64–69

22. Martin KJ, Hruska KA, Freitag JJ, Klahr S, Slatopolsky E (1979) The peripheral metabolism of parathyroid hormone. N Engl J Med 301:1092–1098

23. Martin TJ (1988) Humoral hypercalcemia of malignancy. Bone Miner 4:83–89

24. Mundy GR (1985) Pathogenesis of hypercalcaemia of malignancy. Clin Endocrinol (Oxf) 23:705–714

25. Newman DJ, Thakkar H, Ashby JP (1987) Clinical utility of region-specific parathyroid hormone assays in the investigation of hypercalcaemia. Ann Clin Biochem [Suppl 1] 24:150

26. Nisbet JA (1986) Comparison of three parathyroid hormone assays. Ann Clin Biochem 23:429–433

27. Nussbaum SR, Zahradnik RJ, Lavigne JR, Brennan GL, Nozawa-Ung K, Kim LY, Keutmann HT, Wang C, Potts JT Jr, Segre GV (1987) Highly sensitive two-site immunoradiometric assay of parathyrin, and its clinical utility in evaluating patients with hypercalcemia. Clin Chem 33:1364–1367

28. Oldham SB, Finck EJ, Singer FR (1978) Parathyroid hormone clearance in man. Metabolism 27:993–1001
29. Papapoulos SE, Manning RM, Hendy GN, Lewin IG, O'Riordan JLH (1980) Studies of circulating parathyroid hormone in man using a homologous amino-terminal specific immunoradiometric assay. Clin Endocrinol (Oxf) 13:57–67
30. Raisz LG, Yajnik CH, Bockman RS, Bower BF (1979) Comparison of commercially available parathyroid hormone immunoassays in the differential diagnosis of hypercalcemia due to primary hyperparathyroidism or malignancy. Ann Intern Med 91: 739–740
31. Scharla SH, Minne HW, Sattar P, Mende U, Blind E, Schmidt-Gayk H, Wüster C, Ho T, Ziegler R (1987) Therapie der Tumorhypercalciämie mit Clodronat-Einfluß auf Parathormon und Calcitriol. Dtsch Med Wochenschr 112:1121–1125
32. Schmidt-Gayk H, Schmitt-Fiebig M, Hitzler W, Armbruster FP, Mayer E (1986) Two homologous radioimmunoassays for parathyrin compared and applied to disorders of calcium metabolism. Clin Chem 32:57–62
33. Sokoll LJ, Morrow FD, Quirbach DM, Dawson-Hughes B (1988) Intact parathyrin in postmenopausal women. Clin Chem 34:407–410
34. Suva LJ, Winslow GA, Wettenhall REH, Hammonds RG, Moseley JM, Diefenbach-Jagger H, Rodda CP, Kemp BE, Rodriguez H, Chen EY, Hudson PJ, Martin TJ, Wood WI (1987) A parathyroid hormone-related protein implicated in malignant hypercalcemia: cloning and expression. Science 237:893–896

Chapter 1.2

Clinical Use of Vitamin D Metabolite Assays (Calcidiol and Calcitriol)

R. Bouillon

Vitamin D was recognized at the beginning of this century as a simple vitamin derived either from fatty food or produced in the skin from 7-dehydrocholes-terol under the influence of the shortest waves of ultraviolet light of the sun. After intensive research during the past 2 decades, vitamin D has outgrown its simple status to become a complex series of metabolites, produced in a large number of tissues and displaying an ever-increasing list of effects, not only in the classical calcium endocrine and bone system but also affecting nearly every cell or body system [13, 33, 43]. The complexity of the vitamin D system was initially recognized by the observation of a prolonged lag time between the administration of vitamin D to vitamin D-deficient animals and its subsequent effects (especially intestinal calcium transport). By using radioactive vitamin D (labeled with either ^{14}C or ^{3}H) it soon became apparent that vitamin D was metabolized into more polar metabolites and 25-hydroxyvitamin D was thereby first recognized, identified, and synthesized but was soon also found to be only a mainly biological inert precursor for further activation or inactivation (Fig. 1), depending on several ions, hormones, and humoral factors (Fig. 2). The main series of vitamin D metabolites are represented in Fig. 1 and this clearly shows that the vitamin D endocrine system has at least as many circulating metabolites as the more familiar group of adrenal and sex steroid hormones. In addition, a recent count of all identified vitamin D metabolites ended up with more than 20 genuine metabolites, most of which are probably only inactive degradation products [33]. The crucial metabolites at present recognized as biologically important include:

— Vitamin D (either the plant sterol ergocalciferol or vitamin D_2, which only originates from nutritional intake and usually contributes little to the human vitamin D status, but is used as an important pharmaceutical product in some countries, or vitamin D_3 or cholecalciferol, which can be either derived from food or produced in the skin)
— 25-Hydroxyvitamin D (25-OHD), the main metabolite circulating in plasma (either as 25-hydroxyvitamin D_2 or D_3 depending on its precursor), but with probably little intrinsic biological activity, at least when present in physiolo-gical concentrations

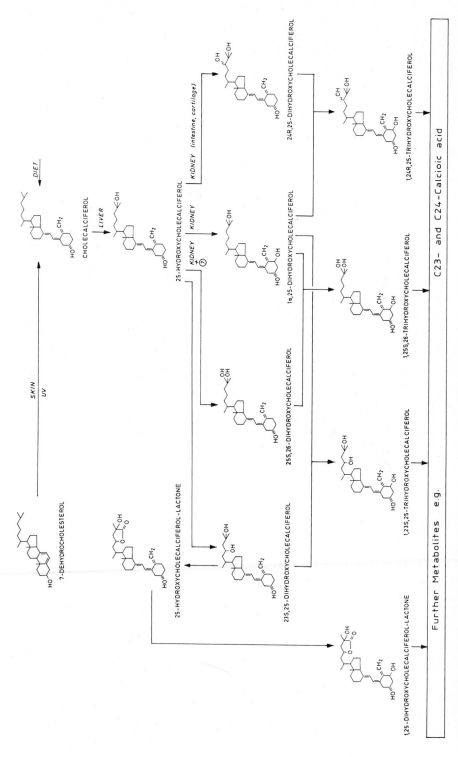

Fig. 1. Pathways and sites of origin of the main vitamin D metabolites

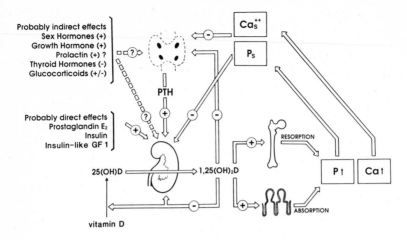

Fig. 2. Regulation of the renal 25-hydroxyvitamin D-1α-hydroxylase activity

— 1,25-Dihydroxyvitamin D_2 or -D_3, which is well recognized as the main
vitamin D hormone, because its production is feedback regulated by specific
regulatory systems (vide infra) and acts, like other steroid hormones, on
peripheral tissues by binding to the vitamin D receptor and subsequent
activation or inactivation of DNA-dependent protein synthesis
— 24,25-Dihydroxyvitamin D_2 or -D_3, probably the most disputed vitamin D
metabolite, either considered as totally inactive (in physiological amounts)
and only the beginning of a degradation system or considered by others as a
metabolite with specific receptors and sui generis biological activity, mainly
on cartilage growth and maturation and as being a dominant vitamin D
metabolite during fetal development
— Several other trihydroxylated vitamin D metabolites with a 1α-hydroxyl
group show biological activity in concentrations that may approach their
physiological concentrations but it is presently unclear whether this is only
due to their resemblance to 1,25-dihydroxyvitamin D [1,25-$(OH)_2$D] or
whether it represents a more specific action profile.

The origin of the different vitamin D metabolites was initially limited to the
skin (photosynthesis of vitamin D itself) but it is now recognized that a fairly
large number of tissues contribute to the metabolism of vitamin D (Table 1).
The list of potential target tissues is also becoming increasingly longer, as was
initially suspected on the basis of the presence of specific vitamin D receptors
and later confirmed by the presence of vitamin D-dependent proteins or
biological responses. A tentative list of these target tissues where vitamin D
might have a biological effect is given in Table 2. From this impressive list of
potential vitamin D target tissues one might conclude that the measurements of
serum concentrations of the main vitamin D metabolites should find applications outside the strict field of calcium and bone metabolism but this has

Table 1. Tissues involved in the origin or metabolism of vitamin D

1. Skin[a]	6. Chorioallantois membrane
2. Liver	7. Intestine
3. Kidney[b]	8. Cartilage
4. Bone[a]	9. Monocyte-lymphocyte[b]
5. Placenta[b]	10. Fibroblast

[a] 1α-Hydroxylase activity demonstrated in vitro only
[b] 1α-Hydroxylase activity demonstrated in vivo and in vitro

Table 2. Distribution of the 1,25-dihydroxyvitamin D receptor and (possible) target tissues for vitamin D

1. Calcium-transporting tissues
   - Intestinal mucosa
   - Bone (osteoblasts and odontoblasts)
   - Kidney (distal and collecting tubules)
   - Placenta
   - Chorioallantois membrane (chick)
   - Yolk sac membrane
   - Mammary glands
2. Endocrine glands
   - Parathyroid gland
   - Thyroid calcitonin cells
   - Endocrine pancreas (insulin-containing β-cells)
   - Hypophyseal gland (especially prolactin-producing cells)
   - Ovary and testes
3. Contractile tissues
   - Skeletal and heart muscle
   - Smooth muscle (vascular cells, uterus)
4. Immune system
   - Thymus
   - Monocyte/macrophages
   - Activated T- and B-lymphocytes
5. Skin epidermal cells
6. Brain
7. Some cancer cells
   (e.g., leukemia, melanoma, mammary cancer, osteosarcoma, gastrointestinal cancers)

yet not been the case, although some studies indicated that measurement of the serum concentration of 1,25-$(OH)_2$D might predict the response to calcium therapy in hypertensive patients.

Clinical Applications of the Measurement
of Vitamins D_2 and D_3

Although vitamins D_2 and D_3 are the basic substrates for all the subsequent metabolites, their measurement has found few clinical applications, partly due to technical reasons and partly due to their limited usefulness. Indeed, the technical measurement of the parent vitamin D is hampered by its very lipophilic character so that interference of other lipids is difficult to avoid in either the subsequent binding assay or spectrophotometry. Moreover, no good natural binding protein with preferential binding for vitamin D itself is available nor have immunization procedures been very successful in raising optimal antibodies. From the available studies [1, 6], however, some initial conclusions can be drawn: the serum concentration of vitamin D will only give information about the recent exposure to either nutritional vitamin D or to recent vitamin D production in the skin. Indeed, nutritional vitamin D is absorbed by the intestine (estimated absorption efficacy of 60%–70%) and then transported by the chylomicron system whereby vitamin D can either reach peripheral storage areas (fat or muscle) or be cleared with the chylomicron remnants in the liver. This vitamin D is therefore quite rapidly (several hours) removed from the circulation but reappears again a few hours later as 25-OHD. The main origin of vitamin D is, however, the skin, where 7-dehydrocholesterol is transformed in previtamin D by ultraviolet light and thereafter slowly (over several days) equilibrates into vitamin D_3 itself. If previtamin D is further irradiated before its thermal transformation into vitamin D it can be photoisomerized into other vitamin D analogs (Fig. 3) that are devoid of intrinsic vitamin D action. This pathway could have physiological sense by avoiding excess production of vitamin D during prolonged or intensive exposure to sunshine [21]. The slow thermal equilibration of previtamin into vitamin D is probably facilitated by the presence of the vitamin D binding protein (DBP), which has a (low but definite) affinity (about $10^5\ M^{-1}$ to $10^6\ M^{-1}$) for vitamin D_3 but not for its previtamin. The end product is, therefore, constantly removed for the equilibrium reaction, thereby facilitating the production of vitamin D itself. Little direct feedback control on this mainly physical photochemical reaction is possible but sunshine-induced or genetically controlled pigmentation can exert important long-term control over the vitamin D synthesis. Moreover, recent data indicate that the active vitamin D hormone [1,25-$(OH)_2D$] can influence the differentiation of melanocytes and increase the skin production of 7-dehydrocholesterol [4]. Due to the slow thermal equilibration of vitamin D, its plasma appearance after a single UV exposure will be gradual over several days and return to basal levels after about 7 days. This again indicates that serum levels of vitamin D will only reflect recent addition of this vitamin and not its overall status. Normal concentrations in healthy adults vary from undetectable to a few nanograms per milliliter but may rise to about 100 ng/ml a few days after intensive exposure to UV light. Low levels have been reported in anephric patients. The separate

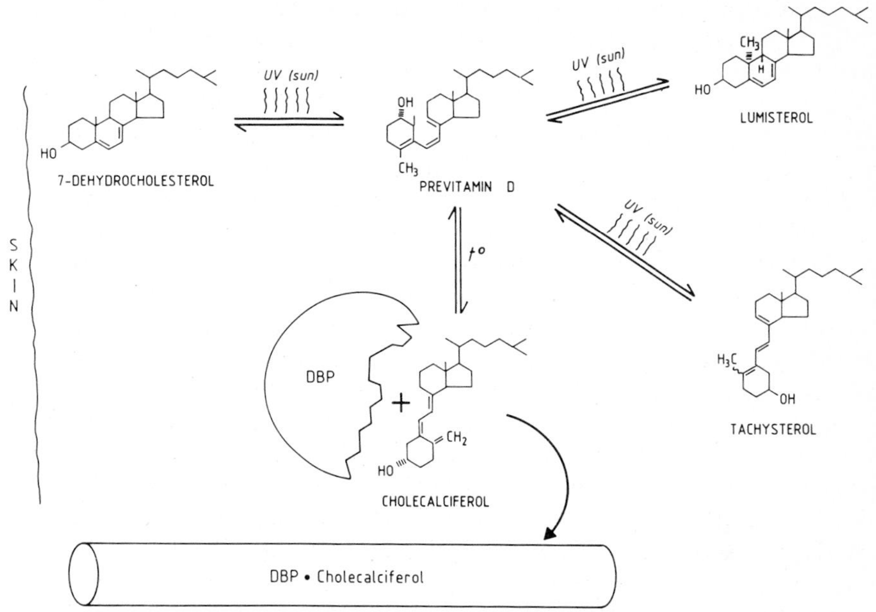

Fig. 3. Photochemical synthesis and transport of vitamin D in the skin

measurement of vitamin D_2 and D_3 may give additional information about the origin (pharmaceutical or otherwise) of the circulating vitamins but this can in general be better evaluated by measuring the 25-hydroxymetabolites. The same rule applies for the global estimation of the vitamin D status. Measurements of vitamin D, of course, do find an application in evaluating the vitamin content of natural or vitamin D-enriched food or pharmaceutical products.

Clinical Applications for the Measurements of 25-Hydroxyvitamin D_2 and D_3

Vitamin D is rapidly converted into 25-hydroxyvitamin D in the liver hepatocytes by a microsomal and/or a mitochondrial vitamin D-25-hydroxylase system both using a P-450 cytochrome. The microsomal enzyme has a low K_m and better specificity than the mitochondrial enzyme, which probably only acts at supraphysiological concentrations of vitamin D and also has less specificity (e.g., it also 25-hydroxylates cholesterol). The end product, 25-OHD, is better bound to the liver-produced DBP than its precursor since its affinity for 25-OHD is about $10^{10} \, M^{-1}$ and therefore exceeds that of its precursor at least 10 000-fold. The removal of the end product might help to explain the rapidity and capacity of this conversion into 25-OHD. The feedback regulation of this 25-hydroxylase activity is not very tight since the 25-OHD level increases in man and animals after increased exposure to either nutritional vitamin D or UV light. The absolute increase in 25-OHD, however, does not parallel the increase in substrate availability, so that some degree of feedback inhibition must exist. More recent studies have shown that 1,25-$(OH)_2$D itself may inhibit the conversion of vitamin D into 25-OHD in the liver. This can explain why some patients with increased 1,25-$(OH)_2$D levels (e.g., in primary hyperparathyroidism and in sarcoidosis) have lower than expected 25-OHD levels. Apart from the liver, which certainly is the major site of 25-OHD production, several other tissues have been shown to be able to 25-hydroxylate vitamin D. The intestine, kidney, placenta, and cartilage can all perform this hydroxylation but their contribution to the systemic availability of 25-OHD is limited as has been shown by studies of the metabolism of radioactive vitamin D after hepatectomy.

The transport of 25-OHD in serum has been extensively studied. All the vitamin D metabolites can bind to three transport systems: chylomicrons transport vitamin D from the intestine to the liver and storage sites but contribute little to the transport of the other D metabolites. Albumin (at least DBP-free albumin) has a low affinity for all D metabolites so that even its large concentration in plasma contributes little to the transport of the hydroxylated D metabolites; moreover, albumin-bound vitamin D metabolites probably behave as free steroid regarding biodisposability for the target tissues. The main transport system for all D metabolites is therefore assured by a specific transport protein, known as vitamin D-binding protein. This protein (DBP) is found in virtually all vertebrate species with a calcified skeleton and is a single-chain protein with a molecular weight slightly smaller than that of albumin, to which it is genetically related. The protein circulates in micromolar concentrations in blood, at least in avian and mammalian species and thus largely exceeds the total concentration of all its ligands. Human and rat DBP has a high affinity binding site (K_a 10^{10} M^{-1} at 4°C) for 25-hydroxyvitamin D_3 whereas its precursor, vitamin D_3, and its active further metabolite, 1,25-dihydroxyvitamin D_3, have a much lower affinity for the same binding site. This phenomenon may play a role in the metabolism of vitamin D, favoring a long half-life of 25-hydroxyvitamin D and creating therefore a role of DBP as protector against sudden vitamin D excess or deficiency.

Since vitamin D is rapidly transformed into 25-OHD after entry in the body and since this 25-OHD is mainly confined to the extracellular compartment, where it is tightly bound to circulating DBP, and since it has in addition a very long half-life in blood, it should be the ideal parameter to indicate the access of the organism to vitamin D. Indeed, many data in animals and men have shown that plasma levels of 25-OHD are the best markers of imminent or existing vitamin D deficiency. Moreover, 25-OHD, being the vitamin D metabolite with the highest serum concentration, is relatively easy to measure so that this assay has found the widest clinical application for the estimation of the vitamin D status or the detection of vitamin D deficiency or excess. A large number of techniques are available [6, 36], varying from the original competitive protein-binding assay (using DBP as binding protein), radioimmunoassay, absorptiometry at 265 or 254 nm, to mass spectrometry after extensive purification [especially high-performance liquid chromatography (HPLC)].

These techniques all agree fairly well with each other and in fact confirm the earlier estimates of the total "vitamin D" content of serum using a bioassay in which serum extracts were given to D-deficient animals and growth plate characteristics were measured as end points. Some assays for 25-OHD, however, do not use proper extraction techniques prior to the assay and some "matrix" components of serum (probably lipids) may then interfere with the assay results, giving rise to spuriously elevated values. In addition, when DBP is used as binding protein, several vitamin D metabolites will compete for the same single binding site so that other metabolites besides 25-OHD will be comeasured. This especially applies to 24,25-$(OH)_2$D and 25,26-$(OH)_2$D, which normally circulate in blood in a relatively fixed ratio (roughly 10% and 2%, respectively) with 25-OHD, so that without purification prior to the assay a mild overestimation of the total 25-OHD concent will be obtained. This small overestimation ($\pm$ 20%) is, however, of little clinical importance in view of the wide biological range of normal 25-OHD levels and therefore in no way hampers the clinical benefit of such nonchromatographic assays when at least nonspecific interference by serum matrix components has been excluded [9].

The exact cutoff points for plasma 25-OHD levels to define vitamin D deficiency and vitamin D excess or intoxication are hard to define but this is not an exception in the field of vitamin assays. Indeed, as for other nonmetabolic substrates, including most vitamins and essential trace elements, low serum levels are the first indication of global tissue store deficits, which later on will result firstly in subtle biochemical defects and only after a more prolonged time will result in organ or whole body diseases. Vitamin D deficiency can therefore be compared with iron deficiency, with which most clinicians are better familiarized: the first sign of iron deficiency is simply a low concentration in plasma. This is later followed by a tissue deficit (using ferritin as marker) and finally by mild to severe anemia and still later there is association with other tissue damage due to failing Fe-containing enzymes. Similarly, vitamin D deficiency will first be recognizable by low circulating stores (especially 25-OHD), by deficiency of the active hormone and the biochemical or hormonal responses to this deficiency (serum ions and hormonal changes, especially secondary hyperparathyroidism), and only in a much later stage, depending on the turnover and growth of bone, will histological and structural (e.g., radiological or clinical) signs of deficient bone mineralization become evident. The same value of 25-OHD deficiency therefore either will be associated with severe rickets or osteomalacia or will be found in a person or animal with no detectable bone abnormalities, depending on the duration of this deficiency. This certainly complicates the definition of the lowest acceptable 25-OHD level compatible with normal mineral (plasma and bone) homeostasis. In clinically evident rickets or osteomalacia due to simple vitamin D deficiency, levels of 25-OHD are usually well *below 5 ng/ml* (12.5 pmol/liter), but frequently are not totally undetectable [37]. Even in animals raised on a D-deficient diet, severe rickets may be found in the presence of a few nanograms of 25-OHD per milliliter. Values above 5 ng/ml are, however, exceptional in clinically evident cases of vitamin D-deficient rickets. Again as for the sequence of events for the clinical expression of vitamin D deficiency, the reverse phenomena might occur in vitamin D repletion, whereby access to vitamin D after prolonged deficiency may result in low-normal 25-OHD levels but still severe signs of rickets or osteomalacia at tissue levels (bone histology).

By the introduction of 25-OHD assays it became evident that low levels of this metabolite are quite frequent in many populations when vitamin D supplementation of food is not the rule and sun exposure is relatively low for climatic or cultural reasons. To define subclinical vitamin D deficiency, we and others have proposed the use of a vitamin D challenge test [11]. If in the absence of histological or biochemical signs (low calcium or phosphorus, secondary hyperparathyroidism) of vitamin D deficiency a rapid (but usually transient) increase in serum $1,25$-$(OH)_2D$ is observed after supplementation with physiological amounts of vitamin D or 25-OHD, then we may conclude that the preexisting substrate availability was considered as insufficient for optimal $1,25$-$(OH)_2D$ production, which is normally well feedback regulated.

By such tests, we demonstrated that serum $1,25$-$(OH)_2D$ increases rapidly and significantly if serum 25-OHD levels are between 5 and 10 ng/ml but does not further increase in young or elderly subjects if their 25-OHD levels are above 10–15 ng/ml [11]. Similar studies by Peacock suggested a similar threshold level above which no further increase in serum $1,25$-$(OH)_2D$ was observed. We therefore consider 25-OHD levels below 5 or 6 ng/ml as severe vitamin D deficiency and values between 6 and 10 ng/ml as relatively low or "subclinical deficiency," whereby bone and mineral homeostasis can be reasonably maintained, at least short term, by adaptive mechanisms (increased renal 1α-hydroxylation, mild secondary hyperparathyroidism, etc.).

Factors Influencing Vitamin D Status or 25-Hydroxyvitamin D Levels in Blood

Nutritional Intake

The daily intake of vitamin D generally recommended is about 400 IU or 10 µg/day. In many countries, however, that intake is not achieved by a large part of the population because vitamin D is mainly present in some fatty food while more commonly used food contains only trace amounts of vitamin D. Fatty fish in general and their liver in particular contain large amounts of vitamin D, probably because these fish consume large amounts of algae [22]. Egg yolk and butter are other rich sources of vitamin D but due to their lipid composition cannot be recommended on the daily menu. Milk, however, is a poor source of vitamin D and this might explain why serum 25-OHD levels usually decrease in early life in breast-fed infants not receiving pharmaceutical vitamin D supplements. Vitamin D supplementation of food is the rule in North America but not in most European countries (except for special margarines with an increased content of polyunsaturated fatty acids) so that serum 25-OHD levels are usually much lower in Europe than in the United States, even when populations living at a similar latitude are compared (e.g., Spain versus Boston). Too high an intake of nutritional vitamin D is exceptional unless pharmaceutical preparations of vitamin D are used. Indeed, vitamin D intoxication due to excess of "natural vitamin" has only been described in Scandinavian fisherman consuming large amounts of broiled fish liver during annual celebrations. Inappropriate and repeated use of pharmaceutical vitamin D (e.g., 5- or 15-mg preparations) can of course increase serum levels of 25-OHD well above 150 ng/ml and such levels are probably sufficient to activate the vitamin D receptor, resulting in hypercalcemia, hyperphosphatemia, kidney stone formation, or metastatic calcification. The duration of such vitamin D intoxication may be surprisingly prolonged and 25-OHD levels can exceed the normal range for more than 1 year after cessation of intake. Moreover, reappearance of vitamin D intoxication (hypercalcemia) has been observed without renewed intake in such patients during severe weight loss, probably because of the release of fat-stored vitamin D (personal observation). In most such cases $1,25\text{-}(OH)_2D$ is low or in the normal range, probably because the associated hypercalcemia results in mild renal failure. Only when renal function remains perfectly normal and/or is associated with parathyroid hyperfunction (primary hyperparathyroidism) will an overload of vitamin D and 25-OHD result in excess $1,25\text{-}(OH)_2D$ levels. Vitamin D intoxication, at least due to vitamin D_2 or D_3 or its 25-hydroxy analogs, therefore, can easily be detected by a screening 25-OHD assay (values well in excess of 100 ng/ml probably indicate imminent or real vitamin D intoxication), but vitamin D intoxication due to dihydrotachysterol excess or supraphysiological amounts of 1α-hydroxylated vitamin D metabolites cannot be detected by measuring 25-OHD levels. Other vitamin D metabolites are also increased during vitamin D intoxication [24,25- and $25,26\text{-}(OH)_2D$ and especially the 25-hydroxyvitamin D lactone, which normally only circulates in picogram quantities, e.g., 40 pg/ml] but may increase into the nanogram range during vitamin D intoxication. Some animals consuming large amounts of fatty fish (e.g., the hooded seal, with an estimated daily vitamin D intake of 10 mg/day) would also be at risk for continuous vitamin D intoxication but they show an adaptive increased metabolism of 25-OHD into $24,25\text{-}(OH)_2D$ [22].

Some studies have revealed that, when exposure to ultraviolet light is limited, 400 IU vitamin D might be sufficient to maintain normal 25-OHD levels, whereas a daily intake of 800 IU/day might slowly increase 25-OHD levels. Most such studies have, however, been performed in the elderly population [20, 28].

Exposure to Sunshine or Ultraviolet Light

Probably the most important source of vitamin D for humans during their evolution and even nowadays is the synthesis in the skin of vitamin D under the influence of the shortest UV waves reaching the earth (280–310 nm). This photochemical reaction requires UVA light, which is most easily filtered through the atmosphere, e.g., through clouds, through air pollution, or even at low angles of the sun. The efficacy of natural sunshine in the most northern areas of the world is therefore virtually nil during winter times (e.g., Siberia, Scandinavia). The importance of sunlight for the human vitamin D supply is further strengthened by the marked seasonal variation of 25-OHD, being highest at the end of summer and autumn (different months in the northern and southern hemisphere) and lowest during early spring [14]. Populations with low sun exposure are therefore at increased risk for vitamin D deficiency if their food intake at least is not rich or enriched in vitamin D. An extreme example is found in the crews of submarines who remain unexposed to natural light for several consecutive months and develop subclinical rickets [37]. More common examples are the elderly population in many west European [11] and maybe also North American countries, and people avoiding the sun for religious reasons or because of traditional beliefs [20, 41]. Paradoxically, clinical vitamin D deficiency is still endemic in many sunny Arabian countries, where the sun is avoided partly because of veiling of the women for religious reasons and because of the traditional belief of the "toxic" effects of the sun (24, 25, 41).

The exact amount of sunshine and the area of skin exposure necessary to maintain a normal 25-OHD level is difficult to define and will depend on the skin pigmentation and energy of the sunlight.

Skin Pigmentation

Skin pigmentation, either because of genetic reasons or by previous sun exposure, decreases the efficacy of UV light for the photochemical production of vitamin D. When, however, vitamin D production is measured after exposure to different amounts of UV energy able to produce the same skin reaction (minimal erythema dose), then nearly the same amount of vitamin D and 25-OHD is subsequently found independently from the skin pigmentation. This clearly demonstrates that skin pigmentation decreases the ability for vitamin D synthesis due to absorption of the UV light by its melanin content. Moreover, recent data indicate that the active vitamin D metabolite might influence the cellular activity of the melanocytes.

Since skin pigmentation decreases in populations living in more northern climates, some authors believe that the white human race originates from a progressive mutational adaptation to decreased sun exposure to avoid endemic vitamin D deficiency [21]. Indeed, populations with increased skin pigmentation (blacks in North America and many immigrants from Mediterranean or Indian origin in western Europe) nearly always have lower 25-OHD levels than the "original" white population living in the same area. This also helps to explain the high frequency of clinical vitamin D deficiency in children of these immigrants in western Europe. The difference in skin pigmentation also explains why the black population of central Africa has 25-OHD levels not much higher than those found during summer in white people of northern Europe and that these blacks show decreasing 25-OHD levels proportional to the duration of their stay in Europe [31].

Age and Sex

The fetus has detectable levels of 25-OHD as soon as 20 weeks onwards. At the time of birth the newborn 25-OHD levels show an excellent correlation with the maternal 25-OHD levels but are usually 40%–50% lower [11]. Indeed, the neonatal: maternal 25-OHD ratio is about 0.5–0.6 in an extremely large number of such studies worldwide. This implies that the neonate starts with vitamin D stores depending on the maternal vitamin D stores but also usually has only half the maternal level. Many infants, especially when born at the end of winter from mothers living in relatively vitamin D-deficient areas, therefore start with 25-OHD hardly above the vitamin D deficiency level (5 ng/ml). The serum level of 25-OHD is similar in children and adults and shows the normal seasonal variation [17, 42]. If older children have somewhat higher levels than young children during wintertime, this might easily be explained by differences in outdoor activity [44].

Calcium Intake and Calcium Requirements

A low vitamin D status will lead to rickets or osteomalacia but the clinical symptoms develop more rapidly in infants than in children, more rapidly during the pubertal growth spurt than before puberty, and much more slowly during adult life. Moreover, some older observations indicate that the sex ratio of rickets (male:female ratio) is 2:1 to 3:1 and this might be related to the higher bone mineral content of boys even at a young age and therefore a higher calcium requirement [30]. Insight into this relationship between calcium requirement or intake and vitamin D deficiency was provided by elegant studies in rats showing that calcium deficiency increased the catabolism of vitamin D and resulted in a depletion of serum levels of 25-OHD [15].

25-Hydroxyvitamin D Levels or Vitamin D Status and Diseases (Table 3)

Low levels of 25-OHD are thus obviously the hallmark and in fact a diagnostic requirement for the formal diagnosis of vitamin D-deficient rickets or osteomalacia. From the preceding chapter it is obvious that several groups are at increased risk from vitamin D deficiency:

1. Infants, especially during the 1st year of life because of their high calcium requirements (increasing the vitamin D catabolism) and the frequently low vitamin D stores received during pregnancy and the low vitamin D content of breast milk. Moreover, due to cultural habits, direct exposure of young

Table 3. Abnormal serum concentrations of 25-hydroxyvitamin D

---

1. Increased 25-OHD levels: vitamin D excess or intoxication[a]
   – (Increased intake of nutritional vitamin D)
   – Increased intake of pharmaceutical vitamin D
   – (Increased exposure to sunshine)
2. Decreased 25-OHD levels: rickets-osteomalacia or subclinical vitamin D deficiency
   a) Decreased availability of vitamin D due to low intake and/or decreased exposure to UV light especially:
      – Infants (especially during the 1st year of life)
      – Women and children of immigrants with pigmented skin living in western Eroupe
      – Elderly population with limited mobility
      – Populations with low exposure to sunshine due to socioeconomic or religious reasons
   b) Decreased intestinal vitamin D absorption due to general intestinal fat malabsorption e.g., biliary cirrhosis, short-bowel syndrome, insufficiency of the exocrine pancreas
   c) Increased metabolism or loss of vitamin D
      – Chronic activation of the liver microsomal P450 enzymes (e.g., barbiturates or antiepileptic drugs)
      – Urinary loss of 25-OHD (nephrotic syndrome)

---

[a] Vitamin D intoxication due to excess exposure to sunshine is virtually impossible while excessively high intake of vitamin D-rich natural food is extremely rare (consumption of large amounts of fatty fish, especially fish liver)

infants to sunlight is frequently avoided. The clinical expression of rickets and the elimination of this subclinical deficiency can only be achieved by continuous and systematic vitamin D supplementation of all infants. If such measures are omitted in temporate climates a rapid reappearance of the nineteenth century endemic rickets is to be expected, as can be seen on a small scale in west European countries among the children of immigrants and in special circumstances (e.g., Arabian countries, vide supra).

2. People with an inappropriate skin pigmentation for the country they live in. Indeed, Asians in Britain and (North) Africans in continental Europe all have an increased incidence of rickets and/or osteomalacia probably due to a number of reasons: low calcium intake or absorption, and lower socioeconomic circumstances with decreased sun exposure especially for the women and young children [16].

3. The steadily increasing group of elderly people is also at increased risk from vitamin D deficiency. This has been better documented in most west European countries than in North America and it seems logical to hold decreased sun exposure as the main responsible factor, as the deficiency is less

pronounced in sunny Spain than in Belgium, The Netherlands, or the United Kingdom at least as long as they are reasonably mobile and healthy [38]. Other contributing factors may be a lower fat intake (and thus vitamin D intake) and decreased efficacy of UV light to produce vitamin D in the skin, because of aging of the responsible cell or due to increased skin pigmentation in old age [34].

4. Several diseases, not primarily involving calcium or bone metabolism, are associated with an increased risk of vitamin D deficiency due to abnormal vitamin D requirements, abnormal vitamin D absorption or excretion, or abnormal vitamin D metabolism [6].

a) All diseases associated with intestinal fat malabsorption frequently result in subclinical or clinical vitamin D deficiency. This is to a great extent due to the loss of nutritional vitamin D as such and may be associated with decreased sun exposure because of a general disease. The contribution of an impaired enterohepatic cycle of vitamin D is less evident. Of course, vitamin D and its metabolites are eliminated in conjugated form (sulfates, glucuronates, etc.) in the bile and can partly be reabsorbed after biliary excretion. It is, however, not evident that these conjugates can be effectively reutilized after reabsorption [23]. Diseases characterized by decreased intestinal fat absorption and vitamin D deficiency include pancreatic deficiency (mucoviscidosis, etc.), gluten enteropathy, short-bowel syndrome, and biliary cirrhosis. Prolonged total parental nutrition without vitamin D supplements can also be counted in this category.

b) Increased urinary loss of vitamin D metabolites, especially 25-OHD, can be observed in many patients with nephrotic syndrome. Indeed, DBP is somewhat smaller than albumin and therefore found in large quantities in the urine of patients with nephrotic syndrome. Due to the high affinity of 25-OHD for DBP this protein loss is associated with loss of 25-OHD. The liver has a remarkably high capacity to resynthesize DBP but the supply of vitamin D substrate is not unlimited so that nephrotic syndrome results in vitamin D deficiency. This was first described by the present editors of this volume as has since been largely confirmed worldwide [2, 40]. The loss of DBP and 25-OHD can also be important during prolonged peritoneal dialysis, again resulting in mild to severe vitamin D deficiency, depending on the general supply (nutritional intake and photochemical synthesis).

c) An increased catabolism of vitamin D into 25-OHD is induced in the liver by many drugs known to enhance microsomal hydroxylase activity [3]. At first sight this should increase 25-OHD levels but unfortunately the same enzymes also seem to enhance the further catabolism of 25-OHD so that low 25-OHD levels may eventually become the rule during prolonged intake of such drugs (e.g., barbiturates, hydantoins, rifampicin). All epileptics treated with such drugs are thus at increased risk for vitamin D deficiency although the clinical expression of antiepileptic osteomalacia is usually limited to persons with additional risk factors (e.g., chronic institutionalization and decreased sun exposure, concomitant diseases such as Paget's disease, or patients requiring higher doses or several antiepileptic drugs in combination).

Clinical Applications for the Measurements of 1,25-Dihydroxyvitamin D

The conversion of 25-OHD into 1,25-$(OH)_2$D was initially thought to be exclusively limited to the kidney (distal tubular cells of the nephron) and this origin remains the main source of circulating 1,25-$(OH)_2$D even now that other cells seem to be able to produce the same metabolite [18, 39]. Indeed, the placenta undoubtedly can synthesize 1,25-$(OH)_2$D (both in vitro and in vivo) but its real contribution seems less than initially thought. Indeed, fetal nephrectomy or congenital anephry is associated with low neonatal 1,25-$(OH)_2$D levels whereas similarly in a patient with severe renal failure 1,25-$(OH)_2$D remained relatively low during subsequent pregnancy. Other cells or tissues have been shown to produce 1,25-$(OH)_2$D in vitro such as bone cells, intestine, and white blood cells. Again, it is doubtful whether these tissues actually contribute to the circulating 1,25-$(OH)_2$D level since in acute situations after bilateral nephrectomy no radioactive 1,25-$(OH)_2$D can be detected after injection of its labeled precursor. Very low levels, however, can be found in anephric subjects loaded chronically with sufficient precursor vitamin D. The renal 25-OHD-1α-hydroxylase activity is under tight feedback control to maintain primarily a normal serum mineral homeostasis and only secondarily to maintain a normal bone homeostasis. The major factors regulating this renal enzyme are given in Fig. 2. PTH is the main stimulator of the renal enzyme; and high serum phosphate, and to a much lesser extent, high serum ionized calcium depress the enzyme. Among the other hormones, only growth hormone and IGF_1 have well-documented stimulatory effects whereas the effects of other hormonal and humoral factors are disputed or limited to some lower species (Fig. 2).

As for other vitamin D metabolites, 1,25-$(OH)_2$D is tightly bound to the serum vitamin D-binding protein and probably only the free hormone is available for cellular entry, receptor occupation, and therefore biological activity. This hypothesis, like that of other free steroid and thyroid hormones, is based on both clinical and experimental observations [8, 10, 46].

Abnormal concentrations of serum 1,25-$(OH)_2$D have been documented in many circumstances and diseases and interpretation of serum measurements therefore requires other clinical and biochemical data. Low levels of 1,25-$(OH)_2$D can be due to deficient substrate concentrations, organic or functional enzyme deficiency, low circulating DBP levels, or other less well defined reasons (Table 4).

Indeed, when the substrate levels (see preceding chapter on 25-OHD) are extremely low, low or undetectable levels of 1,25-$(OH)_2$D are the rule. In clinical

Table 4. Abnormal serum concentrations of 1,25- dihydroxyvitamin D

Decreased concentrations	Increased concentrations
Substrate deficiency e.g., "nutritional" rickets, intestinal malabsorption	(Substrate excess)[a]
25-OHD-1α-hydroxylase *Enzyme deficiency*	25-OHD-1α-Hydroxylase *Enzyme excess*
Inborn: vitamin D-dependent rickets	Functional
Organic: renal insufficiency or anephric patients	Primary or tertiary hyperparathyroidism
Functional: Hypoparathyroidism	Hypothyroidism
Pseudohypoparathyroidism	Glucocorticoid excess
Hypomagnesemia	Acromegaly
Tumoral osteomalacia	Sarcoidosis
Hypercalcemia of malignancy	Idiopathic hypercalciuria
Hyperthyroidism	Hypophosphatemic rickets type 2
Morbus Addison (acute)	(+ hypercalciuria)
Severe insulin deficiency	Pregnancy
X-linked hypophosphatemia	Nutritional calcium deficiency
Rhabdomyolysis	
Tumoral calcinosis	William's syndrome
DBP Deficiency	DBP Excess
Fetus	Pregnancy
Nephrotic syndrome	Estrogens
Liver cirrhosis	End organ resistance
Unknown or disputed origin:	True vitamin D resistance (so-called
primary osteoporosis	vitamin D-dependent rickets type 2)
	Osteopetrosis

[a] Vitamin D excess only increases serum 1,25-$(OH)_2$D when renal function remains normal and/or PTH secretion is elevated. Usually 1,25-$(OH)_2$D levels are low or normal in vitamin D toxicity

vitamin D-deficient rickets or osteomalacia, sometimes near-normal 1,25-$(OH)_2$D levels can be observed and such observations have even confused the crucial role of this metabolite as the main or even only vitamin D hormone. Two possible reasons may explain this apparent discrepancy: firstly, transient access to even very small amounts of vitamin D will immediately result in its conversion into 1,25-$(OH)_2$D by the overstimulated enzymes. Such a transient presence of 1,25-$(OH)_2D_3$ is insufficient to cure longstanding rickets but sufficient to cause difficulties in clinical interpretation of very low 25-OHD levels and near normal 1,25-$(OH)_2$D levels. Secondly, when such vitamin D-deficient humans or animals are treated with physiological amounts of vitamin D, 1,25-$(OH)_2$D immediately rises to very high levels, exceeding the mean normal range 3 to 4-fold. Normal values of 1,25-$(OH)_2$D in the presence of very low 25-OHD levels, secondary hyperparathyroidism, and rickets are thus in fact inappropriately low.

Deficiency of the renal 25-OHD-1α-hydroxylase activity may be simply due to the absence of sufficient kidney tissue as in the case of anephry or severe (acute but especially chronic) renal failure [7]. The deficiency in 1,25-(OH)$_2$D may even precede and contribute to the secondary hyperparathyroidism of renal failure, at least when this hyperparathyroidism is appropriately evaluated by aminoterminal or intact assays ([35] and personal observations). An inborn error of metabolism, known as vitamin D-dependent rickets, is characterized by deficient renal 25-OHD-1α-hydroxylase activity. This has only been documented by indirect means in man but a similar autosomal recessive abnormality has been well evaluated in a pig strain. Whether the human disease is due to a total absence or modification of the enzyme structure (or a mixture of all possible abnormalities) is presently unknown.

All diseases characterized by primary or secondary hypoparathyroidism and pseudohypoparathyroidism are associated with decreased 1,25-(OH)$_2$D levels because PTH is the main hormonal stimulator of the renal 1α-hydroxylase activity (Table 4). Acute or severe chronic insulin deficiency also depresses the formation of 1,25-(OH)$_2$D. This has been well documented in diabetic rats but can also be found in diabetic man when the diabetes is severely out of control [33]. In hypophosphatemic rickets low, normal, and even increased 1,25-(OH)$_2$D levels have been observed. In classical, X-linked dominant hypophosphatemic rickets low or inappropriately low (versus circulating phosphate levels) 1,25-(OH)$_2$D levels are the rule and this may explain the associated low calcium absorption and excretion [12]. Some patients with an autosomal form of hypophosphatemia, however, have a high intestinal calcium absorption, hypercalciuria, and appropriately elevated 1,25-(OH)$_2$D levels and some authors have even suggested that this might be the extreme form of a much more common disease known as idiopathic hypercalciuria [45]. The defect in the phosphate leak may be different in the two forms of rickets and localized either at the serosal site, whereby intracellular phosphate is high and 1,25-(OH)$_2$D synthesis low (X-linked or classical form), or located at the luminal site with subsequent low intracellular phosphate levels and high 1,25-(OH)$_2$D production (hypercalciuric hypophosphatemia).

Low DBP levels can also be the origin of low 1,25-(OH)$_2$D levels but when free plasma levels remain within normal limits no abnormalities in mineral metabolism are to be expected. This is the case during fetal life and in many (mild) cases of impaired DBP synthesis (liver cirrhosis) or DBP loss (nephrotic syndrome) [2].

Whether osteoporosis is associated with low 1,25-(OH)$_2$D is a matter of dispute. In primary osteoporosis type 1, formally known as classical postmenopausal osteoporosis, usually normal, low-normal, or slightly decreased 1,25-(OH)$_2$D levels have been observed but most studies have not used appropriate control groups (e.g., age- and calcium-intake-matched controls). In type 2 or senile osteoporosis, serum 1,25-(OH)$_2$D is more frequently decreased but this is usually due to associated impaired kidney function or subclinical vitamin D deficiency. Abnormalities of 1,25-(OH)$_2$D are thus of doubtful primary importance in both types of osteoporosis. Similarly, in patients with recent hip fractures, serum 1,25-(OH)$_2$D is frequently below the normal mean but this is most often due to decrease in DBP, 25-OHD deficiency, or impaired kidney function [27].

Increased levels of circulating 1,25-(OH)$_2$D are an unusual aspect of vitamin D intoxication (vide supra) and are mostly due to functional overactivity of the renal 1α-hydroxylase, DBP excess, or end organ resistance (Table 4).

Hyperparathyroidism (primary or tertiary) is frequently associated with a mild increase in serum 1,25-(OH)$_2$D. Hypothyroidism and Cushing's disease are also associated with a mild increase in 1,25-(OH)$_2$D maybe (partly) due to associated mild hyperparathyroidism. In active sarcoidosis, ectopic production of 1,25-(OH)$_2$D probably occurs in monocyte-macrocyte noduli which are able to produce more 1,25-(OH)$_2$D than normally required, therefore firstly suppressing the normal renal secretion and finally resulting in excess 1,25-(OH)$_2$D, hypercalciuria, hypercalcemia, and functional hypoparathyroidism [4, 5, 29]. A similar pattern has occasionally been seen in other disorders of monocytes-macrophages (tuberculosis, foreign body granulomatosis, mycosis, and some types of lymphomas). Some patients with idiopathic hypercalciuria have increased 1,25-(OH)$_2$D levels of unknown origin and resemble the hypercalciuric forms of hypophosphatemic rickets (vide supra).

In William's syndrome (a rare form of transient hypercalcemia during childhood associated with supravalvular aortic stenosis and a typical elfin face), increased 1,25-(OH)$_2$D levels have been found during the active phase of the disease [19], but this has not been universally confirmed. The origin of excess 1,25-(OH)$_2$D observed in some cases of tumoral calcinosis (ectopic calcifications or bone formation) is presently unknown.

During pregnancy, 1,25-(OH)$_2$D levels increase in most mammalian species. This is primarily due to an increase in the serum DBP concentration which occurs early in pregnancy due to estrogen impregnation. Only at the end of pregnancy is a real increase in free 1,25-(OH)$_2$D observed at the time of increased maternal calcium need and maternal secondary hyperparathyroidism due to fetal bone mineralization [8]. Outside pregnancy DBP only increases substantially under the influence of estrogens, either used as contraceptive drugs or as prevention or treatment for osteoporosis. Again, this DBP-induced increase in serum 1,25-(OH)$_2$D has frequently been misinterpreted as a physiologically important mechanism of action of estrogens on calcium metabolism, whereas a real increase in free 1,25-(OH)$_2$D during estrogen intake has only been observed when net calcium retention was induced by estrogens (e.g., by increased bone formation induced by estrogens in birds).

When the end organs are partially or totally unresponsive to 1,25-(OH)$_2$D, an increase in circulating hormones might be expected as is the case in other hormone resistance syndromes (e.g., resistance for insulin, thyroid hormones, or androgens). The best known but rare syndrome of true 1,25-(OH)$_2$D resistance is due to abnormal vitamin D receptors (absence, decreased capacity or affinity of receptors, increased lability or loss of binding to DNA or other yet to be defined abnormalities). The hallmark of this abnormality is the presence of (very) high 1,25-(OH)$_2$D concentrations in the presence of rickets and (sometimes) of total alopecia. The formal diagnosis requires the demonstration of abnormal vitamin D receptor [e.g., by measuring receptor affinity, capacity, stability or activity in lymphocytes or fibroblasts in vitro [26]]. Osteopetrosis is a congenital disorder or deficiency of the osteoclast and, since bone resorption is impaired, secondary hyperparathyroidism and high $1,25\text{-}(OH)_2D$ concentrations have been observed. The lack of sufficient thyroid hormone-stimulated bone resorption in hypothyroidism may also contribute to a secondary increase in circulating $1,25\text{-}(OH)_2D$ levels.

Use of Measurements of Vitamin D Metabolites in the Differential Diagnosis of Clinical Syndromes

In real clinical medicine biochemical tests are used for the exploration of symptoms or syndromes and so measurements of the calciotropic hormones, including vitamin D metabolites, can contribute in the differential diagnosis of some common or uncommon syndromes such as rickets, osteopenia, and hyper- and hypocalcemia (Tables 5–7).

Most cases of *rickets* are due to a deficiency of the substrate (vitamin D) and are therefore associated with low 25-OHD levels. Only when 25-OHD levels are within or above the normal range should a further exploration into the etiology of the more exceptional cases of rickets be started especially because it is unlikely that such children would respond to a normal physiological dose of vitamin D or 25-OHD. Measurement of $1,25\text{-}(OH)_2D$ then can help to differentiate vitamin D-dependent rickets from vitamin D-resistant types of rickets, whereas information about calcium intake (rare forms of calcium-deficiency rickets) or renal phosphate handling (hypophosphatemic rickets and its variants) should direct the clinician to the non-vitamin-D-related types of rickets (Table 5).

The differential diagnosis of *osteopenia* always requires the rapid recognition of easily treatable osteomalacia versus the different types of primary or secondary osteoporosis. This can be most easily screened by measurements of alkaline

Table 5. Differential diagnosis of rickets or osteomalacia

	Ca	P	25-OHD	$24,25\text{-}(OH)_2D$	$1,25\text{-}(OH)_2D$	PTH
Vitamin D-deficient rickets	N–↓	↓	↓↓	↓↓	↓N↑	↑
Vitamin D-dependent rickets (I)	↓	↓	N	N	↓	↑
True vitamin D resistance (II)	↓	↓	N	↓–N	↑↑	↑
Calcium-deficient rickets	↓	↓	N	N	↑	↑
Phosphate-deficient rickets	N	↓↓N	N	N	N(↓)	N

Table 6. Differential diagnosis of hypercalcemia

Etiology	PTH(1–84)	25-OHD	1,25-(OH)$_2$D	Other diagnostic tests
Hyperparathyroidism (primary and tertiary)	High	N	(High)	–
Pseudohyperparathyroidism or humoral malignancy-associated hypercalcemia	Low	N	Low	? PTH-related peptide
Granulomatous diseases and lymphoproliferative diseases				
– Sarcoidosis				
– Tuberculosis	Low	N	High	Appropriate test for each disease
– Fungal diseases				
– Berylliosis				
Primary bone involvement due to				
– Bone metastases				
– Hematological cancers				
– Hyperthyroidism	Low	N	Low	Appropriate history and clinical findings
– Addison's disease				
– Immobilization, especially when associated with increased bone turnover (paget's disease, youngsters)				
Drug-induced				
– Vitamin A excess	Low	N	Low	Drug history—vitamin A assay
– Vitamin D excess	?	Very high	?	Drug history—vitamin D assay
– Thiazide diurectics	Low	N	Low	Drug history
– Lithium	High?	N	?	Drug history—Li assay
– Milk-alkali syndrome	Low?	N	Low?	Drug history
Idiopathic hypercalcemia of infancy	?	N	High?	Age and typical elfin face
Familial hypocalciuric (benign) hypercalcemia	N	N	N	Dominant inheritance of benign Hypercalcemia
Hyperproteinemia	N	N	N	Ionized calcium
Laboratory error	N	N	N	Repeat assay of calcium

L, N, H: low, normal, and high serum concentration

Table 7. Hypocalcemia

	PTH	25-OHD	1,25-$(OH)_2$D

Hypoparathyroidism
    Idiopathic
    Postsurgical
	L	N	L

Pseudohypoparathyroidism	H	N	L
Renal failure	H	(N)	L
Vitamin D deficiency	H	L	(L)
Magnesium deficiency	L	N	L
excess	L	N	?
Acute pancreatitis	H	N	?

L, N, H: low, normal, and high serum concentration

phosphatase but 25-OHD measurements give a better degree of certainty about the vitamin D status. Serum 1,25-$(OH)_2$D levels contribute less in this syndrome except in exceptional forms of osteomalacia.

Hypercalcemia is a frequent challenge for rapid and accurate differential diagnosis and measurements of vitamin D metabolites are usually a requisite especially when PTH levels are low. Extremely elevated levels of 25-OHD will immediately prove vitamin D intoxication while high 1,25-$(OH)_2$D levels in the presence of hypercalcemia and low PTH levels are diagnostic for ectopic 1,25-$(OH)_2$D production, usually by active sarcoidosis or other monocyte-macrophage-related diseases (vide supra and Table 6). Low levels of 1,25-$(OH)_2$D and PTH should direct further search in the direction of bone resorption induced by different agents (e.g., bone metastases, hyperthyroidism; Table 6). The most difficult differential diagnosis in hypercalcemia remains the difference between humoral hypercalcemia of malignancy (HHM) and primary hyperparathyroidism, but in addition to low concentrations of both 1,25-$(OH)_2$D and PTH (1-84) high levels of PTH-related peptide should facilitate the correct diagnosis of HHM.

The differential diagnosis of *hypocalcemia* is usually a simpler clinical problem since, after exclusion of hypocalcemia secondary to renal failure, PTH and 25-OHD should be measured: low PTH levels will direct attention to either primary hypoparathyroidism or severe magnesium deficiency, and low 25-OHD levels will confirm vitamin D deficiency (Table 7).

Conclusion

Vitamin D has grown during this century from a single compound (vitamin D), produced in one tissue (skin) and acting on one system (calcium-bone homeostasis), into a complex system where many tissues or cells (Table 1) contribute to the formation of an ever-increasing list of vitamin D metabolites (Fig. 1) active in nearly all tissues even outside the strict field of calcium metabolism (Table 2). Measurement of the main vitamin D metabolites is still confronted with severe technical difficulties but has been improved markedly by the advent of more direct measurements of 25-OHD and 1,25-$(OH)_2$D. These assays certainly contribute to clinical and experimental medicine to allow a better diagnosis and more appropriate therapeutic intervention, especially now that many new drugs are found to be effective in maintaining or restoring normal mineral homeostasis.

References

1. Adams JS, Clemens TL, Parrish JA, Holick MH (1982) Vitamin D synthesis and metabolism after ultraviolet irradiation of normal and vitamin D-deficient subjects. N Engl J Med 306:722–725
2. Auwerx J, De Keyser L, Bouillon R, De Moor P (1986) Decreased free 1,25-dihydroxycholecalciferol index in patients with the nephrotic syndrome. Nephron 42:231–235
3. Baran DT (1983) Effect of phenobarbital treatment on metabolism of vitamin D by rat liver. Am J Physiol 245:E55–E59
4. Bell NH (1985) Vitamin D-endocrine system. J Clin Invest 76:1–6
5. Bell NH, Stern PH, Pantzer E, Sinha TK, DeLuca HF (1979) Evidence that increased circulating 1α,25-dihydroxyvitamin D is the probable cause for abnormal calcium metabolism in sarcoidosis. J Clin Invest 64:218–225
6. Bouillon R (1983) Radiochemical assays for vitamin D metabolites: technical possibilities and clinical applications. J Steroid Biochem 19:921–927
7. Bouillon R (1988) Vitamin D and the kidney: a short review. Contrib Nephrol 64:25–33
8. Bouillon R, Van Assche FA, Van Baelen H, Heyns W, De Moor P (1981) Influence of the vitamin D-binding protein on the serum concentration of 1,25-dihydroxyvitamin D_3. J Clin Invest 67:589–596
9. Bouillon R, Van Herck E, Jans I, Tan BK, Van Baelen H, De Moor P (1984) Two direct (nonchromatographic) assays for 25-hydroxyvitamin D. Clin Chem 30:1731–1736
10. Bouillon R, Van Baelen H, De Moor P (1986) Physiology and pathophysiology of vitamin D-binding protein. In: Forest MG, Pugeat M (eds) Physiology and pathophysiology of vitamin D-binding protein. Libbey, London, pp 333–356
11. Bouillon RA, Auwerx JH, Lissens WD, Pelemans WK (1987) Vitamin D status in the elderly: seasonal substrate deficiency causes 1,25-dihydroxycholecalciferol deficiency. Am J Clin Nutr 45:755–763
12. Broadus AE, Insogna KL, Lang R, Ellison AF, Dreyer BE (1984) Evidence for disordered control of 1,25-dihydroxyvitamin D production in absorptive hypercalciuria. N Engl J Med 311:73–80
13. Brommage R, DeLuca HF (1985) Evidence that 1,25-dihydroxyvitamin D_3 is the physiologically active metabolite of vitamin D_3. Endocr Rev 6:491–511
14. Chesney RW, Rosen JF, Hamstra AJ, Smith C, Mahaffey K, DeLuca HF (1981)

Absence of seasonal variation in serum concentrations of 1,25-dihydroxyvitamin D despite a rise in 25-hydroxyvitamin D in summer. J Clin Endocrinol Metab 53:139–142

15. Clements MR, Johnson L, Fraser DR (1987) A new mechanism for induced vitamin D deficiency in calcium deprivation. Nature 325:62–65

16. Corbeel L, Bouillon R, Deschamps L, Guesens H (1976) Vitamin D sensitive rickets in adolescents. Acta Paediatr Belg 29:103–108

17. Culler FL (1987) Calcitropic hormones in childhood. Pediatr Ann 16:966–973

18. Fraser DR, Kodicek E (1970) Unique biosynthesis by kidney of a biologically active vitamin D metabolite. Nature 228:764–766

19. Garabédian M, Jacqz E, Guillozo H, Grimberg R, Guillot M, Gagnadoux M-F, Broyer M, Lenoir G, Balsan S (1985) Elevated plasma 1,25-dihydroxyvitamin D concentrations in infants with hypercalcemia and an elfin facies. N Engl J Med 312:948–952

20. Heaney RP, Gallagher JC, Johnston CC, Neer R, Parfitt AM, Chir B, Whedon GD (1982) Calcium nutrition and bone health in the elderly. Am J Clin Nutr 36:986–1013

21. Holick MF (1985) The photobiology of vitamin D and its consequences for humans. Ann NY Acad Sci 453:1–13

22. Keiver KM, Draper HM, Ronald K (1988) Vitamin D metabolism in the hooded seal (*Cystophora cristate*). J Nutr 118:332–341

23. Kumar R (1984) Metabolism of 1,25-dihydroxyvitamin D_3. Physiol Rev 64:478–504

24. Ladatan AAD, Adeniyi A (1975) Rickets in Nigerian children, response to vitamin D. J Trop Med Hyg 78:206–210

25. Lapatsanis P, Deliyanni V, Doxiadis S (1968) Vitamin D deficiency in Greece. J Pediatr 73:195–199

26. Liberman UA (1988) Inborn errors in vitamin D metabolism. Their contribution to the understanding of vitamin D metabolism. In: Vitamin D. Molecular, cellular and clinical endocrinology. Norman AW et al. (eds) de Gruyter, Berlin, pp 935–947

27. Lips P, Bouillon R, Jongen MJM, Van Ginkel FC, Van der Vijgh WJF, Netelenbos JC (1985) The effect of trauma on serum concentrations of vitamin D metabolites in patients with hip fracture. Bone 6:63–67

28. Lips P, Van Ginkel FC, Jongen MJM, Rubertus F, Van der Vijgh WJH, Netelenbos JC (1987) Determinants of vitamin D status in patients with hip fracture and in elderly control subjects. Am J Clin Nutr 46:1005–1010

29. Manolagas SC (1987) Vitamin D and its revelance to cancer. Anticancer Res 7:625–638

30. Mazess RB, Cameron JR (1972) Growth of bone in school children: comparison of radiographic morphometry and photon absorptiometry. Growth 36:77–84

31. M'Buyamba-Kabangu JR, Fagard R, Lijnen P, Bouillon R, Lissens W, Amery A (1987) Calcium, vitamin D-endocrine system, and parathyroid hormone in black and white males. Calcif Tissue Int 41:70–74

32. Nyomba BL, Bouillon R, Visser WJ, Einhorn TA, Thomasset M, Dequeker J, De Moor P (1986) Calcium and bone homeostasis in diabetic BB rats. Transplant Proc 18:1502–1503

33. Norman AW, Roth J, Orci L (1982) The vitamin D endocrine system: steroid metabolism, hormone receptors, and biological response (calcium binding proteins). Endocr Rev 3:331–366

34. Parfitt AM, Chir B, Gallagher JC, Heaney RP, Johnston CC, Neer R, Whedon GD (1982) Vitamin D and bone health in the elderly. Am J Clin Nutr 36:1014–1031

35. Pitts TO, Piraino BH, Mitro R, Chen TC, Segre GV, Greenberg A, Puschett JB (1988) Hyperparathyroidism and 1,25-dihydroxyvitamin D deficiency in mild, moderate and severe renal failure. J Clin Endocrinol Metab 67:876–881

36. Porteous CE, Coldwell RD, Trafford DJH, Makin HLJ (1987) Recent developments in the measurement of vitamin D and its metabolites in human body fluids. J Steroid Biochem 28:785–801

37. Preece MA, Tomlinson S, Ribot CA, Pietrek J, Korn HT, Davies M, Ford JA, Dunnigan MG, O'Riordan JLH (1975) Studies of vitamin D deficiency in man. Q J Med 44:575–589

38. Quesada JM, Jans I, Benito P, Jimenez JA, Bouillon R (1989) Vitamin D status of the elderly in Spain. Age Ageing 18:392–397

39. Reeve L, Tanaka Y, DeLuca HF (1983) Studies on the site of 1,25-dihydroxyvitamin D_3 synthesis in vivo. J Biol Chem 258:3615–3617

40. Schmidt-Gayk H, Grawunder C, Tschöpe W, Schmit W, Ritz E, Pietsch V, Andrassy K, Bouillon R (1977) 25-Hydroxyvitamin D in nephrotic syndrome. Lancet II: 105–108

41. Sedrani SH (1987) Are Saudis at risk of developing vitamin D deficiency. Saudi Med J 7:427–433

42. Specker BL, Tsang RC (1986) Vitamin D infancy and childhood: factors determining vitamin D status. Adv Pediatr 33:1–22

43. Stanbury SW (1981) Vitamin D-metamorphosis from nutrient to hormonal system. P Nutr Soc 40: 179–186

44. Taylor AF, Norman ME (1984) Vitamin D metabolite levels in normal children. Pediatr Res 18:886–892

45. Tieder M, Modai D, Samuel R, Arie R, Halabe A, Bab I, Gabizon D, Liberman U (1985) Hereditary hypophosphatemic rickets with hypercalciuria. N Engl J Med 312:611–616

46. Vanham G, Van Baelen H, Tan BK, Bouillon R (1988) The effect of vitamin D analogs and of vitamin D-binding protein on lymphocyte proliferation. J Steroid Biochem 29:381–386

Diagnostic Value of the Peptides from the Calcitonin Gene

F. RAUE, H.-G. SCHNEIDER, and A. GRAUER

Introduction

Calcitonin (CT) was discovered in the 1960s by Copp and colleagues [5], who first recognized the calcium-lowering effect of this hormone which is produced and secreted by the thyroid C-cells. Soon it was regarded as a major calcium-regulating factor, along with parathyroid hormone and vitamin D. Subsequently it was shown that CT protects the skeleton in physiological conditions where much calcium is required, e.g. during growth, pregnancy, and lactation. CT and/or CT receptors are also present in the brain, mediating the inhibition of pain perception, gastric acid secretion, and food intake. This supports a possible role of CT as a neurotransmitter. Despite this progress, the physiological function of CT remains uncertain [3, 42]. But the diagnostic role of CT as a tumor marker of medullary thyroid carcinoma (MTC), a tumor of the C-cells, is indisputable. This diagnostic tool might be extended to the peptides encoded by the calcitonin gene: besides CT, calcitonin gene-related peptide (CGRP) and katacalcin (KC) [2].

Expression of the Calcitonin Gene

Many peptide hormones are synthesized initially as much larger biologically inactive precursors or prohormones, which are subsequently processed in the secretory vesicles to produce a number or family of smaller biologically active polypeptide hormones. Human and rat medullary thyroid carcinoma (MTC) have been the sources of CT-mRNA encoding for the pre-pro-CT (mol wt., 15 000), which could be synthesized by a cell-free translation of this RNA. The human pre-pro-CT, a 136-amino-acid peptide, is cleaved by posttranslational processing to pro-CT (111-amino acid peptide). This generates four different peptides: calcitonin (CT) from the middle region, a 21-amino acid carboxy terminal calcitonin-adjacent peptide [C-CAP = katacalcin (KC) = PDN-21] from the carboxy terminus, and both an amino-terminal peptide (NTP) and an amino-terminal CT-adjacent peptide (N-CAP) from the amino terminus [16] (Fig. 1).

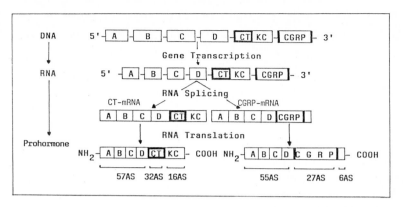

Fig. 1. Organization of the calcitonin gene, the transcription and translation of the RNA to the two prohormones of calcitonin and calcitonin gene-related peptide

The CT gene actually generates another discrete mRNA which encodes the precursor peptide for CGRP. This precursor molecule contains the CGRP at its carboxy terminus and at its amino terminus two larger peptides which are found to be homologous with the amino-terminal peptides of the CT precursor [33] (Fig. 1).

There are two CT/CGRP genes which have been localized to the short arm of chromosome 11 (*Calc I* and *Calc II*). This gene duplication seems to be incomplete, as there are two encoding regions for *CGRP I* (α) and *CGRP II* (β), but in the second human gene the region encoding a CT-like structure seems not to be expressed [37]. The transcription of the CT/CGRP gene is tissue specific. Predominantly CT and only a little CGRP I is expressed in the thyroid C-cell, whereas CGRP II is mainly expressed in the human CNS and in the pituitary gland. Among others the choice of different expression is made by a posttranscriptional event of alternative RNA processing. By splicing the primary transcript two different mRNA's encoding either CT or CGRP are formed. Through gene duplication and alternative splicing new peptides with separate but overlapping biological effects could be involved [7].

Structure and Activity of Peptides from the Calcitonin Family

All known CTs and CGRPs are single-chain peptides with 32 and 37 amino acid residues, respectively. They have in common the amino-terminal ring structures linked by disulfide bridges and the amidated carboxyl termini (Table 1). The CT sequences from different species have been shown to display considerable differences. However, eight residues have been found to be invariant. In contrast CGRP differs only in 8 of the 37 amino acids in chicken, rat, and man. The two

CGRPs (α and β) have been demonstrated to differ in one (rat) and three (man) amino acids, respectively. It can be assumed that CGRP is under stronger evolutionary control than calcitonin [39]. There is no evidence for a second CT in man, while salmon expresses three different CTs. A CT-like molecule has been found in the CNS of mammals.

As a result of 30% homology between the CT and the CGRPs, there is overlapping recognition of the peptides by their receptors and they have some biological targets in common. The difference in the amino acid sequences of the various CTs is not important for their biological response, although salmon CT is more potent, i.e. biologically active, than mammalian CT on a weight basis. The heterogeneity in the amino acid sequences allows development of species-specific antisera which cross-react poorly with the CT molecules of other species.

Katacalcin (KC) has been found to be a 21-amino-acid polypeptide with a molecular weight of 2600. It is situated at the carboxy-terminal end of the pro-CT and separated from CT by a four-amino-acid sequence. In preliminary experiments a plasma calcium-lowering effect could be shown [22], but the same researchers found later that KC had little or no effect on plasma calcium. The physiological role of KC remains to be determined.

Calcitonin is biosynthesized and secreted by the C cells, or parafollicular cells, of the thyroid gland and acts on bone and kidney. The hypocalcemic effect of CT is established by inhibition of bone resorption and reduction in the number and size of osteoclasts and inhibition of Ca reabsorption in the kidney. Binding sites for CT have been demonstrated in osteoclasts and kidney cells. CT receptors are linked to adenylate cyclase activation and cyclic AMP production [18].

Several studies suggest the presence of CT and/or CT receptors in the brain and pituitary [7]. These results support a possible role for CT as a new transmitter, in addition to its calcium-regulating role. CGRP is principally a neuropeptide synthesized throughout the CNS but also by perivascular nerve terminals and to a lesser extent in the C cells of the thyroid. CGRP-binding sites are abundant in the cerebellum and in blood vessels. CGRP modulates arteriolar tone. Intravenous administration of CGRP produces hypotension, while intracerebroventricular injection of CGRP raises the arterial pressure and the heart pulse rate [8].

It also causes dilatation of the coronary vessels in man [21]. Hypocalcemic action of CGRP obtained in high amounts in relation to those of CT is mediated through CT receptors on osteoclasts [9].

Radioimmunoassay

Radioimmunological determination of CT has been performed routinely for clinical use for 15 years [31]. Radioimmunoassays for KC and CGRP have been developed during the past 5 years for research purposes.

Table 1. Amino acid sequences of human calcitonin (hCT) and human calcitonin gene-related peptide I and II (hCGRP I/II, hCGRP α/β)

	hCGRP I/α	hCGRP II/β	hCT	
1	Ala	–	Cys	1
2	Cys	–	Gly	2
3	Asp	Asn	–	3
4	Thr	–	Leu	4
5	Ala	–	Ser	5
6	Thr	–	–	6
7	Cys	–	–	7
8	Val	–	Met	8
9	Thr	–	Leu	9
10	His	–	Gly	10
11	Arg	–	Thr	11
12	Leu	–	Tyr	12
13	Ala	–	Thr	13
14	Gly	–	Gln	14
15	Leu	–	Asp	15
16	Leu	–	Phe	16
17	Ser	–	Asn	17
18	Arg	–	Lys	18
19	Ser	–	Phe	19
20	Gly	–	His	20
21	Gly	–	Thr	21
22	Val	Met	:	
23	Val	–	.	
24	Lys	–	.	
25	Asn	Ser	.	
26	Asn	–	.	
27	Phe	–	–	22
28	Val	–	Pro	23
29	Pro	–	Gln	24
30	Thr	–	–	25
31	Asn	–	Ala	26
32	Val	–	Ile	27
33	Gly	–	–	28
34	Ser	–	Val	29
35	Lys	–	Gly	30
36	Ala	–	–	31
37	Phe	–	Pro	32
	|	|	|	
	NH$_3$	NH$_3$	NH$_3$	

Calcitonin Radioimmunoassay

With commercially available CT-RIA kits results of clinical importance are obtained. But there are several problems concerning the use of CT-RIAs. The major biological problem is the fact that the actual concentration of CT in human plasma appears to be very low. The lower limit of the normal range is undefined, only some healthy persons having measurable CT levels. The upper limit of the normal range varies from 10 to 300 ng/liter [12]. The reason for this variability in the normal levels of CT remains uncertain, but there are several possibilities, such as variability in the purity of the human CT standard, the ability of the antiserum to recognize the regional specificity of the CT molecule, and the immunochemical heterogeneity of circulating CT [4]. Several approaches have been tried to reduce nonspecific effects, including affinity chromatography and immunoextraction. Each of these methods has its limitations and at present they are primarily research techniques. Values of different systems are not directly comparable, as shown in two international quality surveys [26]. The interpretation of radioimmunoassay (RIA) results must be based on normative data developed with the assay in use. "Normal" values from the literature are totally invalid. If the assay is to be used for measuring CT after stimulation of secretion by pentagastrin or calcium (see below), it is absolutely necessary to obtain the appropriate data from stimulation tests in normal volunteers. One has to consider that in both sexes plasma CT values decline with age [6]. The question whether especially osteoporotic postmenopausal women suffer from a decreased CT secretory capacity after stimulation remains open [20].

The recent development of immunoradiometric assays with labeling of a monoclonal antibody [23, 24] or enzymimmunoassays [1, 17] might solve some technical and practical problems of CT assays.

Katacalcin Radioimmunoassay

Antibodies against KC were raised in goats and rabbits by subcutaneous injection of KC conjugated to ovalbumin [13]. In an RIA using [^{125}I]Tyr-KC as a tracer and synthetic KC as standard, a sensitivity of 100 ng/liter was achieved [30]. Extraction of KC onto C_{18} cartridges, followed by its elution and concentration before RIA, permitted the detection of the peptide in normal subjects [14, 39]. CT and KC concentrations are approximately equimolar in samples from MTC patients. Normal C-cells also cosecrete CT and KC in equimolar quantities. Both hormones circulate in higher concentrations in men than in women; the level is reduced at a higher age. There appear also to be ethnic differences: white women show lower KC-levels than black women [38].

Calcitonin Gene-Related Peptide Radioimmunoassay (CGRP RIA)

Antiserum was raised in rabbits against synthetic hCGRP or against synthetic C-terminal analogs of rat CGRP that do not cross-react with a number of other peptides including hCT. The limit of sensitivity of the assay varied from 5 pmol/liter to 21 pmol/liter; the normal serum values are below 10–32 pmol/liter. CGRP circulates at five times the concentration of CT; the most likely origin of plasma CGRP appears to be the perivascular nerves, although a thyroid or pituitary origin cannot be excluded [10]. Recent studies generally found CGRP levels to be 10- to 20-fold lower than CT levels [34]. This apparent discrepancy may reflect differences in the CGRP assays. Clearly further work is necessary in order to define the circulating levels of CGRP in normal subjects accurately.

Diagnostic Value of the Radioimmunoassay

The problem of their inability to measure at/or below the lower limit of normal afflicts all published RIAs for CT, KC, and CGRP. The assays are useful in differentiating between normal and elevated levels. Serum CT is reported to be high in patients with medullary thyroid carcinoma but also in other neoplastic diseases as well as in pancreatitis, pernicious anemia, lung diseases, and renal failure. In MTC the other peptides (KC, CGRP) have been studied.

Medullary Thyroid Carcinoma

In most patients with medullary thyroid carcinoma (MTC), the basal concentration of CT is sufficiently elevated to be diagnostic of the tumor's presence presurgically [27, 28]. There is a positive correlation between the tumor mass and the level of the tumor marker CT. Although CT levels exceed 1000–10 000 times the normal levels and this CT is biologically active in other test systems, no definitive long-term effect of chronic CT excess is observed. Patients with occult C-cell carcinoma may have normal or only slightly elevated CT levels. To identify those patients, provocation tests for CT secretion have been developed. They are highly specific and can differentiate between healthy persons and patients with C-cell hyperplasia or occult MTC. Pentagastrin (0.5 µg/kg body weight, injected i.v. over 15 s) is widely used as a provocative agent for CT secretion in patients with MTC. Within 2–5 min a prompt increase in serum CT is observed, even in patients who formerly had normal basal CT levels, while normal persons show only a slight increase within the normal range. An alternative is the calcium infusion test (3 mg/kg body weight over 10 min i.v.)

which produces an abnormal increase in serum CT in MTC patients within
10–20 min. This test is of importance in the early diagnosis of familial MTC or
of multiple endocrine neoplasia type 2 (Sipple's syndrome; combination of MTC
and pheochromocytoma). In addition, determination of KC can be used as an
independent marker [14, 30]. Katacalcin also responds to i.v. pentagastrin or
calcium. Both peptides are cosecreted from normal C cells as well as from
malignant ones [15, 32]. (Fig. 2).

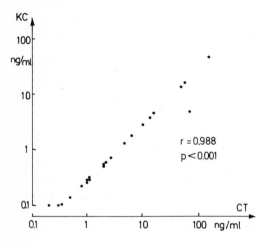

Fig. 2. Correlation between calcitonin and katacalcin in sera of patients with medullary
thyroid carcinoma ($n = 22$)

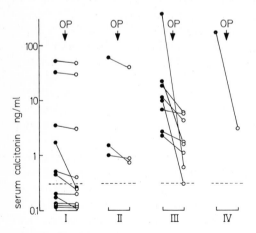

Fig. 3. Calcitonin levels in patients with medullary thyroid carcinoma in relation to the
stage of disease: ●, preoperative; 0, postoperative calcitonin level; *I*, tumor localized to
the thyroid gland; *II*, tumor localized to the thyroid gland and movable regional lymph
nodes; *III*, direct local invasion or fixed cervical lymph nodes; *IV*, distant metastases

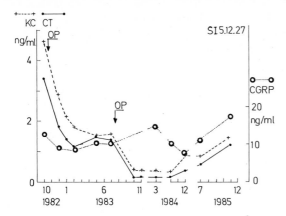

Fig. 4. Long-term follow-up measurement of the tumor marker calcitonin (*CT*), katacalcin (*KC*), and calcitonin gene-related peptide (*CGRP*) in a patient with medullary thyroid carcinoma

Monitoring of serum CT as well as KC is an effective method of evaluating therapy in patients with MTC. Serum CT/KC levels generally fall within days in the immediate postoperative period. Postsurgical determination of CT/KC is valuable for assessing of the radicality of surgery. Elevated basal and/or pentagastrin-stimulated tumor marker levels (CT/KC) are considered to indicate residual tumor and/or metastatic disease (Fig. 3). Localizing investigations are then indicated using selective venous catheterization with determination of CT and KC levels in the various blood samples.

Plasma CGRP levels are usually elevated in MTC, but generally CT values are found to be higher than those of CGRP [19, 34] (Fig. 4); the ratio of the two peptides varies from patient to patient. The results concerning the correlation with CT levels and the release after Ca or pentagastrin infusion are conflicting [19, 29]. The reasons for discrepancies are the different RIAs used for determination of different CGRP (I, II). The importance of CGRP measurement in the management of MTC has to be elucidated further.

Other Diseases and Outlook

Other diseases may be accompanied by elevated levels of CT, particularly cancers (Table 2). A wide variety of tumors besides MTC may cause apparent hypercalcitoninemia by ectopic or eutopic secretion or by nonspecific interference with the assay. Some of the tumors are of neuroectodermal origin like the C-cells, e.g., pheochromocytoma, carcinoid, endocrine tumors of the pancreas, and perhaps oat cell carcinoma of the lung [11, 35]. On the other hand, osteolytic tumors can induce hypercalcemia, which might stimulate CT secretion [36]. Interestingly, chronic hypercalcemia of primary hyperparathyroidism

Table 2. Conditions associated with an elevated serum calcitonin concentration

Origin of CT	Condition	Disease
Eutopic		
Thyroid	Increased production	Medullary thyroid carcinoma, hypercalcemia of malignancy, hypergastrinemia (Zollinger–Ellison syndrome, pernicious anemia)
	Altered metabolism	Chronic renal failure
?	?	Pancreatitis
Ectopic		
Malignant tumor	Increased production	Lung tumor, carcinoid, leukemia
Benign tumor		Pheochromocytoma

is not associated with elevated CT levels. It should be pointed out that when plasma from a patient with a paraneoplastic CT-producing tumor is subjected to gel filtration, CT immunoreactivity is frequently found to occur with larger molecular weight forms of the hormone, and the levels of authentic CT monomer may not be elevated in this condition. The structural differences between the various CT species (heterogeneity) and the specificity of the different antisera in recognizing the higher molecular forms of CT are causes for the different results concerning the elevated CT levels in malignancy. Some authors recommend the routine use of CT measurement in posttreatment follow-up of patients with lung cancer; measurement of CT may be useful in studying therapeutic response or recurrence in these conditions. In our view this recommendation is premature at present, primarily because sensitivity, specificity, and utility of the parameter in relation to other methods have not been established adequately.

Apart from paraneoplastic secretion, other mechanisms may account for hypercalcitoninemia, including hypergastrinemia (Zollinger–Ellison syndrome) and decreased metabolic clearance in renal failure. High CT levels found in some patients with pancreatitis have not been explained. Hypercalcitoninemia of these conditions must be taken into account before an MTC is suspected. In the future nucleotide probes (complementary DNA to the mRNA) that encode CT will determine whether CT is synthesized ectopically or by the C cells. Parallel measurement of CT and KC will also help to differentiate between hypercalcitoninemia induced by nonspecific interference with the CT assay or by eutopic or ectopic CT secretion.

Measurement of CGRP in serum has been performed in patients with acute leukemia [25]; elevated CGRP levels were found in 51% and significantly correlated to more immature forms of leukemia. It might be speculated that tumors of the brain or nerve tissue express CGRP. This could not be confirmed for pheochromocytoma; mRNA for CGRP has been detected in the tissue of a pheochromocytoma from a patient who had multiple endocrine neoplasia type II [41]. To evaluate the indications for CGRP measurement, further studies are required.

Acknowledgments. This study was supported by the Deutsche Forschungsgemeinschaft, grant Ra 371/1-2, and the Tumorzentrum Heidelberg/Mannheim. We are indebted to Dr. Maria C. Jockers-Scherübel for helpful suggestions and to Mrs. Doris Skalecki for help in preparing the manuscript.

References

1. Aikawa R, Ohyama K, Mori E, Hironakal SK, Miyake M, Morishita M (1985) Enzyme immunoassay for eel-calcitonin, a synthetic analogue of calcitonin, in plasma. J Pharm Sci 74:300–303
2. Amara SG, Jonas V, Rosenfeld MG, Ong ES, Evans RM (1982) Alternative RNA processing in calcitonin gene expression generates mRNAs encoding different polypeptide products. Nature 298:240–244
3. Austin LA, Heath H III (1981) Calcitonin, physiology and pathophysiology. N Engl J Med 304:269–278
4. Body JJ, Heath H III (1983) Estimates of circulating monomeric calcitonin: physiological studies in normal and thyroidectomized man. J Clin Endocrinol Metab 57:897–903
5. Copp DH, Cameron CE, Cheney BA, Davidson AGF, Henze KG (1962) Evidence for calcitonin—a new hormone from the parathyroid that lowers blood calcium. Endocrinology 70:638–649
6. Deftos LJ, Weisman MH, Williams GW, Karpf DB, Frumar AM, Davidson BJ, Parthemore JG, Judd HL (1980) Influence of age and sex on plasma calcitonin in human beings. N Engl J Med 302:1351–1353
7. Fischer JA, Born W (1987) Calcitonin gene products: evolution, expression and biological targets. Bone Mineral 2:347–359
8. Fisher LA, Kikkawa DO, Rivier JE, Amara SG, Evans RM, Rosenfeld MG, Vale WW, Brown MR (1983) Stimulation of noradrenergic sympathetic outflow by calcitonin gene-related peptide. Nature 305:534–536
9. Frank K, Fidorra K, Raue F, Minne HW, Ziegler R (1988) Interaction of calcitonin gene-related peptide with the calcitonin receptor in fetal rat osteoclasts. Acta Endocrinol (Copenh) 117 [Suppl 287]: (abstr 98, p. 84)
10. Girgis SI, MacDonald DWR, Stevenson JC, Bevis PJR, Lynch C, Wimalawansa SJ, Self CH, Morris HR, MacIntyre I (1985) Calcitonin gene-related peptide: potent vasodilator and major product of calcitonin gene. Lancet II:14–16
11. Gropp C, Havemann K, Pflüger KH (1980) Calcitonin als Tumormarker beim Bronchialkarzinom. Dtsch Med Wochenschr 105:1175–1178
12. Heath H III, Sizemore GW (1982) Radioimmunoassay for calcitonin. Clin Chem 28:1219–1226
13. Hillyard CJ, Myers C, Abeyasekera G, Stevenson JC, Craig RK, MacIntyre I (1983) Katacalcin: a new plasma calcium-lowering hormone Lancet I:846–848

14. Hurley DL, Katz HH, Tiegs RD, Calvo MS, Barta JR, Heath H III (1988) Cosecretion of calcitonin gene products: studies with a C_{18} cartridge extraction method for human plasma PDN-21 (Katacalcin). J Clin Endocrinol Metab 66:640–644

15. Ittner J, Dambacher MA, Born W, Ketelslegers JM, Buysschaert M, Albert PM, Lambert AE, Fischer JA (1985) Diagnostic evaluation of measurements of carboxyl-terminal flanking peptide (PDN-21) of the human calcitonin gene in human serum. J Clin Endocrinol Metab 61:1133–1137

16. Jacobs JW, Goodman RH, Chin WW, Dee PC, Habener JF (1981) Calcitonin messenger RNA encodes multiple polypeptides in a single precursor. Science 213:457–459

17. Lynch C, Seth R, Bates DL, Self CH (1988) Calcitonin determination by a fast and highly sensitive enzyme amplified immunoassay. J Immunoassay 9:179–192

18. Marx SJ, Woodward CJ, Aurbach GD (1972) Calcitonin receptors of kidney and bone. Science 178:999–1001

19. Mason RT, Shulkes A, Zajac JD, Flecher AE, Hardy KJ, Martin TJ (1986) Basal and stimulated release of calcitonin gene-related peptide (CGRP) in patients with medullary thyroid carcinoma. Clin Endocrinol (Oxf) 25:675–685

20. McDermott MT, Kidd GS (1987) The role of calcitonin in the development and treatment of osteoporosis. Endocr Rev 8:377–390

21. McEwan J, Larkin S, Davies G, Chierchia S, Brown M, Stevenson J, McIntyre I, Maseri A (1986) Calcitonin gene-related peptide: a potent dilator of human epicardial coronary arteries. Circulation 74:1243–1247

22. MacIntyre I, Hillyard CJ, Murphy PK, Reynolds JJ, Gaines Das RE, Craig RK (1982) A second plasma calcium-lowering peptide from the human calcitonin precursor. Nature 300:460–462

23. Motté P, Ait-Abdellah M, Vauzelle P, Gardet P, Bohuon C, Bellet D (1987) A two-site immunoradiometric assay for serum calcitonin using monoclonal antipeptide antibodies. Henry Ford Hosp Med J 35:129–132

24. Motté P, Vauzelle P, Gardet P, Ghillani P, Caillou B, Parmentier C, Bohuon C, Bellet D (1988) Construction and clinical validation of a sensitive and specific assay for serum mature calcitonin using monoclonal anti-peptide antibodies. Clin Chim Acta 174:35–54

25. Pflüger KH, Köppler H, Jaques G, Havemann K (1988) Peptide hormones in patients with acute leukaemia. Eur J Clin Invest 18:146–152

26. Raue F (1982) Interlaboratory comparison of radioimmunological calcitonin determination. J Clin Chem Clin Biochem 20:157–161

27. Raue F, Schmidt-Gayk H, Ziegler R (1983) Tumormarker beim C-Zell-Carcinom Dtsch Med Wochenschr 108:283–287

28. Raue F (1985) Diagnostik des medullären Schilddrüsenkarzinoms. Dtsch Med Wochenschr 110:1334–1337

29. Raue F, Girgis S, Boden M, Ziegler R (1986) Tumormarker beim C-Zell-Karzinom der Schilddrüse: Katacalcin, Calcitonin, Calcitonin gene-related Peptide und carcinoembryonales Antigen. In: Wüst G (ed) Tumormarker. Steinkopff, Darmstadt, pp 258–259

30. Raue F, Boden M, Girgis S, Rix E, Ziegler R (1987) Katacalcin—Ein neuer Tumormarker beim C-Zell-Karzinom der Schilddrüse. Klin Wochenschr 65:82–86

31. Raue F, Minne HW, Ziegler R (1987) Calcitonin. In: Pesce AJ, Kaplan LA (eds) Methods in clinical chemistry. Mosby, St Louis, pp 695–701

32. Roos BA, Huber MB, Birnbaum RS, Aron DC, Lindall AW, Lips K, Baylin SB (1983) Medullary thyroid carcinomas secrete a noncalcitonin peptide corresponding to the carboxyl-terminal region of preprocalcitonin. J Clin Endocrinol Metab 56:802–807
33. Rosenfeld MG, Mermod JJ, Amara SG, Swanson LW, Sawchenko PE, Rivier J, Vale WW, Ewans RM (1983) Production of a novel neuropeptide encoded by the calcitonin gene via tissue-specific RNA processing. Nature 304:129–135
34. Silva OL, Broder LE, Doppmann JL, Snider RH, Moore CF, Cohen MH, Becker KL (1979) Calcitonin as a marker for bronchogenic cancer: a prospective study. Cancer 44:680–684
35. Schifter S, Williams ED, Craig RK, Hansen HH (1986) Calcitonin gene-related peptide and calcitonin in medullary thyroid carcinoma. Clin Endocrinol (Oxf) 25:703–710
36. Schwartz KE, Wolfsen AR, Forster B, Odell WD (1979) Calcitonin in non-thyroidal cancer. J Clin Endocrinol Metab 49:438–444
37. Steenbergh PH, Höppener JWM, Zandberg J, Visser A, Lips CJM, Jansz HS (1986) Structure and expression of the human calcitonin/CGRP genes. FEBS Lett 209:97–103
38. Stevenson JC, Myers CH, Ajdukiewicz AB (1984) Racial differences in calcitonin and katacalcin. Calcif Tissue Int 36:725–728
39. Woloszczuk W, Schuh H, Kovarik J (1986) Determination of circulating monomeric katacalcin and calcitonin: physiological studies in normal subjects. J Clin Chem Clin Biochem 24:451–455
40. Zaidi M, Breimer LM, MacIntyre I (1987) Biology of peptides from the calcitonin genes. Q J Exp Physiol 72:371–408
41. Zajac JD, Penschow J, Mason T, Tregear G, Coghlan J, Martin TJ (1986) Identification of calcitonin and calcitonin gene-related peptide messenger ribonucleic acid in medullary thyroid carcinomas by hybridization histochemistry. J Clin Endocrinol Metab 62:1037–1043
42. Ziegler R, Deutschle I, Raue F (1984) Calcitonin in human pathology. Horm Res 20:65–73

Chapter 1.4

An Immunoassay Vial for Improved Assay Performance

H. Schmidt-Gayk, H. J. Limbach, and S. Walch

This chapter describes briefly a widely used immunoassay vial and some of the immunoassays in which it has been used. Immunoassays are performed today in nearly every clinical laboratory. They may be radioimmunoassays (RIA), immunoradiometric assays (IRMA), enzyme immunoassays (EIA), fluoroimmunoassays (FIA), enzyme-linked immunosorbent assays (ELISA), and others, and we can extend this list to include the second antibody hot avidin radioassay (SAHARA) and the second antibody radioassay with ^{3}H (SARAH), as described in Chaps. 2.7, 4.3, and 4.6. Immunoassays are performed in endocrinology, clinical chemistry, pharmacology, hematology, oncology, virology, and numerous other areas. In this chapter we focus mainly on RIA and IRMA, as used in the methods described below.

To perform these assays, the following substances are required:

1. Specific antibodies against the substance to be measured.
2. Standards (the substances to be measured in known concentrations).
3. Radioactive-labeled antigen (in the case of RIA) or radioactive-labeled antibody against a second epitope on the molecule to be measured, or, in the case of the biotin-avidin system, labeled avidin. The isotope used in most assays today is ^{125}I; however, as for sterols like vitamin D metabolites and as for cyclic AMP, tritium (^{3}H) is used, since in this case the labeled and unlabeled molecules are very similar. Most antibodies do not discriminate between ^{3}H-labeled and unlabeled antigen.

The term "radioimmunoassay" is used if labeled and unlabeled antigen compete for a limited number of binding sites on an antibody, and the term "competitive protein-binding assay" is used if labeled and unlabeled ligand compete for a limited number of binding sites on naturally occurring binding proteins, as used for cyclic AMP or 25-hydroxyvitamin D determination.

After incubation has been completed, the "bound" fraction is separated from the "free" fraction, in the case of RIA usually by the addition of a second, precipitating antibody, and in the case of competitive protein-binding assay by the addition of charcoal. The main disadvantage of charcoal separation is the disruption of the equilibrium obtained, necessitating critical timing of the charcoal addition. After centrifugation has been performed in these methods, the bound fraction is usually counted. Therefore the supernatants have to be transferred to new vials if charcoal is used for separation.

Charcoal separation is used mainly in RIAs for steroids, cyclic nucleotides, vitamins, drugs, and other low molecular weight substances. Often, dextran-coated charcoal is used to decrease the binding capacity of charcoal or to decrease the binding of larger molecules. For peptides and proteins, second antibody separation is often employed. This method has a high specificity and is nondisruptive. As shown in Chaps. 4.3 and 4.6, we now use second antibody separation also for the separation of 1,25-dihydroxyvitamin D with good results. In addition to these methods there are numerous other methods for separating bound and free, such as double-antibody solid-phase (DASP), magnetizable particles, antibody- or second antibody-coated tube, cellulose-bound anti-bodies, proximity scintillation reagent (Amersham Buchler, Frankfurt/Main, FRG) and others.

Comparing the accuracy of RIAs in different vials we have noted marked differences and we have then tried to develop a new vial optimized for the purpose of immunoassay [1]. If possible, the assay should be performed in the same vial from the beginning to counting. Such a vial has the following advantages:

1. The tube need not be numbered; the position on the rack is indicated by the aluminum rack.
2. Easy closure of the tube with self-adhesive tape.
3. Ease of centrifugation and of loading and unloading the centrifuge.
4. Firm adherence of the sediment in second antibody separation.
5. Easy aspiration of supernatants with a rack.
6. Low nonspecific binding.
7. Compatible with existing gamma counters.
8. Useful for liquid scintillation counting.
9. Low volumes of radioactive waste.
10. High adsorptive capacity for immunoglobulin G under certain circum-stances.
11. Immunoextraction and immunoconcentration are possible.
12. High accuracy; this could depend on the shape of the tube, especially that of the bottom.

Results

In preliminary experiments we found that in commercially available tubes with a flat or round bottom the sediment after second antibody separation was sometimes washed away or aspirated because it did not adhere firmly to the bottom. Therefore we compared different experimental vials (manufactured by W. Sarstedt, D-5223 Nümbrecht-Rommelsdorf, Federal Republic of Germany) with a conical lower end until low coefficients of variation were obtained with the vial shown in Fig. 1.

Figure 2 shows a commercially available Styrofoam rack (Dynatech, Plochingen, FRG) for 96 immunoassay vials. As the Styrofoam rack may be used only a few times, a solid aluminum rack was designed and made by W. Sarstedt, which bears the letters "A–H" on the left-hand side and the numbers "1–12" on the upper end (Fig. 3). The tubes may be closed with adhesive tape (3M company St. Paul, MN, USA, 55144-100).

As the vial is also used for liquid scintillation counting, experiments were performed with ^{3}H-containing tracer (10 μl and 250 μl of scintillation fluid) and a firmly placed stopper (W. Sarstedt). In these experiments it was noted that optimum counting efficiency in liquid scintillation counters with racks for 20-ml tubes was obtained if the immunoassay vial was placed in a central position and

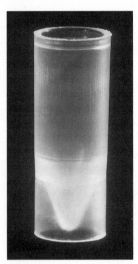

Fig. 1. Immunoassay vial, external diameter 9 mm, internal volume 600 μl

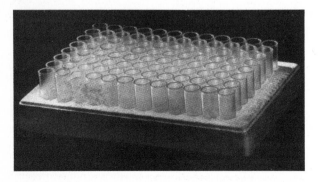

Fig. 2. Styrofoam rack for 96 immunoassay vials

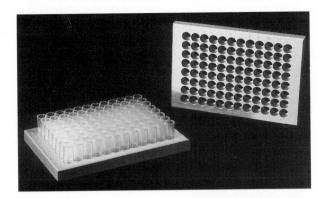

Fig. 3. Aluminum rack for 96 immunoassay vials

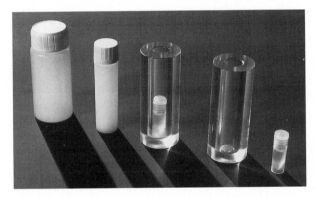

Fig. 4. Polyacrylamide adapters for the immunoassay vial designed for liquid scintillation counters with racks for 20-ml tubes

elevated by 3 mm. For this purpose, polyacrylamide adapters were prepared in our institute (Fig. 4).

If the liquid scintillation counter is equipped with racks for 6-ml tubes (second from left in Fig. 4), the 6-ml tube is used as a container for the immunoassay tube and no adapter is necessary.

In some experiments, a supernatant from protein precipitation with ethanol or acetonitrile has to be evaporated with nitrogen; therefore an adapter was built for simultaneous evaporation of 96 tubes, as shown in Fig. 5.

Shape of the Vial and Immunoassay Accuracy

Reproducibility was determined in triplicate samples in a calcitonin assay. Charcoal separation was performed in a volume-reduced assay in a microtiter plate (300 µl total volume), and second antibody separation was performed in Removawell tubes (Dynatech, Plochingen, FRG) U-shaped like the microtiter

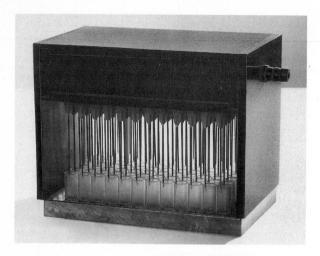

Fig. 5. Device for the simultaneous evaporation of 96 extracts (supernatants from protein precipitation with ethanol or acetonitrile)

Table 1. Immunoassay accuracy: Mean coefficient of variation (%)

Charcoal separation Microtiter plate	Second antibody Removawell vial	Second antibody Immunoassay vial	Second antibody Eppendorf vial
2.88	8.52	2.16	4.28

plate; in addition second antibody separation was performed in the immuno-assay vial and Eppendorf reaction vial (Eppendorf-Gerätebau, 2000 Hamburg, FRG, 600 µl volume) for comparison. The latter vial has a narrow lower part but a rounded bottom. The means, standard deviations, and coefficients of variation ($CV\%$) were determined for 32 triplicates; the mean coefficients of variation were then calculated (Table 1).

As shown in Table 1, the immunoassay vial is the most accurate. Experiments have shown that different angles at the bottom of the vial have a major influence on accuracy. The aspiration device (initially prepared by ourselves, now available from W. Sarstedt) is mounted to leave 5–10 µl fluid in the bottom of the tube. Twelve supernatants are aspirated simultaneously. The nonspecific bound (NSB) values are less than 1% of total activity added initially if the sediments are washed once with 500 µl 0.15 mol/liter NaCl. The results may be improved such as by addition of polyethyleneglycol and detergents like Tween

20 to the washing solution; however, this has to be tested for each assay for results to be optimized.

Other separation methods such as charcoal, DASP, magnetizable particles, proximity scintillation reagent or cellulose-coated antibodies may be used successfully in the immunoassay vial. As the storage costs of radioactive waste depend on volume in many countries, these costs can be considerably reduced by using this vial. The immunoassay vial has been used for more than one million determinations over 10 years. If robotic pipetting is introduced, the same coordinates may be used for microtiter plates and immunoassay racks.

Conclusions

A new vial has been developed for improved immunoassay performance. It fits into a microtiter plate format rack and may contain a volume of up to 600 μl. The conical lower end has been optimized for the separation of bound and free ligands.

This vial offers several advantages:

1. The tube need not be numbered; the position on the rack is indicated by the aluminum rack.
2. Easy closure of 96 tubes with self-adhesive tape.
3. Ease of centrifugation—loading and unloading—of 4 × 96 tubes in commercially available centrifuges equipped with a microtiter-plate rotor; or 8 × 96 tubes in the Beckman J-6 centrifuge (Beckman Instruments Inc., Irvine, CA 92713, United States).
4. Firm adherence of the sediment during second antibody separation or other separation methods (magnetic particles, charcoal, cellulose-coupled antibodies).
5. Easy aspiration of supernatants with a rack (aspiration of 96 supernatants in less than 1 min).
6. Low nonspecific binding (high-volume ratio of aspirated supernatant to the remaining sediment).
7. Compatible in diameter to nearly all existing gamma-counting equipment.
8. In RIAs with ^{3}H-labeled antigens and second antibody separation, only 250 μl scintillation fluid is necessary for liquid scintillation counting, resulting in a dramatic cost reduction (as shown in Chaps. 4.3, 4.6).
9. Low volume of radioactive or nonradioactive waste; 1000 tubes yield about 1 liter.
10. High binding of immunoglobulin G under certain conditions, permitting the use of solid-phase methods (as shown in Chap. 2.9).
11. Immunoextraction and immunoconcentration methods may be easily performed by adding cellulose-coupled antibodies to relatively large sample volumes. After incubation and centrifugation, the supernatant may

be aspirated and discarded. The assay is then performed in a small volume in the conical lower part of the vial. In contrast to the usual RIA procedure, a tenfold concentration may be achieved (as shown in Chap. 2.8).

12. The accuracy of the assays is markedly improved.

Reference

1. Schmidt-Gayk H, Wahl HM, Limbach HJ, Walch S (1979) Ein spezielles Gefäß zur Durchführung des Radioimmunoassay (RIA). Medizintechnik 99:103–104

2 Parathyroid Hormone Assays
and Clinical Application

Chapter 2.1

Homologous Radioimmunoassay for Human Parathyroid Hormone (Residues 53-84) with Tyrosylated Peptide as Tracer

W. HITZLER

Introduction

Measurement of carboxyl-terminal fragments of human parathyroid hormone (hPTH) helps to distinguish patients with primary hyperparathyroidism from healthy controls [12, 22]. In renal failure, the greatly increased concentration of circulating carboxyl-terminal fragments results from hypersecretion of the hormone by the parathyroid glands and its inadequate removal from the circulation [14]. The main disadvantage of existing carboxyl-terminal PTH assays is that sometimes the results for healthy individuals, patients with tumor hypercalcemia, and patients with proven primary hyperparathyroidism overlap [2]. This overlapping could be related to (e.g.) differences in the structure of bovine, porcine, and human hormone, resulting in incomplete recognition of the structure of the human hormone by the antibody. Therefore we have tried to develop a largely homologous radioimmunoassay (RIA) system for measurement of PTH in human serum, based on the use of a commercially available synthetic fragment of human PTH (residues 53-84).

Materials and Methods

Reagents and Standards

Mix 800 ml of 67 mmol/liter Na_2HPO_4 (No. 6587) with 200 ml of 67 mmol/liter KH_2PO_4 (No. 4875; both from Merck AG, Darmstadt, FRG) to obtain a pH 7.4 buffer. To this buffer add 1 g human serum albumin (Behringwerke AG, Marburg, FRG), 1000 mg sodium azide (No. 6688, Merck AG), and 400 mg ethylenediaminetetraacetic acid (EDTA) (No. 2426 Merck AG) to prepare buffer A. Antisera are obtained by immunizing guinea pigs with partly purified hPTH extract from adenomas, similar to the procedure of Bouillon et al. [3] as described below. Dilute 200 µl antiserum with 1000 ml buffer A. Add 3.8 ml normal guinea pig serum to this antiserum solution, resulting in a total of 4.0 ml guinea pig serum/liter antiserum solution.

Assay Standards

Human plasma was rotary mixed with charcoal [1 liter serum with 120 g Norit A (Serva, Heidelberg FRG)] overnight at room temperature. The mixture was then centrifuged (Sorvall RC2-B centrifuge, 5000 rpm, 1 h, rotor GS3). The supernatant serum was filtered through filter No. 311651 (Schleicher & Schüll, Dassel, FRG), then centrifuged overnight at 6000 rpm and 4 °C. The supernate was again filtered through the same material. Bovine serum was treated in the same way. N-terminal hPTH(1-34) fragment (synthetic, structure according to Niall et al. [13] was obtained from Beckman Instruments Inc., Palo Alto, CA 94304 (Cat. No. 337751). C-terminal hPTH(53-84) fragment was obtained from Paesel, Frankfurt/Main, FRG. Tyr^{52}-hPTH(52-84) was obtained from Bachem AG, Bubendorf, Switzerland. Both peptides contained aspartic acid at position 76. Goat anti-guinea-pig gamma globulin was purchased from Deutsche Wellcome GmbH, Burgwedel, FRG (Cat. No. RD18). To obtain material for eliciting guinea pig anti-PTH antibody, we homogenized 100 g human parathyroid adenoma tissue in 400 ml glycine hydrochloride (pH 3.0, 0.1 mol/liter), centrifuged it in a Sorvall RC-2B for 1 h, and reextracted the sediment with the glycine buffer. The supernate was applied to a 100 × 5-cm column of Sephadex G50 and eluted with the glycine buffer. We collected 10 ml fractions and measured their absorbance at 280 nm (for protein content) and their PTH content by a heterologous immunoassay according to Bouillon et al. [3]. We then injected about 10–20 µg of this partly purified hPTH six times, at monthly intervals, into guinea pigs. The antiserum used in these experiments was that which produced the most sensitive standard curve (serum from guinea pig 7).

Iodination

We radiolabeled 1 µg Tyr^{52}-hPTH(52-84) with 0.5 mCi $Na^{125}I$ (Amersham Buchler, Frankfurt/Main, FRG) by a modification of the Hunter and Greenwood [10] procedure, as follows: Combine 1 µg Tyr^{52}-hPTH(52-84) in 10 µl pH 7.4 phosphate buffer 0.06 mol/liter, 5 µl (0.5 mCi) $Na^{125}I$ and 10 µl (1 µg) chloramine-T dissolved in water. Let this mixture react for 60 s at room temperature and stop the reaction by adding 10 µl (2.5 µg) sodium metabisulfite dissolved in water. Next 200 µl buffer A with 20 g/liter bovine serum albumin (BSA) is added for protection against radiolysis. Purification follows immediately with Sep-Pak C_{18} cartridges (Waters Association, Eschborn, FRG) according to Schöneshöfer et al. [14]. The reaction mixture was transferred onto a Sep-Pak C_{18} cartridge and free ^{125}I was eluted with 2 ml 0.05 mol/liter trifluoroacetic acid solution. The labeled peptide was eluted with 2 ml of a 60/40 (by volume) mixture of 0.05 mol/liter trifluoroacetic acid solution and acetonitrile and 3 ml buffer A. The tracer was further diluted in buffer A with 20 g/liter BSA to about 30 000 cpm/100 µl. The specific activities were about 420–550 Ci/g. These tracers were stable for at least 8 weeks. In addition, hPTH(53-84) was labeled in a similar procedure; however, the oxidation time with chloramine-T was prolonged to 30 min and chloramine-T and sodium metabisulfite were increased tenfold in concentration.

Radioimmunoassay

We routinely assayed each standard curve concentration and each sample in triplicate. Individual non-specific count measurements were checked in one assay, but this step was later omitted because all samples exhibited the same low nonspecific binding. The incubation mixture (100 µl standard or sample, 100 µl buffer A, and 100 µl first antibody) was incubated in "radioimmunoassay vials" (Sarstedt, Nümbrecht, FRG) (see Chap. 1.4). After preincubation with the antiserum for 24, 48, 72, or 240 h, 100 µl ^{125}I-labeled Tyr^{52}-hPTH(52-84) or hPTH(53-84) containing about 30 000 cpm (1100 Bq) was added, and the incubation was continued for another 48 h. Then 100 µl second antibody was added and incubated for 5–6 h. Thereafter the tubes were centrifuged (10 min, 2000 g) to separate bound from free peptide. The supernate was aspirated and discarded, and the sediment washed again with 500 µl buffer A. The tubes were again centrifuged for 10 min at 2000 g and the supernates again aspirated and discarded. The radioactivity of the sediment was counted until 10 000 counts were reached. The nonspecific counts (average of one triplicate in each assay) were subtracted from the average of each triplicate determination of sample and standard. The bound radioactivity (linear scale, y-axis) was graphed versus the concentration of the competitor [(hPTH(53-84) or adenoma extract, logarithmic scale, x-axis)].

Serum calcium was determined routinely with an SMA 12/60 (Technicon Instruments Corp., Tarrytown, NY 10591), and by an automated selective analyzer (Hitachi 737, Hitachi Corp., Kobe, Japan).

Results

Results Obtained with [^{125}I]hPTH(53-84) as Tracer

We prepared hPTH(53-84) standards in plasma or bovine serum, both previously stripped with charcoal (Norit A). Then hPTH(53-84) was added in a concentration of 2000 pmol/liter. This standard was serially diluted (1000, 500, 250, 125, 62, and 31 pmol/liter) and used to prepare two different sets of standard curves, one with the standard in human plasma and the other in bovine serum. Euparathyroid controls and hyperparathyroid samples were measured as described below. The results (not shown) demonstrated that charcoal-treated bovine serum was superior for our purposes because hypoparathyroid patients yield counting rates near that of the zero standard. In contrast, charcoal-treated human plasma contained immunoreactive material, and hypoparathyroid patients demonstrated more binding of the tracer than the zero standard. Therefore, we performed all further experiments with charcoal-treated bovine serum.

Two further standard curve experiments were performed: (a) with hPTH(53-84) diluted in charcoal-treated bovine serum and (b) with bovine parathyroid hormone (1-84) (bPTH, donated by Prof. O'Riordan, Middlesex Hospital, London, UK) diluted in charcoal-treated bovine serum. In addition to labeling hPTH(53-84), for the following experiment we also labeled bPTH(1-84) by the chloramine-T method at pH 7.4 according to Hunter and Greenwood [10]: 2 µg bPTH(1-84), 10 µg chloramine-T, oxidation for 30 s. In experiment (a), hPTH(53-84) standard or human parathyroid gland extract was incubated with the antiserum for 48 h, and ^{125}I-labeled hPTH(53-84) was added as tracer and again incubated for 48 h at 4 °C.

In experiment (b), bPTH(1-84) standard or human parathyroid gland extract was incubated with the antiserum, and ^{125}I-labeled bPTH(1-84) was added as tracer under the same conditions. The results of these experiments are shown in Figs. 1 and 2. As can be seen from Fig. 1, extracted hPTH is as competitive as hPTH(53-84), the lines being nearly parallel; such is not the case with bPTH(1-84) (Fig. 2). Therefore we concluded that the use of hPTH(53-84) as standard and tracer could improve the assay for the carboxyl-terminal

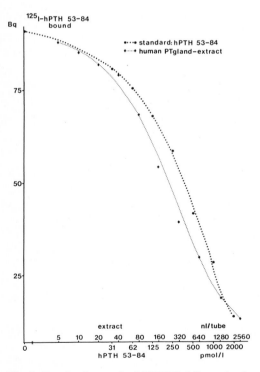

Fig. 1. Standard curve for hPTH(53-84) standards and tracer. Human parathyroid gland extract in several dilutions(◆) and hPTH(53-84) fragment chemically synthesized (●). Asp[76]-hPTH(53-84) was used.

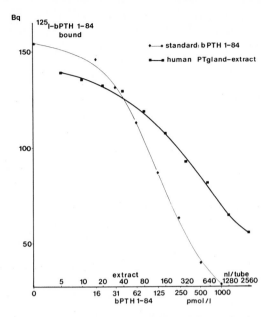

Fig. 2. Standard curve for bPTH(1-84) standards and tracer. Human parathyroid gland extract in several dilutions (■) and bPTH(1-84) standards (◆)

fragments of hPTH in serum, as compared with heterologous assays involving ^{125}I-labeled bPTH(1-84) as tracer.

Analytical Variables

Sensitivity. The most sensitive standard curve is produced by the use of 100 µl standard and 48 h of preincubation (Fig. 3). Fifty percent displacement is at 270 pmol/liter with this procedure, in contrast to 680 pmol/liter when 50 µl standard and 24 h preincubation are used. The results of these and other experimental conditions are shown in Table 1.

Specificity. Synthetic hPTH(1-34) yields no displacement of ^{125}I-labeled hPTH(53-84). Human parathyroid gland extract displaces hPTH(53-84) tracer in parallel to hPTH(53-84). Therefore we conclude that only the carboxyl-terminal portion of hPTH is recognized in this assay system.

Linearity. Hyperparathyroid serum from a patient with primary hyperpara-thyroidism was diluted serially with charcoal-treated bovine serum. Undiluted hyperparathyroid serum and different serum dilutions were measured in the hPTH(53-84) and the bPTH(1-84) assay systems. The results are shown in Fig. 4, which illustrates that both assay systems yield nearly linear results with serum dilutions. However, the concentration of PTH determined with the

W. Hitzler

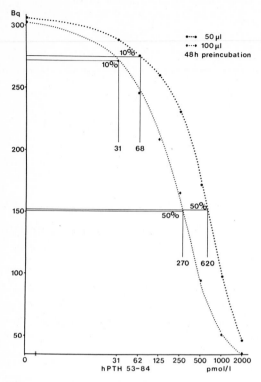

Fig. 3. Sensitivity of the assay. Standard (50 or 100 µl) was incubated with the antiserum for 48 h, and ^{125}I-labeled hPTH(53-84) was added as tracer and again incubated for 48 h at 4°C

Table 1. Sensitivity of the hPTH(53-84) assay: effect of different preincubation periods

Vol. of standard (µl)	% bound (B/B_0)	Preincubation (h)			
		24	48	72	240
			hPTH(53-84) (pmol/liter)		
50	90	75	68		
	50	680	620		
100	90	45	31	32	32
	50	400	270	220	200
200	90			33	
	50			155	
100 $(B_0 - 2\,SD)$			58	20	24

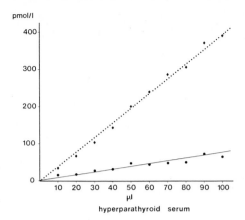

Fig. 4. Serum from a patient with primary hyperparathyroidism was diluted serially with charcoal-treated serum to test the linearity of the hPTH(53-84) (dotted line) and the bPTH(1-84) (solid line) assay systems

hPTH(53-84) assay system is about fivefold that determined with the bPTH(1-84) assay system. Figure 2 shows nonparallelism in the bPTH(1-84) assay if human parathyroid adenoma extract is determined at different dilutions.

Clinical Use

We evaluated healthy persons, healthy persons after calcium infusion, and patients with primary hyperparathyroidism. Sera from 32 ostensibly healthy blood donors were assayed for carboxyl-terminal PTH, using 100 µl standard and 48 h of preincubation.

A healthy subject was given a calcium infusion according to Kyle et al. [11]. Table 2 gives the results of serum calcium and hPTH(53-84) determination. As can be seen, 145 min after the start of the infusion, serum PTH as determined with the hPTH(53-84) system was undetectable. From a patient with 1° hyperparathyroidism, blood samples were taken every 30 min before, during and after

Table 2. Serum calcium and hPTH(53-84) before, during and after calcium infusion (10 mg Ca^{2+}/kg)[a]

Time (min)	Serum calcium (mmol/liter)	hPTH(53-84) (pmol/liter)
0	2.13	69
70	2.82	41
145	3.24	< 30
220	3.28	< 30
300	3.05	37

[a] Calcium was infused from min 1 to min 220

surgical removal of parathyroid adenoma. The resection started at 9 a.m. The serum PTH level decreased rapidly after resection and remained nearly constant in the upper normal range after 3–4 h. Serum calcium decreased continuously (see Fig. 5).

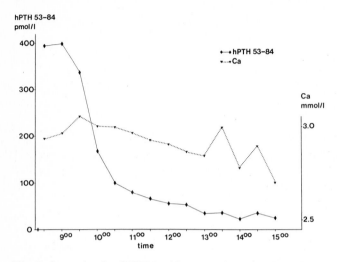

Fig. 5. Serum levels of PTH (residues 53-84) and calcium after resection of a parathyroid adenoma in a patient with primary hyperparathyroidism

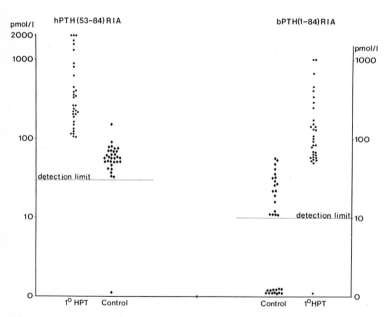

Fig. 6. Serum levels of PTH fragments determined with the hPTH(53-84) and the bPTH(1-84) assay in 32 healthy controls and 32 patients with surgically confirmed primary hyperparathyroidism

When the speed of the assay was increased it was no longer possible to distinguish suppressed PTH values from normal ones. Therefore further investigations were performed with 48 h of preincubation and 100 μl standard. The results for 32 healthy control persons and for 32 patients with surgically confirmed primary hyperparathyroidism are shown in Fig. 6. It can be seen that the mean value for patients with primary hyperparathyroidism is about fivefold higher in the hPTH(53-84) assay than in the bPTH(1-84) assay. One case of primary hyperparathyroidism was undetectable in the bPTH(1-84) assay; this was confirmed in a further experiment.

Results Obtained with [^{125}I]Tyr^{52}-hPTH(52-84) as Tracer

Figure 7 depicts a typical standard curve showing the binding of [^{125}I]Tyr^{52}-hPTH(52-84) and its displacement by increasing concentrations of hPTH(53-84). In addition, a standard curve with the previously described [^{125}I]hPTH(53-84) as tracer is shown (Fig. 7).

Figure 7 demonstrates that in the carboxyl-terminal assay for hPTH the radioiodinated tyrosylated fragment is far better suited as tracer. The specific

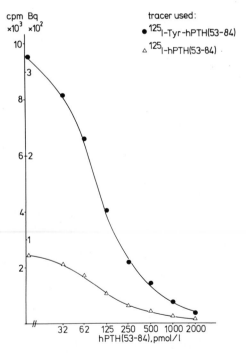

Fig. 7. Binding of [^{125}I]Tyr^{52}-hPTH(52-84) and its displacement by increasing concentrations of hPTH(53-84). In addition, a standard curve with [^{125}I]hPTH(53-84) as tracer is shown

activities were 420 and 50 Ci/g, respectively. Further iodinations with the tyrosylated peptide produced specific activities of 420–550 Ci/g.

Temperature Dependency of the Binding of Tyr^{52}-hPTH(52-84) to the Antiserum MS7

We performed the assay at both 4 °C and 22 °C, all other incubation conditions being identical. The results are shown in Fig. 8.

It can be seen that the binding of the tracer is markedly temperature dependent, with far better binding at 4 °C.

Sensitivity. As the tyrosylated fragment as tracer yields a much higher sensitivity (steeper standard curve) than the hPTH(53-84) fragment, sensitivity was again determined by equilibrium incubation (48 h) and sequential saturation (24 h + 24 h). The results are shown in Fig. 9, which shows that sensitivity is higher with sequential saturation. However, the useful concentration range of patient samples is small; samples above 250 pmol/liter have to be diluted. With equilibrium incubation, a better binding of the tracer is obtained (> 10 000 cpm compared to 7000 cpm at standard zero) and samples up to 500 pmol/liter do not have to be diluted and reassayed.

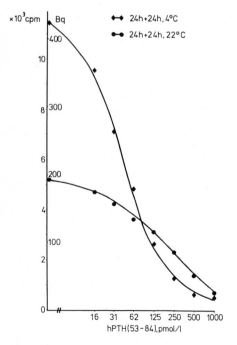

Fig. 8. Temperature dependency of the binding of [^{125}I]Tyr^{52}-hPTH(52-84) to the antiserum MS7. The assays were performed at 4° and 22 °C

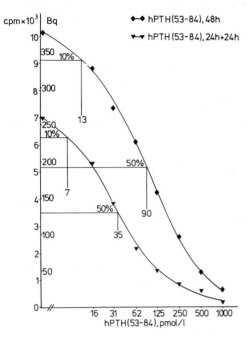

Fig. 9. Determination of assay sensitivity with [^{125}I]Tyr^{52}-hPTH(52-84) as tracer. Equilibrium incubation (48 h) and sequential saturation (24 h + 24 h) were employed

Clinical Use of the Carboxyl-Terminal Assay with Tyrosylated Peptide as Tracer

The concentration of PTH was determined in 30 healthy controls and 20 patients with surgically proven primary hyperparathyroidism. Incubation conditions were as shown in Fig. 9; equilibrium incubation was compared with sequential saturation. In addition to 100 μl standard and sample volume, the assay was also run with 50 μl sample under equilibrium conditions. The results are given in Fig. 10, which shows that only equilibrium incubation for 48 h permits the distinction of healthy controls from patients with primary hyperparathyroidism. In addition, the values were in many cases below the detection limit in the assay with the 50 μl sample.

Discussion

[^{125}I]hPTH(53-84) as Tracer

Before 1981, parathyroid hormone in human serum was mainly determined by RIAs in which ^{125}I-labeled bPTH was used as tracer [3, 4, 6–8, 12, 16, 20]. We have advocated the necessity for a homologous RIA for hPTH because with the

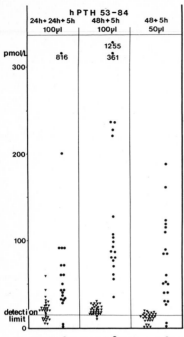

Fig. 10. Concentration of carboxy-terminal PTH fragments in the serum of 30 healthy controls and 20 patients with surgically proven primary hyperparathyroidism. Equilibrium incubation was compared with sequential saturation. In addition, 100 µl standard and sample volume was compared with 50 µl. [^{125}I]Tyr^{52}-hPTH(52-84) was used as tracer

various heterologous RIAs, hyperparathyroid patients were not distinguished clearly from healthy controls [18]. An assay using ^{125}I-labeled bPTH(1-84) was improved by using standards of hPTH extracted from human adenomatous glands and antiserum against this extracted hPTH [20]. As we have shown, synthetic hPTH(53-84) may also be used as the standard, and these standard curves are superimposable on curves of various dilutions of hPTH extracted from adenomas. Antisera against hPTH can be produced by immunizing guinea pigs with partly purified hPTH(1-84) or by immunizing rabbits with synthetic hPTH(53-84) conjugated to thyroglobulin according to Sofroniew et al. [15]. Relatively little ^{125}I is incorporated into hPTH(53-84) as compared to Tyr^{52}-hPTH(52-84). This may be caused by the absence of tyrosine and the presence of only one histidine in hPTH(53-84). Shortening of the oxidation time yielded hPTH(53-84) tracer of low specific activities. Use of the lactoperoxidase-labeling technique [17] resulted in insufficient incorporation of ^{125}I into hPTH(53-84) (results not shown).

When hPTH(53-84) was used for labeling, high sensitivity was only achieved by 2 or 3 days of preincubation followed by the addition of tracer, similar to the incubation procedure of Di Bella et al. [6] and Mallette [12]. The concentrations of hPTH in the serum of healthy controls and patients with primary hyperparathyroidism demonstrated that the homologous RIA for hPTH(53-84) was superior to the heterologous RIA: more healthy controls are identified as such and there is less overlap with results for hyperparathyroid patients. The question has to be resolved whether a homologous assay with hPTH(53-84) or with hPTH(1-34) is more useful in the diagnosis of primary hyperparathyroidism [5].

We show the results of the hPTH(1-34) RIA later in this volume (Chap. 2.7).

$[^{125}I]$ Tyr^{52}-hPTH(52-84) as Tracer

Further improvement of the assay was achieved by attaching a tyrosine to the hPTH(53-84) molecule for improved radioiodination.

The specific activities obtained were about eight- to tenfold higher with Tyr^{52}-hPTH(52-84) (420–550 Ci/g) than with hPTH(53-84). In addition, very mild oxidation conditions with chloramine-T were sufficient to yield high incorporation of ^{125}I. The high specific activity of the tracer improved the sensitivity of the assay: 90% B/B_0 was obtained at 13 pmol/liter hPTH(53-84) standard under equilibrium conditions, whereas with the nontyrosylated tracer 90% B/B_0 was obtained at 31 pmol/liter after 2 days of preincubation (sequential saturation). This means that with the tyrosylated tracer, the assay is more than twice as sensitive and the turnaround time is 2 days (4 days with nontyrosylated tracer).

Temperature dependency has to be tested for every antiserum: an opposite result with better binding is shown later in the assay of hPTH(44-68) (see Chap. 2.4).

The incubation mode was very important: whereas with 48 h under equilibrium conditions with 100 µl of sample a clear separation of controls and patients with primary hyperparathyroidism is obtained, with 24 h + 24 h sequential saturation a large overlap is observed. This was found despite the higher sensitivity shown in Fig. 9. However, as also shown in Fig. 9, the binding is not complete after 24 h: B_0 is more than 10000 cpm in 48 h compared with 7000 cpm with 1-day tracer incubation. The binding kinetics of $[^{125}I]$Tyr^{52}-hPTH(52-84) to the antibody (data not shown) showed complete binding after 48 h; further prolongation to 72 h or 96 h did not improve the binding. This may explain the clinically useful results obtained with 48 h equilibrium incubation: the reaction proceeded to completion. As a general rule in immunoassays, reproducibility is improved when the reaction proceeds to completion. Unfortunately, industrial companies try to sell quick assays; their clinical usefulness is sometimes severely compromised [9, 19].

We would highly recommend the tracer purification procedure (modified method according to Schöneshöfer et al. [14]); it is rapid, convenient, and produces only small volumes of radioactive waste.

For the preparation of standards we recently observed that dilution of hPTH(53-84) in buffer A with BSA (20 g/liter) and 10% hypoparathyroid serum was superior to charcoal-treated bovine serum.

In conclusion, we describe a double-antibody RIA for carboxyl-terminal fragments of hPTH in serum. Standards are prepared with synthetic hPTH (residues 53-84), in buffer A with BSA (20 g/liter) containing 10% hPTH-free serum. Antisera are obtained by immunizing guinea pigs with partly purified hPTH extracted from adenomatous glands. Tracer is prepared by labeling Tyr^{52}-hPTH(52-84) with ^{125}I by the chloramine-T method followed by rapid purification on Sep-Pak C_{18} cartridges. Dilution curves for hPTH extracted from adenomas are superimposable on dilution curves for the synthetic hPTH(53-84) fragment. Dilution of sera from hyperparathyroid patients showed linearity of response with concentration in the present assay. In contrast to the heterologous system which distinguished 28 of 32 patients with primary hyperparathyroidism from 32 normals, the present assay separated these groups with less overlap. To obtain clinically valid results, the importance of the incubation mode (equilibrium versus sequential saturation) and temperature is demonstrated. Separation of patients with primary hyperparathyroidism from healthy controls is only obtained with 48 h equilibrium incubation at 4 °C.

References

1. Arnaud CD, Goldsmith RS, Bordier PJ, Sizemore GW (1974) Influence of immuno-heterogeneity of circulating parathyroid hormone on results of radioimmunoassays of serum in man. Am J Med 56:785–793
2. Ashby JP, Thakkar H (1988) Diagnostic limitations of region-specific parathyroid hormone assays in the investigation of hypercalcemia. Ann Clin Biochem 25:275–279
3. Bouillon R, Koninckx P, De Moor P (1974) A radioimmunoassay for human serum parathyroid hormone: methods and clinical evaluation. In: Radioimmunoassay and related procedures in medicine. International Atomic Energy Agency, Vienna, pp 353–365
4. Boyd JC, Lewis JW, Slatopolsky E, Ladenson JH (1981) Parathyrin measured concurrently with free or total calcium in the differential diagnosis of hypercalcemia. Clin Chem 27:574–579
5. Desplan C, Jullienne A, Moukhtar MS, Milhaud G (1977) Sensitive assay for biologically active fragment of human parathyroid hormone. Lancet ii:198–199
6. Di Bella FP, Kehrwald JM, Laakso K, Zitzner L (1978) Parathyrin radioimmuno-assay: diagnostic utility of antisera produced against carboxyl-terminal fragments of the hormone from the human. Clin Chem 24:451–454
7. Di Bella FP, Gilkinson JB, Flueck J, Arnaud CD (1978) Carboxyl-terminal frag-ments of human parathyroid hormone in parathyroid tumors: unique new source of immunogens for the production of antisera potentially useful in the radioimmuno-assay of parathyroid hormone in human serum. J Clin Endocrinol Metab 46:604–612
8. Di Bella FP, Hawker CD, McCann DS, Martin KJ, Heath H III, Anast CS, Forman

DT (1982) Parathyrin (parathyroid hormone): radioimmunoassay for intact and carboxyl-terminal moieties. Clin Chem 28:226–235

9. Gorog RH, Hakim MK, Thompson NW, Rigg GA, McCann DS (1982) Radioimmunoassay of serum parathyrin: comparison of five commercial kits. Clin Chem 28:87–91

10. Hunter WM, Greenwood FC (1962) Preparation of iodine-131-labelled human growth hormone of high specific activity. Nature 194:495–496

11. Kyle LH, Canary JJ, Mintz DH, De Leon A (1962) Inhibitory effects of induced hypercalcemia on secretion of parathyroid hormone. J Clin Endocrinol Metab 22:52–58

12. Mallette LE (1980) Sensitivity of the antibovine parathyroid hormone serum 211/32 to synthetic fragments of human parathyroid hormone. J Clin Endocrinol Metab 50:201–203

13. Niall HD, Sauer RT, Jacobs JW, Keutmann HT, Segre GV, O'Riordan JLH, Aurbach GD, Potts JT Jr (1974) The amino-acid sequence of the amino-terminal 37 residues of human parathyroid hormone. Proc Natl Acad Sci USA 71:384–388

14. Papapoulos SE, Hendy GN, Tomlinson S, Lewin IG, O'Riordan JLH (1977) Clearance of exogenous parathyroid hormone in normal and uremic man. Clin Endocrinol 7:211–225

15. Schöneshöfer M, Kage A, Kage R, Fenner A (1982) A convenient technique for the specific isolation of ^{125}I-labelled peptide molecules. Fresenius Z Anal Chem 311:429–430

16. Sofroniew MV, Madler M, Müller OA, Scriba PC (1978) A method for the consistent production of high quality antisera to small peptide hormones. Fresenius Z Anal Chem 290:163

17. Solling H (1981) A rapid and inexpensive radioimmunoassay for parathyroid hormone utilizing the Wide-principle in combination with an improved separation technique. Clin Chim Acta 116:349–359

18. Thorell JI, Johansson BG (1971) Enzymic iodination of polypeptides with iodine-125 to high specific activity. Biochim Biophys Acta 251:363–369

19. Voll R, Schmidt-Gayk H, Wiedemann J, Hüfner M, Bouillon R, Keutmann H, Hehrmann R (1978) Radioimmunoassay for parathyrin. Characterization of six different antigens and antisera. J Clin Chem Clin Biochem 16:269–277

20. Wood WG (1983) A comparison of six commercial kits for the determination of parathyrin (PTH) levels in serum. Ärztl Lab 29:311–316

21. Wood WG, Butz R, Casaretto M, Hehrmann R, Jüppner H, Marschner I, Wachter C, Zahn H, Hesch RD (1980) Preliminary results on the use of an antiserum to human parathyrin in a homologous radioimmunoassay. J Clin Chem Clin Biochem 18:789–795

22. Zillikens D, Armbruster FP, Stern J, Schmidt-Gayk H, Raue F (1987) Sensitive homologous radioimmunoassay for human parathyroid hormone to diagnose hypoparathyroid conditions. Ann Clin Biochem 24:608–613

Sensitive Homologous Radioimmunoassay for Human Parathyroid Hormone (Residues 53-84) to Diagnose Hypoparathyroid Conditions: Guidelines for the Establishment of Highly Sensitive Assays*

D. ZILLIKENS

Introduction

Several sensitive parathyroid hormone (PTH) assays have been published, but differentiation between hypoparathyroid and healthy subjects remains a problem [7, 15, 16, 17, 18, 22, 23]. The main difficulty of the PTH radioimmunoassay (RIA) is the lack of assay sensitivity. This causes hypoparathyroid sera to be mistakenly placed within the normal range or PTH to remain undetectable in normal subjects. We have developed a procedure which is able to differentiate between normal and hypoparathyroid sera [26]. We used the same antiserum as for the "rapid assay" which has been described previously [25]. Guidelines are given for the establishment of highly sensitive assays.

Materials and Methods

Buffer A

Buffer A, composed of phosphate, human serum albumin, sodium azide, and ethylenediaminetetraacetic acid (EDTA), is described in Chap. 2.1.

Standards

The standards were prepared by dissolving synthetic hPTH fragments (1-34), (28-48), (44-68), (53-84) (all Bachem AG, Bubendorf, Switzerland) and synthetic intact hPTH(1-84) (Peptide Institute Inc., Osaka, Japan) in buffer A and 10 g/liter human serum albumin (HSA) (Behringwerke AG, Marburg, FRG).

Antiserum

The antiserum (first antibody) was generously provided by Prof. Dr. O'Riordan, Middlesex Hospital, London. It was raised by immunizing goats (H4) with human parathyroid extracts. Further details have been described elsewhere [17,

*This study was supported by Deutsche Forschungsgemeinschaft (Schm/7-1). Parts of this chapter have been published in Annals of Clinical Biochemistry.

25]. The antiserum was diluted in buffer A (1:6000) and normal goat serum was added to give a final concentration of 4 ml/liter. Anti-goat IgG (second antibody) was raised by immunizing a donkey. A six-fold dilution in buffer A completely precipitated the first antibody.

Tracer

The preparation of $[^{125}I]$ Tyr^{52}-hPTH(52-84) was performed by modifying a method of Hunter and Greenwood [12]. Sep-Pak C_{18} cartridges were used to separate labeled peptide from free ^{125}I; for details see Chap. 2.1. Specific activity was about 500 µCi/µg. Incorporation of a single iodine atom into each peptide would have resulted in a specific activity of about 559 µCi/µg. Standards and tracer contained aspartic acid at position 76. The tracer was diluted in buffer A with HSA, 20 g/liter, resulting in 30000 cpm/100 µl.

Assay Procedure

The procedure for the assay with antiserum H4 is shown in Table 1. Each sample was measured in duplicate. The *standard assay* for the C-terminal fragment of PTH used in our laboratory is a homologous procedure of incubating for 48 h under equilibrium conditions and has been described previously [11, 25]. It works with an antiserum raised in guinea pigs (code MS 7), $[^{125}I]$ Tyr^{52}-hPTH(52-84) as a tracer and synthetic hPTH(53-84) as a standard, as described in Chap. 2.1.

Serum Calcium

Serum calcium was determined by calcein fluorometry.

Table 1. Flow diagram of the assay

First day:	−100 µl standard or sample
	− 50 µl first antibody (H4, 1:6000)
	− 10 µl normal goat serum diluted in buffer A (1:50)
	Incubate for 24 h at 4°C
Second day:	− 50 µl $[^{125}I]$ Tyr^{52}-hPTH(52–84) with PEG 50 g/liter (Serva Feinbiochemica, Heidelberg, FRG)
	Incubate for at 24 h at 4 °C
Third day:	−100 µl second antibody (1:6)
	−100 µl PEG 50 g/liter in buffer A
	Incubate for 30 min at room temperature
	Centrifuge the tubes for 10 min at 2000 g
	Aspirate the supernatants
	Determine the radioactivity of the pellets in a gamma counter

Affinity and Maximum Binding Capacity

Calculations of affinity constant and maximum binding capacity were performed by Scatchard plot and saturation analysis as described by Zettner [24].

Results

Analytical Variables

The characteristics of the antiserum in terms of *tracer binding* and *specificity* are described within the procedures for the "rapid assay," Chap. 2.3. Additional experiments with intact hPTH(1-84) demonstrated that in a range from 8 to 250 pmol/liter the displacement curve with intact hormone as a standard ran parallel to the one with hPTH(53-84) as a standard. The binding affinity of intact hormone was reduced four times at low concentrations and three times at high concentrations when compared with the C-terminal fragment.

To examine the *binding kinetics* of the first antibody (1:6000) we varied incubation time (2–72 h) and temperature (room temperature, 4 °C). At 4 °C the plateau of the curve (12 000 cpm with a total tracer activity of 30 000 cpm) was reached after 24 h. At room temperature less binding was achieved. The incubation was completed after 8 h (10 000 cpm), whereby 8000 counts were detected after 2 h. Because of these results we used two different approaches in the following experiments:

1. Development of a sensitive assay with a long incubation time (24 h) at 4 °C
2. Development of a rapid assay at room temperature, which is described in Chap. 2.3

Examining the *mode of saturation* we found the sequential assay (24 h + 24 h) to be more sensitive and to be able to distinguish between normal and hypoparathyroid sera. This was not possible for the equilibrium assay (24 h).

Studying the *effect of polyethylene glycol (PEG)* on the assay we obtained the best differentiation between normal and hypoparathyroid sera using PEG 50 g/liter in the tracer buffer along with a PEG solution of 50 g/liter given with the second antibody (Table 1). The final PEG concentration in the assay tube was 20 g/liter.

Table 2 shows data of standard curves with 50, 100, 150, and 200 µl standard solution, each with 100 µl antiserum and 100 µl tracer. In addition, there is the standard curve containing 100 µl standard, 50 µl tracer, and 50 µl antiserum. Thereby the proportion in terms of *volumes of standard, tracer, and antiserum* is 2:1:1. The standard curve with reduced volumes of tracer and antiserum lies between the 150- and 200-µl standard curves.

Measuring PTH levels in normal, hypoparathyroid, and hyperparathyroid sera the three sensitive versions (middle and right part of the table) yielded better distinction between normal and hypoparathyroid sera.

Table 2. Antiserum H4: standard curves with 50, 100, 150, and 200 μl standard. Data in B/B₀% and pmol/liter. Sequential saturation (24 h + 24 h), 100 μl first antibody, 100 μl tracer with 50 g/liter PEG, 100 μl second antibody, 100 μl 50 g/liter PEG solution. One curve with 100 μl standard, 50 μl tracer with 50 g/liter PEG, 50 μl antiserum and 10 μl 1:50 diluted normal goat serum. Otherwise as above

		50 μl	100 μl	150 μl	200 μl	50 μl antiserum 50 μl tracer 100 μl standard	
B/B₀	90%	11	4	3	2	2	pmol/liter
	80%	20	9	5	5	4.5	pmol/liter
	50%	44	25	16	14	15	pmol/liter
	20%	180	70	50	37	45	pmol/liter
	10%	450	180	130	80	130	pmol/liter

The assay with decreased volumes of tracer and antiserum had almost the same sensitivity and an identical clinical utility compared to the version with 200 μl standard. But here the advantage of decreased radioactivity, saving of antiserum and saving of sample was given.

The *detection limit* of the assay ($B_0 - 2$ SD) was 2 pmol/liter hPTH(53-84), which equals 2×10^{-16} mol/tube.

Figure 1 compares antiserum H4 with the standard antiserum of our laboratory (MS 7) regarding their *sensitivity*. The sensitive assay with antiserum H4 placed seven out of eight hypoparathyroid sera lower than the normal range (5–15 pmol/liter). One hypoparathyroid patient had a PTH level of 5 pmol/liter. Despite a very steep standard curve the sensitive assay with antiserum MS 7 was not able to distinguish between normal and hypoparathyroid sera. The PTH levels of all hypoparathyroid sera were within the normal range. Using the less sensitive assay with antiserum H4 (using 100 μl of all reagents), six patients with hypoparathyroidism had PTH concentrations lower than the normal range, and two were falsely placed within the normal range.

Washing the precipitate with normal saline considerably reduced the unspecific binding (from 420 to 70 cpm). But differentiation between normal and hypoparathyroid sera did not improve. To eliminate possible mistakes caused by different matrices of standards (dissolved in buffer A) and samples (serum) we tried to dissolve the standards in serum free of PTH. To separate PTH from serum we used Sep-Pack C_{18} cartridges. But the majority of the serum PTH did not stay on the column surface; the first fractions being eluted contained the highest PTH levels in both the H4 and the MS 7 assay. For this reason the cartridges were not suitable for eliminating PTH from serum.

The calculation of the *affinity constant* of H4 was based on the results of a 24-h equilibrium assay. With Scatchard plots we obtained a maximum affinity constant (C_{max}) of 1.7×10^{10} liter/mol, the mean affinity constant (C_{mean}) being

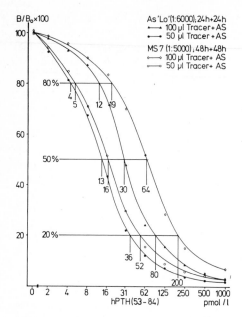

Fig. 1. Sensitive assays with antisera H4 and MS7. H4 with sequential saturation (24 h + 24 h): 50 µl tracer and 50 µl antiserum (●) and 100 µl tracer and 100 µl antiserum (▲). MS7 with sequential saturation (48 h + 48 h): 50 µl tracer and 50 µl antiserum (○) and 100 µl tracer and 100 µl antiserum (◇)

0.7×10^{10} liter/mol. The results obtained by Scatchard plot correlated well with those obtained by saturation analysis.

Antiserum MS 7 only has a C_{max} of 0.7 and a C_{mean} of 0.4×10^{10} liter/mol.

Clinical Use

To examine the *linearity* of the assay we diluted the sera of a normal subject and of a patient with 1° hyperparathyroidism in series. The PTH levels of the different dilutions are presented in Fig. 2. The serum of the patient with 1° hyperparathyroidism was diluted in hypoparathyroid serum. The serum of the normal subject diluted in buffer A since hypoparathyroid serum was not totally free of PTH and would have falsified measurements of very low concentrations. The assay produces linear results within a range of 3 to 60 pmol/liter. Linearity decreases beyond this range, which can be explained by the shape of the standard curve: 80% B/B_0 is reached at 4 pmol/ liter and 20% B/B_0 at 45 pmol/liter. We consider 80% B/B_0 and 20% B/B_0 to be the limits of the linear range for our RIAs. To stay within this linear range sera with PTH concentrations above 60 pmol/liter should be diluted and redetermined. For dilution we used hypoparathyroid serum. If this is not available, buffer A with 20 g BSA/liter may be tested as a substitute.

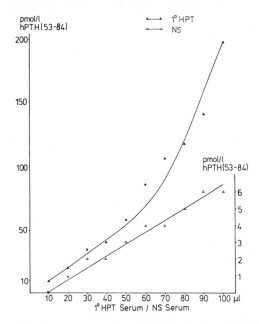

Fig. 2. Antiserum H4: PTH levels in serial dilutions of a normal (△) and hyper-parathyroid serum (▲). *Left ordinate* relates to the patient with 1° hyperparathyroidism; *right ordinate* indicates the normal subject

Determination of PTH levels in samples which had been drawn shortly before, during, and over a 2-h period after *surgical removal of a parathyroid adenoma* revealed a decrease in PTH from 160 pmol/liter to 52 pmol/liter, suggesting a half-life of the C-terminal fragment of about 40 min. Serum calcium declined from 2.9 to 2.5 mmol/liter during the same period.

Figure 3 shows the results of determining the PTH levels in patients and healthy control persons. Normal subjects ($n = 36$) had concentrations ranging from 5 to 12 pmol/liter. Of 14 hypoparathyroid patients (3 idiopathic, 10 surgical, 1 patient with pseudohypoparathyroidism) 11 had levels below the normal range, and 2 had concentrations at the lower limit of normal (5 pmol/liter). One patient had laboratory parameters suggesting hypoparathyroidism; however, a significantly elevated PTH level was found. He proved to be a patient with pseudohypoparathyroidism. All hypoparathyroid patients received high doses of vitamin D. The PTH levels of 13 patients with hypercalcemia of malignancy were within the normal range. There was no overlap between the normal range and patients with surgically confirmed primary hyperparathyroidism (1° HPT, $n = 36$) or secondary (renal) hyperparathyroidism (2° HPT, $n = 19$). Sera with PTH levels higher than 60 pmol/liter were diluted and redetermined. Concentrations up to 4000 pmol/liter were obtained by multiplication with the dilution factor.

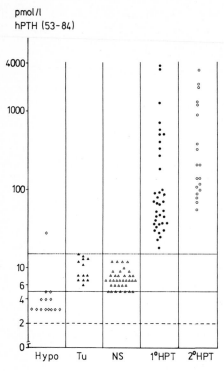

pmol/l
hPTH (53-84)

Fig. 3. Antiserum H4: hPTH (53-84) levels in sera from 14 patients with hypoparathyroidism (*Hypo*), 13 patients with tumor hypercalcemia (*TU*), 36 normal subjects (*NS*), 36 patients with surgically confirmed 1° HPT, and 19 patients with 2° HPT. *Dashed line* represents the detection limit; *dotted lines* mark the normal range

Reproducibility

The intra- and interassay variances were examined by repeated measurements of both a plasma pool obtained from healthy blood donors and another pool obtained from hyperparathyroid subjects. The results are shown in Tables 3 and 4. The assay proved to be very stable.

Table 3. Intraassay variance. The numbers for mean ($\bar{X}$) and coefficient of variation (CV) result from 21 duplicate determinations within the same assay

	n	$\bar{X}$ (pmol/liter)	CV (%)
Normal individuals	21	7.2	5.9
Primary hyperparathyroidism	21	37.8	3.8

Table 4. Interassay variance. The figures are from duplicate determinations in seven assays over a period of 11 weeks. The upper part of the table shows control sera data, the lower part shows data in relation to the shape of the standard curves

	n	$\bar{X}$ (pmol/liter)	CV (%)
Normal individuals	7	7.6	8.8
Primary hyperparathyroidism	7	36.5	5.9
80% B/B_0	7	4.2	9.3
50% B/B_0	7	12.8	15.9
20% B/B_0	7	44.3	11.2

Discussion

A few assays for the differentiation of normal and hypoparathyroid subjects have been published [7, 15, 17, 18, 22, 23]. None of the assays achieved a completely accurate differentiation. In some cases there was an overlap of up to 70% between normal and hypoparathyroid sera.

Cytochemical bioassays have been reported to show better results [1, 8, 13]. But this technique is too cumbersome as a standard procedure [2]. The first studies on other highly sensitive procedures such as two-step immunochemical assays for PTH(1-84) do not contain enough data on the differentiation between normal and hypoparathyroid subjects [10, 14]. However, as shown in Chaps. 1.1, 2.8, and 2.9, two-site immunoradiometric and immunoluminometric assays have recently differentiated between normal and hypoparathyroid sera [4, 5].

Three sensitive immunoradiometric assays and RIAs were described. They are homologous assays specific for N-terminal [18], mid-region [7], and C-terminal fragment of hPTH [17]. There is a significant overlap of normal and hypoparathyroid sera in all three assays.

Some older assays achieve a better differentiation between normal and hypoparathyroid subjects despite the heterologous nature of the systems [15, 22, 23]. In the assay described here there is only a small spread of PTH concentrations in 36 healthy subjects (5–12 pmol/liter), suggesting a high specificity of the antiserum. It discriminates well between normal and hypoparathyroid sera. Of 13 patients with true hypoparathyroidism, 11 had PTH levels below the normal range and 2 had concentrations at the lower limit of normal (5 pmol/liter). The PTH levels in 13 patients with hypercalcemia of malignancy were within the normal range even though lower concentrations were expected. But most of these patients had impaired renal function (serum creatinine > 1.5 mg/dl) so that the glomerular filtration of the C-terminal fragment was decreased [6, 21].

The high sensitivity of the assay permits small PTH increases within the normal range (serial dilution of the serum of a normal subject) to be detected.

After removal of the parathyroids in a patient with primary hyperparathyroidism PTH levels dropped continuously, suggesting a half-life of the C-terminal fragment of 40 min. Reports on the half-life of the C-terminal fragment range from 20 min to 3 h [17]. This discrepancy is probably secondary to differences in the specificity of the antisera used.

The assay detects small amounts of PTH even in hypoparathyroid sera, which could be due to the use of PEG. The standards are dissolved in buffer A, and the medium of the samples is serum. The increase of precipitation by PEG is more effective in buffer A than in serum, leading to falsely high concentrations in serum samples.

To eliminate this problem it would be ideal to dissolve the standards in serum that is free of PTH. Experiments using Sep-Pak C_{18} cartridges to separate PTH from serum were not successful. The small cartridges were quickly loaded with serum components so that there was not enough surface left for binding of PTH. Sep-Pak C_{18} cartridges are useful for separating labeled peptide from free ^{125}I when purifying the tracer [20]. In this case there are no competing serum components and enough surface for the binding of labeled peptide is available. For the separation of PTH from serum, experiments with larger reverse-phase columns or affinity chromatography could be performed. However, the latter would require large amounts of antiserum.

For this assay we used the same antiserum as for the rapid assay described in Chap. 2.3. Here the assay conditions are very different, though. Decreasing the volumes of tracer and antiserum in relation to the standard resulted in a more sensitive displacement curve and there was a better discrimination of normal and hypoparathyroid sera.

Similar changes applied to the standard assay of our laboratory with antiserum MS 7 yielded highly sensitive standard curves, but the clinical utility in terms of differentiation between normal subjects and patients with hypoparathyroidism did not improve. This is due to the lower affinity of antiserum MS 7 (C_{max} H4 $= 1.7 \times 10^{10}$ liter/mol, C_{max} MS 7 $= 0.7 \times 10^{10}$ liter/mol). PTH concentrations determined with the assay described here are lower in relation to other C-terminal assays [9, 11, 17]. The results correspond to those determined with assays for N-terminal fragment or intact hormone [3, 18]. The low levels in our assay are probably due to the fact that the antiserum H4 is more specific. A detection limit as low as 2 pmol/liter is unusual for PTH radioimmunoassays. In the first place this is due to the extraordinary affinity of the antiserum H4. In generating such an antiserum the human origin of the immunogen was definitely a precondition; furthermore the long intervals between booster injections (6 months) might have been important. So far all assays for the differentiation of normal and hyperparathyroid subjects have been using antisera raised in goats [7, 15, 17, 18, 22, 23]. But there is no real proof that antisera from goats are of higher affinity for hPTH than antisera generated in other species.

As a guideline for high sensitivity, several components of the assay are important: a high-affinity antiserum, a fully homologous assay system, a tracer with about one iodine atom per molecule, small volumes of tracer and antiserum in relation to the volume of standard or sample, sequential saturation at the optimum temperature, and an optimized concentration of PEG during incubation and separation of bound and free hormone. In the future, even more sensitive assays may be established on the basis of the immunoradiometric principle, that is now generally introduced for the measurement of thyroid-stimulating hormone and is shown in this volume in Chaps. 1.1, 2.8, and 2.9.

In conclusion, a sensitive RIA for hPTH to diagnose hypoparathyroid conditions is described. The antiserum was raised in goats against extracted hPTH. The working dilution of the antiserum is 1:6000. Synthetic human PTH fragment (53-84) is used as a standard and $[^{125}I]Tyr^{52}$-hPTH (52-84) as a tracer. After a two-step incubation (24 h + 24 h) at 4°C, the bound and free fractions are separated by a mixture of second antibody and PEG solution. To achieve a more sensitive assay we use smaller volumes of tracer and first antibody in relation to the volume of standard solution commonly used (ratio 2:1:1, standard:first antibody:tracer). The lowest concentration detectable is 2 pmol/liter hPTH(53-84), which equals 2×10^{-16} mol/tube. The PTH level in 36 healthy subjects was 5-12 pmol/liter. Of 14 patients with hypoparathyroidism (3 idiopathic, 10 surgical), 11 patients had PTH concentrations below normal, and 2 patients had levels at the lower limit of the normal range (5 pmol/liter). The concentration of one patient with pseudohypoparathyroidism was markedly elevated. Interassay variation (CV 6%–9%) and intraassay variation (3.8%–6%) were acceptable. This assay is capable of detecting low PTH levels, which has been difficult in the past. It is a good instrument for the differentiation of hypocalcemic conditions and for studying changes of PTH concentrations within the normal range. It is suggested that in the future even more sensitive assays for the measurement of carboxyl-terminal fragments of human parathyroid hormone (residues 53–84) may be established if standards and tracer contain asparagine at position 76. These peptides (residues 53-84, asparagine at position 76) are now commercially available (Sigma, Deisenhofen, FRG; Bachem, Heidelberg, FRG; Peptide Institute, Osaka, Japan; Peninsula Laboratories Ltd. St. Helens Cheshire, England).

References

1. Allgrove J, Chayen J, O'Riordan JLH (1983) The cytochemical bioassay of parathyroid hormone: further experience. J Immunoassay 4:1–19
2. Armitage EK (1986) Parathyrin (parathyroid hormone): metabolism and methods for assay. Clin Chem 32:418–424
3. Atkinson MJ, Wong CC, Jüppner H (1982) Intact human PTH(h1-84) radioimmunoassay using the h 28–48 peptide. Acta Endocrinol [Suppl] (Copenh) 246:138
4. Blind E, Schmidt-Gayk H, Scharla S, Flentje D, Fischer S, Göhring U, Hitzler W (1988) Two-site assay of intact parathyroid hormone in the investigation of primary hyperparathyroidism and other disorders of calcium metabolism compared with a midregion assay. J Clin Endocrinol Metab 67:353–360

5. Brown RC, Aston JP, Weeks I, Woodhead JS (1987) Circulating intact parathyroid hormone measured by a two-site immunochemiluminometric assay. J Clin Endocrinol Metab 65:407–414
6. Fogh-Andersen N, Ladefoged J, Moller-Petersen J (1984) Renal and hepatic extraction of carboxyl-terminal immunoreactive parathyrin in normal man. J Clin Chem Clin Biochem 22:479–482
7. Gleed JH, Hendy GN, Nussbaum SR, Rosenblatt M, O'Riordan JLH (1986) Development and application of a mid-region specific assay for human parathyroid hormone. Clin Endocrinol (Oxf) 24:365–373
8. Goltzman D, Henderson B, Loveridge N (1980) Cytochemical bioassay of parathyroid hormone. Characteristics of the assay and analysis of circulating hormonal forms. J Clin Invest 65:1309–1317
9. Gorog RH, Hakim MK, Thompson NW, Rigg GA, McCann DS (1982) Radioimmunoassay of serum parathyrin: comparison of five commercial kits. Clin Chem 28:87–91
10. Hackeng WHL, Lips P, Netelenbos JC, Lips CJM (1986) Clinical implications of estimation of intact parathyroid hormone (PTH) versus total immunoreactive PTH in normal subjects and hyperparathyroid patients. J Clin Endocrinol Metab 63:447–453
11. Hitzler W, Schmidt-Gayk H, Spiropoulos P, Raue F, Hüfner M (1982) Homologous radioimmunoassay for human parathyrin (residues 53-84). Clin Chem 28:1749–1753
12. Hunter WM, Greenwood FC (1962) Preparation of iodine-131-labelled human growth hormone of high specific activity. Nature 194:495–496
13. Klee GG, Preissner CM, Schloegel IW, Kao PC (1988) Bioassay for parathyrin: analytical characteristics and clinical performance in patients with hypercalcemia. Clin Chem 34:482–488
14. Lindall AW, Eltring J, Ells J, Roos BA (1983) Estimation of biologically active intact parathyroid hormone in normal and hyperparathyroid sera by sequential N-terminal immunoextraction and midregion radioimmunoassay: J Clin Endocrinol Metab 57:1007–1013
15. Mallette LE, Tuma SN, Berger RE, Kirkland JL (1982) Radioimmunoassay for the middle region of human parathyroid hormone using an homologous antiserum with a carboxy-terminal fragment of bovine parathyroid hormone as radioligand. J Clin Endocrinol Metab 54:1017–1024
16. Mallette LE, Wilson DP, Kirkland JL (1983) Evaluation of hypocalcemia with a highly sensitive, homologous radioimmunoassay for the midregion of parathyroid hormone. Pediatrics 71:64–69
17. Manning RM, Adami S, Papapoulos SE, Gleed JH, Hendy GN, Rosenblatt M, O'Riordan JLH (1981) A carboxy-terminal specific assay for human parathyroid hormone. Clin Endocrinol (Oxf) 15:439–449
18. Papapoulos SE, Manning RM, Hendy GN, Lewin IG, O'Riordan JLH (1980) Studies of circulating parathyroid hormone in man using a homologous amino-terminal specific immunoradiometric assay. Clin Endocrinol (Oxf) 13:57–67
19. Schmidt-Gayk H, Schmitt-Fiebig M, Hitzler W, Armbruster FP, Mayer E (1986) Two homologous radioimmunoassays for parathyrin compared and applied to disorders of calcium metabolism. Clin Chem 32:57–62
20. Schöneshöfer M, Kage A, Kage R, Fenner A (1982) A convenient technique for the specific isolation of ^{125}I-labelled peptide molecules. Fresenius Z Anal Chem 311:429–430

21. Slatopolsky E, Martin K, Morrissey J, Hruska K (1982) Current concepts of the metabolism and radioimmunoassay of parathyroid hormone. J Lab Clin Med 99:309–316

22. Streibl W, Minne H, Raue F, Ziegler R (1979) Radioimmunoassay for human parathyroid hormone for differentiation between patients with hypoparathyroidism, hyperparathyroidism and normals. Horm Metab Res 11:375–376

23. Wood WG, Butz R, Casaretto M, Hehrmann R, Jüppner H, Marschner I, Wachter C, Zahn H, Hesch RD (1980) Preliminary results on the use of an antiserum to human parathyrin in a homologous radioimmunoassay. J Clin Chem Clin Biochem 18:789–795

24. Zettner A (1973) Principles of competitive binding assays (saturation analyses). I. Equilibrium techniques. Clin Chem 19:669–705

25. Zillikens D, Armbruster FP, Hitzler W, Horn J, Schmidt-Gayk H (1985) Schneller homologer Radioimmunoassay für human-Parathormon (hPTH) zur Differenzierung der hyperkalzämischen Krise. Ärztl Lab 31:151–156

26. Zillikens D, Armbruster FP, Stern J, Schmidt-Gayk H, Raue F (1987) Sensitive homologous radioimmunoassay for human parathyroid hormone to diagnose hypoparathyroid conditions. Ann Clin Biochem 24:608–613

Chapter 2.3

Rapid Homologous Radioimmunoassay for Human Parathyroid Hormone (Residues 53-84) as a Diagnostic Aid in Hypercalcemic Crisis

D. ZILLIKENS

Introduction

The most frequent cause of hypercalcemia is primary hyperparathyroidism (HPT). Primary HPT is found in 55% of all hypercalcemic patients, while 35% of them suffer from malignancy [1]. Malignancies, which are occasionally associated with hypercalcemia, are divided into three groups: (a) hematopoetic malignancies, (b) solid tumors with bone metastases and (c) solid tumors without bone metastases [2]. Less frequent causes of hypercalcemia are sarcoidosis, vitamin D intoxication, thiazide intake, hyperthyroidism, Addison's disease, and familial hypocalciuric hypercalcemia. There is some variation in reports of the frequency of disease which causes hypercalcemia [3]. The underlying disease in patients who develop hypercalcemic crisis (serum calcium > 4.0 mmol/liter) is most often primary HPT [3]. However, another group has reported somewhat different data [4]. Hypercalcemic crisis is an acute disease with high lethality. Therefore, rapid diagnostic procedures are mandatory. The search for a malignancy must parallel measures to reveal hyperparathyroidism (anamnesis, laboratory results, hand and skull X-rays). It is important to perform surgery in a patient with primary HPT while therapy of other causes of hypercalcemic crisis does not include surgery of the parathyroid glands.

Rapid measurement of parathyroid hormone (PTH) in the serum is necessary to confirm the diagnosis of parathyrotoxic crisis. The PTH radioimmunoassays (RIAs) which are available either have long incubation times [5, 6] or become unreliable with shorter ones [4, 7]. We have developed a rapid procedure to measure PTH in serum which allows reliable differentiation between normal and elevated PTH levels.

Materials and Methods

Buffer A (pH 7.4) was prepared as indicated in Chap. 2.1. The antiserum (generously provided by Prof. Dr. O'Riordan, Middlesex Hospital, London, UK) was prepared by immunizing goats (H4) with human parathyroid extracts.

(See ref. [8] for details.) The antiserum was diluted in buffer A. Normal goat serum (No. 13770, Merck AG) was added to a final concentration of 4 ml/liter. The standards were prepared by dissolving chemically synthesized hPTH(53-84) (Bachem Heidelberg, FRG) in buffer A and 1% human serum albumin (HSA). Anti-goat IgG was obtained by immunizing a donkey. Dilution was in buffer A.

The tracer was prepared by modifying a method of Hunter and Greenwood [9]. To 1 μg Tyr^{52}-hPTH(52-84) (Bachem AG) the following were added: 5 μl (0.5 mCi) Na^{125}I (No. IMS 30, Amersham Buchler GmbH, Gieselweg 1, 3300 Braunschweig, FRG), 5 μl phosphate buffer (pH 7.4, 0.06 mol/liter), and 10 μl (1 μg) chloramine-T-solution. Oxidation time was 60 s. To terminate the reaction 10 μl (2.5 μg) Na$_2$S$_2$O$_5$ solution and 200 μl buffer A with 2% HSA were added. Sep Pak C$_{18}$ cartridges (No. 51910, Waters GmbH, Herzog-Adolf-Str. 4, 6240 Königstein/Ts., FRG) served to separate the mixture. Free iodine was eluted after addition of 2 ml 0.05 mol/liter trifluoroacetic acid (TFA) (No. 8262, Merck AG). Subsequently, the peptide was eluted with 2 ml 0.05 mol/liter TFA/acetonitrile No. 3; Merck AG) (60:40). Protein concentration was increased with 3 ml buffer A and 2% HSA. The tracer was further diluted in buffer A and 2% HSA to yield an activity of 30 000 cpm in a volume of 100 μl. Specific activity was 450–500 μCi/μg. Standards and tracer contained aspartic acid at position 76. The assay procedure is shown in Table 1. The samples were measured in duplicate or triplicate. Iodination of Tyr^{27}-hPTH(27-48), Tyr^{34}-hPTH(1-34) (Peptide Institute Inc., 476 Ina, Minoh-shi, Osaka 562, Japan) was performed in an analogous fashion.

The standard PTH assay in our laboratory is a homologous C-terminal assay with an incubation time of 48 h. [^{125}I] Tyr^{52}-hPTH(52-84) is the tracer. The antiserum (code MS 7) in the standard assay binds the amino acids 69-84; the peptide hPTH(44-68) does not compete with the tracer for antibody binding. (For details see ref. [17]). Serum calcium was determined by calcein fluorometry. Serum creatinine was determined by the kinetic method of Jaffe.

Table 1. Flow diagram of the rapid assay

100 μl	Standard or sample
100 μl	[^{125}I] Tyr^{52}-hPTH(52-84)
100 μl	First antibody (1:4000). Working dilution
	2 h incubation at room temperature
100 μl	Second antibody (1:6)
100 μl	PEG 10% in buffer A
	30 min incubation at room temperature
	10 min at 1800 g
	Aspiration of the supernatant
	Determination of radioactivity of pellet in a gamma counter

Results

Tracer Binding and Specificity

Tracer binding experiments, employing the C-terminal fragment, yielded binding of 12 000 cpm at an antiserum dilution of 1:4000 and an incubation time of 24 h (30 000 cpm total activity). The labeled fragments hPTH(27-48) and hPTH(43-68) were examined under similar conditions. Binding was 9000 cpm and 6000 cpm, respectively. The labeled fragment hPTH(1-34) was not bound. Intact hormone and C-terminal fragment competed with C-terminal tracer for antibody binding. Competition by intact hormone was slightly weaker at low concentrations than competition by the C-terminal fragment. Other hPTH fragments (1-34, 28-48, 44-68) were not able to compete with the C-terminal tracer for antibody binding, even at high concentrations.

Binding Kinetics

After a 2-h incubation, the antibody bound more C-terminal fragment than other fragments. Therefore, the C-terminal fragment was considered to be most appropriate for a rapid assay. The first antibody yielded 70–75% of its maximal binding within 2 h of incubation time. The binding characteristics of the antibody were not markedly altered by temperature (22 °C or 4 °C) or by the presence of polyethylene glycol (PEG) in the tracer. Further experiments were carried out at room temperature and without PEG during the incubation step between first antibody and antigen.

Incubation Conditions

Calibration curves at different incubation conditions are shown in Fig. 1. PTH levels of normal subjects, of patients with hypercalcemia of malignancy, and of patients with primary HPT (documented by surgery) and with secondary HPT were determined simultaneously. A comparison of the different methods demonstrated that the PTH levels of the different patient groups were determined correctly, regardless of the incubation time (1, 2, and 4 h). However, the longer assay version was slightly more sensitive. Sequential saturation analysis yielded a very sensitive calibration curve in spite of a short incubation time. However, the use of this method was restricted by its limited dose range, which does not allow the reliable determination of PTH levels higher than 200 pmol/liter. The assay variation with very short incubation times (30 min, 15 min) did not yield enough counts per minute. In addition the calibration curve was not sensitive enough. This assay could not distinguish the PTH levels of normal subjects from the standard 0. Thus, the incubation time of 1–2 h could not be shortened further.

Another series of experiments demonstrated that the assay was not significantly dependent on temperature (37 °C, 22 °C, 4 °C). Subsequently, the assay was

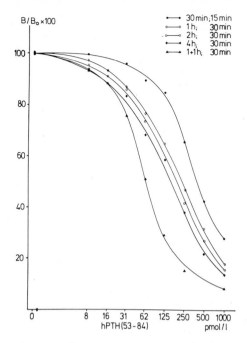

Fig. 1. Calibration curves at different incubation times of first antibody: equilibrium technique: 30 min (●), 1 h (◇), 2 h (○), 4 h (◆), and sequential saturation: 1 h + 1 h (▲). The second incubation time was 30 min in each experiment except in the version with a 30-min first and a 15-min second incubation

carried out at room temperature because of convenience and slightly higher sensitivity. The assay with an incubation time of 1 h reliably distinguished normal individuals from either patients with hypercalcemia of malignancy or primary HPT. However, the lower detection limit varied so that occasionally normal subjects could not be distinguished from standard 0. Therefore, the assay with the 2-h incubation time was preferred to the 1-h assay due to its higher reliability at the lower dose range. The total time for finishing the assay after the arrival of serum samples was 3 h. This assay time is suitable for emergency diagnosis since other preoperative measures (ECG, X-ray, etc.) take a comparable amount of time.

Polyethylene Glycol Concentration

Two hours were required to complete precipitation of the second antibody. We tried to reduce this time by adding PEG. Several PEG concentrations in the tracer were tested. Also, we tested several PEG concentrations during the second incubation in order to accelerate the reaction of the second antibody (with the first antibody-antigen) and combinations of both variations. The best results were obtained without PEG in the tracer and 100 µl 10% PEG solution after addition of the second antibody. The PEG did not influence the sensitivity of the assay and the accuracy of the results. However, the PEG made it possible to reduce the second incubation time from 2 h to 30 min. A second incubation time of 30 min without PEG was not appropriate for accurate measurements.

Detection Limits

The lower detection limit (B_0-2 s) was 8 pmol/liter. The upper detection limit was 800 pmol/liter (20% B/B_0) with undiluted serum. By dilution of the serum this limit could be arbitrarily increased.

Comparison of Sensitivity

The calibration curves of the rapid assay in comparison with a longer assay version (24 h incubation, identical conditions) and with the routine assay in our laboratory (48 h, 1 h) are shown in Fig. 2.

The calibration curve of the rapid assay is very similar to the curves of the other assays. The antiserum "London" (H4) bound 13 000 cpm of 30 000 cpm total activity after 24 h of incubation. The activity of the rapid assay was slightly lower with 10 000 cpm bound of 30 000 cpm total activity.

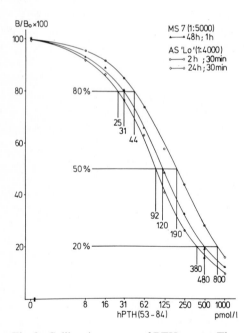

Fig. 2. Calibration curves of PTH assays: The *upper curve* represents the rapid assay, the *middle curve* the routine assay with antibody MS7, and the *lower curve* the assay with a longer incubation time, employing antiserum London

Clinical Applications

To examine the linearity of a dilution series, the serum of a patient with primary hyperparathyroidism was serially diluted in hypoparathyroid serum. The PTH levels of the different dilutions were determined with both the rapid assay and the routine assay. Both assays gave linear increases of PTH concentrations. The values of the rapid assay were slightly higher. Furthermore, we used the rapid assay and the routine assay to determine PTH levels in sera which had been drawn immediately before, during, and over 2 h after surgical removal of parathyroid adenoma. Initially, a clear increase in PTH levels was detected with both assays (routine assay 180 pmol/liter, rapid assay 170 pmol/liter). This was possibly due to intraoperative manipulations of the parathyroid glands. Both assays yielded similar values in the further course. Two hours after surgery the values of the routine assay had declined somewhat more (50 vs. 70 pmol/liter).

The PTH levels of a larger patient group were determined with the rapid assay. The results are shown in Fig. 3.

Normal subjects ($n = 36$) had PTH concentrations between 10 and 30 pmol/liter. The PTH levels of normal subjects did not overlap with the levels of

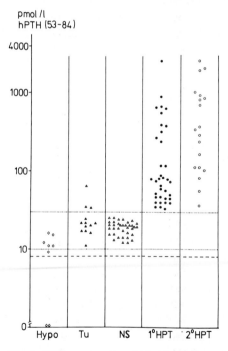

Fig. 3. Human parathyroid hormone(53-84) was measured in the serum of eight hypoparathyroid patients (*Hypo*), 13 patients with malignancy-associated hypercalcemia (*Tu*), 36 normal subjects (*NS*), 36 patients with surgically confirmed 1° HPT, and 19 patients with 2° HPT. The *dashed line* indicates the lower detection limit. The *dotted lines* mark the normal range

patients with primary ($n = 36$) or secondary ($n = 19$) HPT. The PTH and calcium concentrations in the serum of 21 patients with primary hyperparathyroidism correlated significantly ($r = 0.95$; $P < 0.005$). Furthermore, the PTH levels of 13 patients with hypercalcemia of malignancy were determined. Ten patients had normal concentrations of PTH and three patients had elevated PTH levels. The serum creatinine in these three patients was between 180 and 280 µmol/liter, demonstrating reduced kidney function. The PTH levels did not exceed 79 pmol/liter. In contrast patients with primary HPT and PTH concentrations below 100 pmol/liter had a serum calcium below 3.2 mmol/liter. Therefore, differential diagnosis of hypercalcemic crisis in these patient subgroups could be made unambiguously. A comparison of PTH and calcium levels was performed in eight patients with hypoparathyroidism, nine normal subjects, ten patients with primary HPT, and ten patients with secondary HPT. The characteristic features associated with each disease are shown in Fig. 4: primary HPT with elevated calcium and PTH, malignancy-associated hypercalcemia with elevated calcium and normal or slightly elevated PTH, and secondary HPT with high PTH and normal or decreased calcium. Patients with hypoparathyroidism were distinguished from normal subjects by their decreased serum calcium levels. This could not be achieved with the PTH assay since the sensitivity was too low. However, the assay yielded the essential information: It could reliably discriminate primary HPT from malignancy-associated hypercalaemia in patients with severe hypercalcemia.

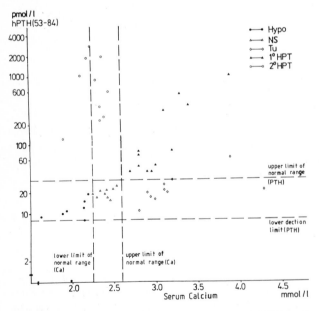

Fig. 4. Relationship between serum calcium and PTH in the serum of 8 patients with hypoparathyroidism (*Hypo*), 9 normal subjects (*NS*), 10 patients with hypercalcemia of malignancy (*Tu*), 12 patients with primary HPT, and 10 patients with secondary HPT

Table 2. Some laboratory parameters of two patients with hypercalcemic crisis at the time of hospital admittance

		Female 61 years	Female 47 years
Serum calcium	(mmol/l normal 2.2–2.6)	4.0	4.0
Serum creatinine	(μmol/liter, normal 50–120)	180	115
PTH	(pmol/liter, normal 10–30)	350	450

Since the rapid PTH assay was established two patients were admitted with hypercalcemic crisis. Some laboratory parameters of the two patients are shown in Table 2.

Both patients were found to have clearly elevated PTH levels employing the rapid assay. Surgery was performed within hours. A solitary parathyroid adenoma was detected in both of the patients.

Reproducibility

The intra- and interassay variances of the rapid PTH assay were examined by measuring PTH in control sera with normal or elevated PTH (see Tables 3, 4).

The PTH concentrations were reproducible and the shape of the calibration curve did not change over several months.

Discussion

Only a few assays for the rapid measurement of PTH have been published. Older methods [4, 7, 10] include heterologous assays with low sensitivity and only limited reliability. Recently, a homologous midregional assay with an

Table 3. Intraassay variance. Means and coefficients of variation were determined from 16 triplicate measurements.

	n	Mean (pmol/liter)	CV (%)
Normal individuals (serum)	16	13.8	4.8
Primary hyperpara- thyroidism (serum)	16	72.8	2.9

Table 4. Interassay variance. Means and coefficients of variation were
determined from duplicates in nine assays over 10 weeks. The upper part of
the table shows control sera data. The lower part shows data from the
calibration curves

		Mean (pmol/liter)	CV (%)
Normal individuals	9	19.8	15.1
Primary hyperparathyroidism	9	75.6	9.7
80% B/B_0	9	45.6	8.9
50% B/B_0	9	185	6.8
20% B/B_0	9	767	4.8

incubation time of 6 h was developed [11]. The conditions of this assay are
different from our assay in terms of specificity, standard medium, separation
procedure, and total length.

Experiments with more concentrated antiserum showed that only 75% of
our tracer was bound although the antiserum was present in great abundance.
We assumed that iodination changed the immunological properties of a part of
the peptide. Thus, an improved assay seemed possible by separation of immunologically changed from unchanged tracer. This could be achieved by high-
performance liquid chromatography (HPLC) [12].

The antiserum was shown to be polyvalent. However, the subpopulation
which bound hPTH(53-84) had a high specificity for this fragment.

The use of 100 µl 10% PEG (in addition to second antibody in order to
accelerate precipitation) shortened the second incubation time from 2 h to
30 min. Similar effects of PEG have been reported previously [13]. A comparison of the rapid assay with the routine assay revealed similar calibration
curves and equivalent clinical usefulness. The advantage of the rapid assay is its
considerably shorter incubation time. The PTH levels of 13 patients with
malignancy-associated hypercalcemia were lower in the rapid assay than in the
routine assay. Both assays were able to detect changes in serum PTH concentration in the first 2 h after surgical removal of a parathyroid adenoma.

In some patients with malignancy-associated hypercalcemia PTH-like compounds were detected (see Chap. 3.1, parathyroid hormone-related protein,
PTH-rP). However, it can be assumed that humoral tumor products do not
interfere with the results of the PTH RIA [2, 14].

The danger of erroneously diagnosing primary HPT in patients with
reduced kidney function has been described repeatedly [15, 16]. Similarly, this is
relevant for the differential diagnosis of hypercalcemic crisis since patients with
malignancy-associated hypercalcemia may also have some kidney damage. Our
rapid assay was able to distinguish these patients from patients with primary
HPT. The PTH levels of patients with primary HPT were markedly higher than

the PTH levels of patients with malignancy and reduced kidney function. Therefore our newly developed rapid PTH assay is a reliable and safe diagnostic aid to clarify the cause of a hypercalcemic crisis.

Conclusion

A rapid RIA for parathyroid hormone (PTH) is described. This assay can serve as a diagnostic aid in hypercalcemic crises. The antiserum was prepared by immunizing goats with extracted human PTH. The working dilution of the antiserum is 1:4000. Synthetic human PTH fragment (53-84) is utilized as a standard. The tracer is ^{125}I-Tyr^{52}hPTH(52-84), which is labeled by the chloramine-T technique and separated from free iodine on Sep-Pak C_{18} cartridges. After a one-step incubation at room temperature, the bound and free fractions are separated by a solution of second antibody and PEG. The total assay time is 3 h. The PTH levels in 36 healthy subjects were 10–30 pmol/liter. Elevated PTH levels were found in 36 patients with primary and 19 patients with secondary hyperparathyroidism. PTH was normal in 10 of 13 patients with malignancy-associated hypercalcemia. The three remaining patients had impaired renal function and PTH levels up to 70 pmol/liter. Patients with hypercalcemic crisis caused by primary hyperparathyroidism had PTH levels above 100 pmol/liter. These data demonstrate that the 'rapid assay' can reliably identify patients with hyperparathyroidism in the case of a hypercalcemic crisis. This information can be important in the attempt to initiate therapy as rapidly as possible.

References

1. Mundy GR, Martin TJ (1982) The hypercalcemia of malignancy: pathogenesis and management. Metabolism 31:1247–1277
2. Mundy GR, Ibbotson KJ, D'Sousa SM, Simpson EL, Jacobs JW, Martin TJ (1984) The hypercalcemia of cancer. Clinical implications and pathogenic mechanisms. N Engl J Med 310:1718–1727
3. Ziegler R, Minne H, Bellwinkel S, Fröhlich D (1973) Hypercalciämie-Syndrom und hypercalciämische Krise. Dtsch Med Wochenschr 98:276–283
4. von Lilienfeld-Toal H, Schulz D, Vogerl F, Vaerst R (1981) Hyperkalzämische Krise: Diagnose akuter Hyperparathyreoidismus durch Parathormon-Schnell-Assay. Intensivmedizin 18:232–235
5. Hitzler W, Schmidt-Gayk H, Spiropoulos P, Raue F, Hüfner M (1982) Homologous radioimmunoassay for human parathyrin (residues 53-84). Clin Chem 28:1749–1753
6. Gorog RH, Hakim MK, Thompson NW, Rigg GA, McCann DS (1982) Radioimmunoassay of serum parathyrin: comparison of five commercial kits. Clin Chem 28:87–91

7. Wood WG, Marschner I, Scriba PC (1979) Tests on three antisera and subsequent development of radioimmunoassay for different regions of human parathyrin. Horm Metab Res 11:309–317
8. Manning RM, Adami S, Papapoulos SE, Gleed JH, Hendy GN, Rosenblatt M, O'Riordan JLH (1981) A carboxy-terminal specific assay for human parathyroid hormone. Clin Endocrinol (Oxf) 15:439–449
9. Hunter WM, Greenwood FC (1962) Preparation of iodine-131-labelled human growth hormone of high specific activity. Nature 194:495–496
10. Hehrmann R (1980) Plasma-Parathormon: Entwicklung einer radioimmunologischen Bestimmungsmethode und klinisch-pathophysiologische Untersuchungen. Urban and Schwarzenberg, Munich
11. Wood WG (1983) A rapid homologous radioimmunoassay for the mid-region of human parathyrin using a high-affinity antiserum directed against the 44-68 sequence. Ärztl Lab 29:307–310
12. Schöneshöfer M, Kage A, Kage R, Fenner A (1982) A convenient technique for the specific isolation of ^{125}I-labelled peptide molecules. Fresenius Z Anal Chem 311:429–430
13. Wood WG, Stalla G, Müller OA, Scriba PC (1979) A rapid and specific method for separation of bound and free antigen in radioimmunoassay systems. J Clin Chem Clin Biochem 17:111–114
14. Minne HW, Ziegler R (1984) Hyperkalzämie bei Malignomen-vermitteln humorale Tumorprodukte? Klinikarzt 13:448–455
15. Mallette LE, Tuma SN, Berger RE, Kirkland JL (1982) Radioimmunoassay for the middle region of human parathyroid hormone using an homologous antiserum with a carboxy-terminal fragment of bovine parathyroid hormone as radioligand. J Clin Endocrinol Metab 54:1017–1024
16. Hehrmann R (1982) Parathormon-Radioimmunoassay: methodische Entwicklungen, klinische Indikationen und Wertigkeit. Nuklearmediziner 5:165–177
17. Schmidt-Gayk H, Schmitt-Fiebig M, Hitzler W, Armbruster FP, Mayer E (1986) Two homologous radioimmunoassays for parathyrin compared and applied to disorders of calcium metabolism. Clin Chem 32:57–62

Chapter 2.4

Homologous Radioimmunoassay for Human Parathyroid Hormone (Residues 44-68) with Tyrosylated Peptide as Tracer

H. Schmidt-Gayk and G. Kunst

Introduction

Along with the steroid hormone 1,25-dihydroxyvitamin D_3 and the peptide hormone calcitonin, the polypeptide parathyroid hormone (parathyrin) (PTH) is responsible for maintaining calcium and phosphorus homeostasis in vertebrates. A decrease in the concentration of calcium in serum is followed by the release of the 84-amino-acid polypeptide PTH and some of its fragments from the secretory granules of the parathyroid glands into the bloodstream. These peptides undergo rapid proteolytic cleavage in the liver and kidneys to yield the N- and C-terminal fragments of PTH. The half-life of the C-terminal fragment, which is believed to be biologically inert, is about 20–40 min, whereas the N-terminal fragment and the intact hormone disappear much faster from the circulation ($t_{1/2} < 5$ min) [1–3]. Thus, N-terminal assays reflect the secretory state of the parathyroid glands at the time of blood sampling. For the diagnosis of hyperparathyroidism, however, these results might be misleading if PTH secretion has temporarily been suppressed [3]. In contrast, assays for both the middle region (residues 44-68) and the C-terminal region (53-84) of PTH will give an integrated value for immunoreactive PTH (iPTH), reflecting the chronic state of parathyroid gland function [3]. Because circulating PTH is heterogeneous, both assays will probably detect several fragments of PTH, each of which contains the respective amino acid sequence; these fragments are mainly derived from the peripheral metabolism of native PTH, but in part they also appear to be secretory products of the parathyroid glands [4, 5].

Several heterologous [6–8] and homologous [9–11] RIAs for hPTH(44-68) have been developed. Here we describe a homologous sensitive radioimmunoassay (RIA) system for the midregion of hPTH, in which we use a guinea pig antiserum raised against a partly purified extract from human parathyroid adenomas, radioiodinated tyrosylated hPTH(44-68) as tracer, and hPTH(44-68) as standard. We also describe a rapid tracer purification technique in which we use Sep-Pak C_{18} cartridges to purify the iodinated form of hPTH(44-68).

Materials and Methods

Specimens

Blood was sampled, and the serum was stored at $-30\,°C$. Control samples from apparently healthy volunteers, from patients with primary hyperparathyroidism and from patients with renal failure were divided into 1-ml aliquots and stored at $-30\,°C$ until use. Storage of the samples for 18 months did not measurably change the iPTH concentration, nor did repeated freezing and thawing as often as three times change the iPTH concentration measured. Thawing the samples and storing them for 48 h at room temperature also did not alter the concentration of iPTH.

Reagents

To prepare 1 liter assay buffer (pH 7.4) we combined 800 ml of 67 mmol/liter Na_2HPO_4, 200 ml of 67 mmol/liter KH_2PO_4, and 200 ml of 67 mmol/liter KH_2PO_4 (Merck AG, Darmstadt, FRG), then added 1 g sodium azide (Merck AG), 400 mg ethylenediaminetetraacetic acid (EDTA), and 1 g human serum albumin (Behringwerke AG, Marburg, FRG). Antiserum MS6 was obtained by immunizing guinea pigs with partly purified hPTH that had been extracted from adenomas and passed through a column of Sephadex G50 [12]. The specificity of the antiserum obtained was determined. We diluted 100 µl antiserum with 996 ml assay buffer, then added 3.9 ml normal guinea pig serum to each preparation.

Standards

Standards were prepared by diluting the synthetic fragments hPTH(44-68), hPTH(1-34), hPTH(28-48), hPTH(53-84), hPTH(64-84), and hPTH(1-84) in PPPNE buffer in which the human serum albumin had been increased to 10 g/liter. hPTH(1-84) was purchased from Peptide Institute Inc., Osaka, Japan; the other PTH peptides were from Bachem Co., Bubendorf, Switzerland. Antiserum to guinea pig IgG was obtained by immunizing a goat with guinea pig IgG. A 31-fold dilution of this antiserum in assay buffer completely precipitated the first antibody (antiserum MS6) and was therefore a suitable second antibody in the RIA.

Radioiodination Procedure

We radiolabeled 1 µg of either Tyr^{43}-hPTH(44-68) or hPTH(44-68) with 0.5 mCi $Na^{125}I$ (Amersham Buchler, Frankfurt/M., FRG) by a modification of the procedure described by Hunter and Greenwood [13], as follows: Dissolve 1 µg of the respective peptide in 10 µl phosphate buffer (pH 7.4), then add 5 µl (0.5 mCi) $Na^{125}I$ solution and 10 µl (1 µg) of chloramine-T. After 60 s at room temperature, stop the reaction by adding 10 µl (2.5 µg) sodium metabisulfite. Next add 1 ml assay buffer and 1 ml of a 50 mmol/liter solution of trifluoro-acetic acid. Transfer this mixture onto a Sep-Pak C_{18} cartridge (Waters Associates, Eschborn, FRG) and elute free ^{125}I with 2 ml of the trifluoroacetic acid solution. Elute the labeled peptide with 2 ml of a 60/40 (by vol) mixture of the trifluoroacetic acid and acetonitrile [14]. Add to the tracer solution 3 ml assay buffer in which the human serum albumin content has been increased to 20 g/liter. Further dilute the tracer in assay buffer (to which 19 g human serum albumin and 60 g polyethylene glycol has been added per liter) to about 30 000 cpm/100 µl.

Improved Radioiodination Procedure (Iodogen Method)

Since June 1985, Tyr^{43}-hPTH(44-68) has been labeled routinely with the Iodogen technique; for details see "Materials and Methods", p. 117. The improved quality of this tracer is also described in detail in the article on monoiodinated tyrosylated parathyrin fragments (see p. 116). The results that follow were obtained by the chloramine-T technique as described above.

Radioimmunoassay

Place 100 µl synthetic hPTH(44-68) (the PTH peptide standard) or the patient's sample, 100 µl tracer [30 000 cpm ^{125}I-Tyr^{43}-hPTH (44-68) or radioiodinated native hPTH(44-68)/100 µl assay buffer] to which 60 g/liter polyethylene glycol (mol. wt. 6000: Serva Chemicals, Heidelberg, FRG) and 19 g human serum albumin have been added per liter, and 100 µl first antibody (antiserum MS6, diluted 10 000-fold in assay buffer containing normal guinea pig serum, 3.9 ml/liter into immunoassay vials (Chap. 1.4) (Fa. Sarstedt, Nümbrecht, FRG), mix, and incubate at room temperature (22 °C) for 48 h. Then, after adding 100 µl second antibody (goat anti-guinea pig IgG), mix the vial contents again and incubate for another 60 min at 4 °C. Centrifuge the vials (2000 g, 10 min) to separate bound from free peptide. Discard the supernates and count the radioactivity of the pellets. For this we used a Searle 1285 gamma counter (Fa. Zinsser, Frankfurt/M., FRG) and performed determinations in triplicate.

Calculations

To construct the assay standard curves, we plotted the concentration of the respective hPTH peptide, in picomoles per liter, versus specifically bound tracer in counts per minute. Alternatively, decays per second (Becquerels, Bq) can be calculated (e.g., see Figs. 1, 3). The sensitivity of the system was defined as the B_0 value less 3 SD (determined, in turn, from 12 triplicate measurements of the zero-hPTH sample). Relative binding affinity was determined as the ratio of the molar concentrations of the various hPTH fragments to that of hPTH(44-68) at 50% displacement of the respective tracer.

Results

Radioiodination of hPTH(44-68) Versus Tyr[43]-hPTH(44-68)

We used Sep-Pak C_{18} cartridges to separate the labeled peptides from free ^{125}I. The specific radioactivity for the labeled peptides obtained was 450 Ci/g for Tyr[43]-hPTH(44-68) and 67 Ci/g for hPTH(44-68). Figure 1 depicts a typical standard curve showing the binding of ^{125}I-labeled Tyr[43]-hPTH(44-68) and its displacement by increasing concentrations of hPTH(44-68). Analogously, ^{125}I-labeled hPTH(44-68) was applied as a tracer in the RIA for hPTH(44-68). As Fig. 1 shows, in our midregion assay for hPTH the radioiodinated tyrosylated fragment is the only suitable tracer. ^{125}I-labeled hPTH(44-68) bound only weakly to the antiserum and was not displaced by hPTH(44-68); the binding was therefore nonspecific.

Characteristics of hPTH Assay (44-68)

Sensitivity and Specificity of hPTH(44-68) RIA. Figure 1 depicts a typical displacement curve of the homologous RIA for hPTH(44-68). The smallest detectable concentration in the assay, defined as the point 3 SD below the B_0, was 6 fmol/tube, corresponding to a detection limit of 15 pmol/liter. The range of hPTH(44-68) concentrations covered by the displacement curve was

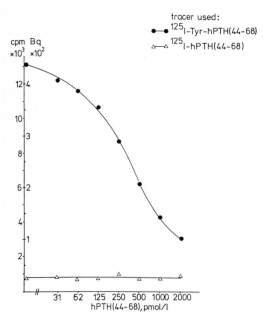

Fig. 1. Standard curves for hPTH(44-68) RIA, prepared with either ^{125}I-labeled Tyr[43]-hPTH(44-68) (●) or ^{125} I-labeled hPTH(44-68) (△) as the assay tracer

6 fmol/tube to 660 fmol/tube. Synthetic fragments of hPTH, representing other regions of the intact hormone—such as hPTH(1-34), hPTH(28-48), and hPTH(64-84)—were not recognized by antiserum MS6 (Fig. 2). In contrast, hPTH(53-84) was 100% cross-reactive with hPTH(44-68).

Also, a dilution curve for hPTH extracted from human parathyroid adenomas paralleled the standard curves for hPTH(1-84) and hPTH(44-68) (Fig. 2).

Precision of hPTH(44-68) RIA. The between-run and within-run *CVs*, estimated by the repeated measurement of both a pool of normal (iPTH concentration 37.1 pmol/liter) and hyperparathyroid human serum (iPTH concentration 202 pmol/liter), were 12% ($n = 12$) for the latter, and 21% ($n = 11$) for the former.

Temperature Dependency of the Binding of Tyr^{43}-hPTH(44-68) to Antiserum MS6. We performed the assay at both 4° and 22°C, all other incubation conditions being identical (see "Materials and Methods"). The binding of tracer at standard zero and the sensitivity of the assay carried out at 22°C were superior to those in the assay performed at 4°C (Fig. 3). As expected, a prolonged incubation (96 h) of the 4°C assay mixture resulted in a standard curve identical to the assay performed with incubation at 22°C for 48 h (data not shown). The reason for this finding is that in the assay at 22°C and 4°C, equilibrium was reached after 48 and 96 h, respectively, as evaluated by equilibrium kinetic experiments (data not shown).

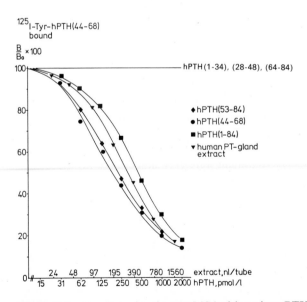

Fig. 2. Cross-reaction of antiserum MS6 with various PTH peptides and with extract of human parathyroid gland in hPTH(44-68) RIA

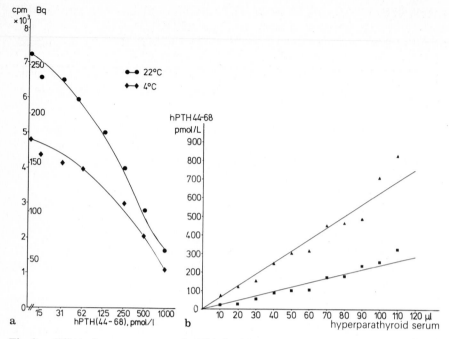

Fig. 3. a Effect of temperature on the RIA for hPTH(44-68). **b** Linearity of the RIA for hPTH(44-68)

Clinical Results

The normal range in the hPTH(44-68) assay is < 15 up to 40 pmol/liter based on data for 124 normal adults. In patients with primary hyperparathyroidism, iPTH values were above normal; there was nearly no overlap with the upper limit of the normal range (Fig. 4). For 12 patients with malignancy-associated hypercalcemia the iPTH values were within the normal range. In a group of patients with renal failure not requiring dialysis, iPTH values were increased. The mean iPTH value is 408 (SD, 368) pmol/liter ($n = 146$). iPTH values for patients on chronic hemodialysis treatment were even higher than for the former group: the mean for hPTH(44-68) was 732 (SD, 628) pmol/liter ($n = 38$). A subgroup of these patients with renal failure is shown in Fig. 5.

Discussion

Sep-Pak C_{18} cartridges were used by Schöneshöfer et al. [14] in the purification of the radiolabeled peptides human gastrin, porcine insulin, and human corticotropin (1-34). Here we report the adaptation of this method to the

hPTH 44-68
pmol/L

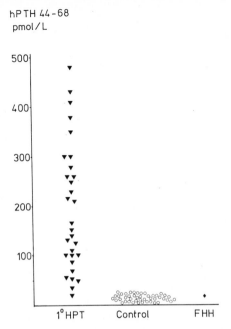

Fig. 4. Immunoreactive parathyroid hormone concentrations in serum of patients with primary hyperparathyroidism, healthy controls and a person with familial hypercalcemia and hypocalciuria (FHH) as measured by the hPTH(44-68) RIA

preparation of radiolabeled PTH peptides for use as RIA tracers. We found that Sep-Pak C_{18} cartridges are well suited for use in the purification of ^{125}I- labeled Tyr^{43}-hPTH(44-68). This method is less time-consuming than the conventional Sephadex G-10 column chromatography applied for tracer purification.

We describe here a homologous RIA for hPTH(44-68) in which ^{125}I-labeled Tyr^{43}-hPTH(44-68) is used as tracer and guinea pig antiserum MS6 as binding protein. This system was sensitive to 6 fmol hPTH(44-68)/tube. hPTH(1-34) and hPTH(28-48) showed no cross-reactivity up to a concentration of 660 fmol/tube, indicating no N-terminal PTH-reactivity of the system. Also, hPTH(64-84) was not recognized by the antibody. Therefore this RIA is selective for the midregion of PTH. Further, hPTH(53-84) was almost equicompetitive to hPTH(44-68), indicating that the amino acid sequence of PTH recognized by antiserum MS6 is located between amino acid residues 53 and 63. The standard curve for hPTH(1-84) was about 2.4 times less sensitive.

Using a sheep antiserum raised against partly purified extract from human parathyroid adenoma, Jüppner et al. [10, 11] developed a midregion assay for hPTH which recognized intact hPTH about ten times less well than hPTH(44-68). These authors concluded that conformational differences must exist that result in the lower affinity for hPTH(1-84). In our study, this difference in affinity between the intact hormone and the hPTH(44-68) fragment was much

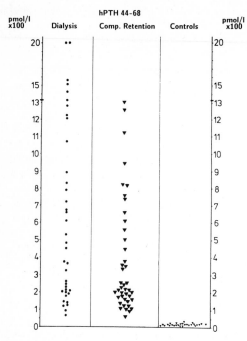

Fig. 5. Immunoreactive parathyroid hormone concentrations in serum of patients receiving chronic dialysis treatment and patients with renal failure not requiring dialysis (comp. retention), as measured by the hPTH(44-68) RIA

(2.4 times) less pronounced than in their study, indicating possible species differences. As already pointed out, our antiserum was raised in a guinea pig; that applied by Jüppner et al. was derived from sheep. This midregional assay is useful in the diagnosis of parathyroid and calcium disorders. It may also be used advantageously for side-location of parathyroid adenomas, as shown before (p. 16). This midregional assay was compared with a C-terminal assay. Both assays were useful for the diagnosis of primary and secondary hyperparathyroidism (15).

Conclusions

This 48-h homologous equilibrium RIA for hPTH is based on an antiserum (MS6) raised in a guinea pig against human parathyroid adenoma extract. For the assay with MS6, Tyr^{43}-hPTH(44-68) and hPTH(44-68) were radioiodinated for use as the tracer. Labeled peptides were separated from free iodine by passage through Sep-Pak C_{18} cartridges. This RIA appears to be midregion specific: hPTH(28-48) and hPTH(64-84) were not recognized, whereas hPTH(53-84) was 100% cross-reactive with hPTH(44-68). Thus, the PTH recognition site of antiserum MS6 must be between amino acid residues 53 and 63. This midregional assay is useful in the diagnosis of parathyroid and calcium disorders.

References

1. Arnaud CD (1983) Hormonal regulation of calcium homeostasis. In: Bikle DD (ed) Assay of calcium regulating hormones. Springer, Berlin Heidelberg New York, pp 1–20
2. Segre GV (1983) Amino-terminal radioimmunoassays for human parathyroid hormone. In: Frame B, Potts JT (eds) Clinical disorders of bone and mineral metabolism. Excerpta Medica, Amsterdam pp 14–17
3. Slatopolsky E (1983) Comparison of amino- and carboxyl-terminal assay methods. In: Frame B, Potts JT (eds) Clinical disorders of bone and mineral metabolism. Excerpta Medica, Amsterdam, pp 20–21
4. Flueck JA, DiBella FP, Edis AJ, Kehrwald JM, Arnaud CD (1977) Immunohetero-geneity of parathyroid hormone in venous effluent serum from hyperfunctioning parathyroid glands. J Clin Invest 60:1367–1375
5. Morrisey JJ, Cohn DV (1979) Secretion and degradation of parathormone as a function of intracellular maturation of hormone pools: modulation by calcium and dibutyryl cyclic AMP. J Cell Biol 83:521–526
6. Mallette LE, Tuma SN, Berger RE, Kirkland JL (1982) Radioimmunoassay for the middle region of human parathyroid hormone using an homologous antiserum with a carboxy-terminal fragment of bovine parathyroid hormone as radioligand. J Clin Endocrinol Metab 54:1017–1024
7. Roos BA, Lindall AW, Aron DC et al. (1981) Detection and characterization of small midregion parathyroid hormone fragment(s) in normal and hyperparathyroid glands and sera by immunoextraction and region-specific radioimmunoassays. J Clin Endocrinol Metab 53:709–721
8. Mallette LE (1981) A radioimmunoassay for human parathyroid hormone using a goat anti-bovine PTH serum. Acta Endocrinol 96:215–221
9. Marx SJ, Sharp ME, Krudy A, Rosenblatt M, Mallette LE (1981) Radioimmuno-assay for the middle region of human parathyroid hormone: studies with a radio-iodinated synthetic peptide. J Clin Endocrinol Metab 53:76–84
10. Jüppner H, Rosenblatt M, Segre GV, Hesch RD (1983) Discrimination between intact and mid-C-regional PTH using selective radioimmunoassay systems. Acta Endocrinol (Copenhagen) 102:543–548
11. Atkinson MJ, Niepel B, Jüppner H et al. (1981) Homologous radioimmunoassay for human midregional parathyroid hormone. J Endocrinol Invest 4:363–366
12. Hitzler W, Schmidt-Gayk H, Spiropoulos P, Raue F, Hüfner M (1982) Homologous radioimmunoassay for human parathyrin (residues 53–84). Clin Chem 28:1749–1753
13. Hunter WM, Greenwood FC (1962) Preparation of iodine-131 labeled human growth hormone of high specific activity. Nature 194:495–496
14. Schöneshöfer M, Kage A, Kage R, Fenner A (1982) A convenient technique for the specific isolation of ^{125}I-labeled peptide molecules. Fresenius Z Anal Chem 311:429–430
15. Schmidt-Gayk H, Schmitt-Fiebig M, Hitzler W, Armbruster FP, Mayer E (1986) Two homologous radioimmunoassays for parathyrin compared and applied to disorders of calcium metabolism. Clin Chem 32:57–62

Chapter 2.5

Purification of ^{125}Iodine-Labeled Tyrosylated Human Parathyroid Hormone Fragment (Residues 44-68), Optimized by Reverse-Phase High-Performance Liquid Chromatography

G. VOGEL

Introduction

In 1986 a homologous assay for the biologically inactive midregion fragment of human parathyroid hormone (hPTH) was published [11]. This assay differentiated well between patients with hyperparathyroidism and normal subjects. Due to a lack of sensitivity the normal range of the assay was located on the shallow part of the standard curve, leading to poor reproducibility of results when assessing PTH levels in healthy subjects.

The most important factors contributing to the sensitivity of radioimmunoassays (RIAs) are affinity of the antibody, specific activity, and purity of the radiolabeled antigen. With any of the labeling techniques used the tracer has to be purified from free iodine, nonlabeled peptide, and immunologically damaged peptide. The chloramine-T method, first described by Hunter and Greenwood [5], has been the conventional technique for labeling purposes. But damage of the peptide by oxidizing and reducing agents is significant. The use of Iodogen has decreased this damage [1, 18]. Different techniques for the purification of labeled peptides have been described. The method most commonly used for purifying labeled hPTH fragments has been gel filtration [4, 7–9, 14, 16, 17]. Other techniques for tracer purification include hydrophobic interaction chromatography (HIC) [3], ion-exchange chromatography [2], immunoaffinity chromatography [15], reverse-phase chromatography [6, 11, 12, 19], and reverse-phase high-performance liquid chromatography (HPLC) [13]. Gel filtration, HIC, and ion-exchange chromatography separate free iodine from peptide but have so far not been reported to remove immunologically damaged peptide. Immunoaffinity chromatography requires large quantities of antisera which are usually provided by monoclonal antibody production. This technique has not been available for PTH so far. Reverse-phase chromatography using Sep-Pak C_{18} cartridges is an easily performed method but again there is no removal of nonimmunoreactive peptide. The best purification of the tracer is achieved by reverse-phase HPLC. It separates immunoreactive and even monoiodinated peptide [12].

The separation of iodine-labeled PTH fragments on reverse-phase HPLC and the utility of the purified tracer is demonstrated. With this method we increased the sensitivity of our earlier described midregion PTH assay [11].

Materials and Methods

Chemicals

Tyr^{43}-hPTH(44-68), Tyr^{27}-hPTH(28-48), and Tyr^{52}-hPTH(53-84) were purchased from Bachem AG (Bubendorf, Switzerland) and Na^{125}I (specific activity, 15 mCi/µg) from Amersham Co. (Amersham, UK). Iodogen (Pierce Chemical Company, Rockford/Ill, United States) was prepared for use by dissolving 1 mg in 25 ml CH$_2$Cl$_2$; 50 µl of this solution was transferred to a vial and dried under nitrogen. Chloramine-T, Na$_2$S$_2$O$_5$, acetonitrile, and trifluoroacetic acid were obtained from Merck Co. (Darmstadt, FRG) and water (HPLC grade) from Baker Co. (Deventer, Holland). Phosphate buffer (pH 7.4) was prepared from 800 ml of 67 mmol/liter Na$_2$HPO$_4$ and 200 ml of 67 mmol/liter KH$_2$PO$_4$ (Merck Co.). 1 g sodium azide (Merck Co.), 400 mg ethylenediaminetetraacetic acid (EDTA) (Merck Co.), and 1 g human serum albumin (Behringwerke Ag, Marburg, FRG) were added to prepare 1 liter assay buffer. Bovine serum albumin (purest form) was purchased from Serva Co. (Heidelberg, FRG).

Radioiodination Procedure

With Chloramine-T. Using a modification of the procedure described by Hunter and Greenwood [5], 1 µg Tyr^{43}-hPTH(44-68) was radiolabeled with 0.5 mCi Na^{125}I. To 1 µg peptide dissolved in 10 µl phosphate buffer were added 5.0 µl (0.5 mCi) Na^{125}I solution and 10 µl (1 µg) chloramine-T. After mixing for 60 s at room temperature, 10 µl (2.5 µg) sodium metabisulfite was added to stop the reaction. Next 200 µl assay buffer with 20 g/liter bovine serum albumin (BSA) was added for protection against radiolysis. Purification was performed immediately.

With Iodogen. Using a modification of the procedure described by Wood et al. [18], 1 µg Tyr^{43}-hPTH(44-68) was radiolabeled with 0.5 mCi Na^{125}I. 1 µg peptide dissolved in 10 µl phosphate buffer was added to 0.5 mCi Na^{125}I, and this solution was transferred to an Iodogen vial. After mixing for 240 s at room temperature the mixture was decanted from the vial to stop the reaction. Purification was performed immediately.

Purification Procedure

With Sep-Pak C$_{18}$ (Modified Method of Schöneshöfer et al. 1982). The reaction mixture was transferred onto a Sep-Pak C$_{18}$ cartridge (Waters Assoc., Eschborn, FRG) and free ^{125}I was eluted with 2 ml 0.05 M trifluoroacetic acid solution. The labeled peptide was eluted with 2 ml of a 60/40 (by vol.) mixture of 0.05 M trifluoroacetic acid solution and acetonitrile and 3 ml assay buffer. The tracer was further diluted in assay buffer with 20 g/liter BSA to about 30 000 cpm/100 µl.

By HPLC. The reaction mixture—in the case of chloramine-T labeling without the last step (without assay buffer containing BSA)—was filled into a gas-tight syringe (Hamilton Co., Reno, United States) and subsequently subjected to HPLC (gradient controller model 680; model 6000A solvent delivery system; model U6K injection system; RCM-100 radial compression separation system equipped with a radial Pak liquid chromatography C_{18} cartridge, particle size 5 μm, 8 mm internal diameter; model 440 detector monitoring ultraviolet absorbance at 280 nm); all purchased from Waters Assoc., Milford, MA, United States. A fraction collector model Frac-3000 was purchased from Pharmacia Fine Chemicals, Uppsala, Sweden.

A gradient elution (Fig. 1) was performed at a constant flow rate of 1 ml/min. Initial conditions: 5% acetonitrile, 95% 0.05 M trifluoroacetic acid solution; after 30 min: 50% of each. 70 fractions (2 min) were collected and 0.5 ml assay buffer containing 2% BSA was applied to each tube before fractioning. Ten microliters of each fraction were pipetted into tubes, and the radioactivity was counted in a Searle 1285 gamma counter (Zinsser, Frankfurt/M, FRG). The fractions containing the monoiodinated tracer were pooled and diluted in assay buffer containing 2% BSA to about 30000 cpm/100 μl.

Radioimmunoassay. We used a homologous midregion assay incubating sample, tracer, and first antibody for 48 h at room temperature under equilibrium conditions. Details are given in Chap. 2.4 [11]. The antiserum was raised in guinea pigs (code MS6); [^{125}I]Tyr^{43}-hPTH(44-68) was used as tracer and synthetic hPTH(44-68) as standard. The bound and free fractions were separated by use of a second antibody (raised in sheep).

Results

Four different parathyroid hormone fragments were chromographed and their retention times determined to calibrate our separation system (Table 1). After labeling 1 μg Tyr^{43}-hPTH(44-68) with 1 μg chloramine-T or 2 μg Iodogen (oxidation times 60 and 240 s, respectively), the reaction mixtures were separated by HPLC and fractionated. The upper part of Fig. 1 shows the radiochro-

Table 1. Retention times of HPLC-separated PTH fragments and free ^{125}I

Nle^{8,18}, Tyr^{34}-hPTH(1-34)	r_f: 23.0 min
Tyr^{27}-hPTH(28-48)	r_f: 21.6 min
Tyr^{43}-hPTH(44-68)	r_f: 16.6 min
Tyr^{52}-hPTH(53-84)	r_f: 17.8 min
^{125}I	T_f: 3.5 min

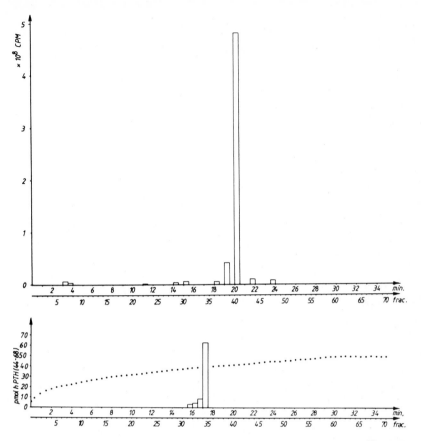

Fig. 1. *Upper*, reverse-phase C_{18}-HPLC radiochromatogram: 1 µg Tyr^{43}-hPTH (44-68) was iodinated with 0.5 mCi ^{125}I using the Iodogen method. Oxidation time: 240 s. *Lower*, eluents: *A*, 005 mol/liter aqueous trifluoroacetic acid solution; *B*, acetonitrile; nonlinear gradient from 5% B to 50% B over a period of 30 min. Flow rate, 1 ml/min. Nonlabeled Tyr^{43}-hPTH (44-68) during the same chromatography. (For conditions see Fig. 1, *upper*)

matogram of the iodination mixture after being labeled with Iodogen. It demonstrates a rather complete incorporation of iodine into the peptide. Only 2% of the initial iodine amount was found as free iodine. With the midregion assay using antiserum MS6 the quantity of nonradioactive free Tyr^{43}-hPTH(44–68) was evaluated. The lower part of Fig. 1 shows that 80 pmol (25% of the initial quantity of peptide) were found in fractions 32–35. The fractions with higher radioactivity were diluted with assay buffer containing 20 g/liter BSA to about 30 000 cpm/100 µl and were used as tracer in the RIA. The iodinated material in fraction 41 showed the highest tracer binding related to the total activity (47% B/T) (Fig. 2).

We then compared three different tracers: labeled with chloramine-T and purified on HPLC; labeled with Iodogen and purified on HPLC; labeled with

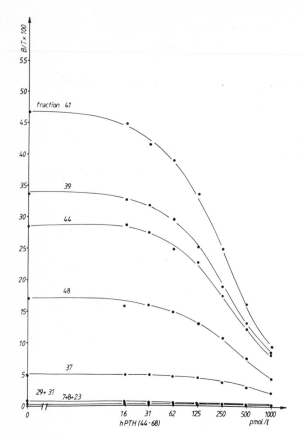

Fig. 2. MS6 assay: standard curves with fractions 7, 8, 23, 29, 31, 37, 39, 41, 44, 48 as tracers. Total activity of each tracer was about 30 000 cpm/100 μl

chloramine-T and purified on Sep-Pak C_{18} cartridges (formerly used routine tracer). Material of fraction 41 was used as HPLC tracer. Samples of all three were diluted to give a total activity of about 30 000 cpm/100 μl.

Figure 3 shows that the Iodogen HPLC tracer provides similar binding: Iodogen HPLC tracer = 47% B_0/T; chloramine-T HPLC tracer = 44% B_0/T. The chloramine-T Sep-Pak tracer had a B_0/T of only 30%.

Tracer binding was slightly higher with Iodogen labeling, and there was no need to use reducing agents. We therefore decided to perform further experiments with tracer labeled with the Iodogen method. The use of diiodinated peptide as a tracer led to a more sensitive standard curve. Ninety percent binding was reached at 25 pmol/liter hPTH(44-48) with the monoiodinated tracer versus 18 pmol/liter with the diiodinated tracer.

When increasing the amount of ^{125}I up to 0.6 mCi (315 pmol) in the iodination process, we found the amount of free peptide to be only 6% (Fig. 4). In this experiment we used nearly equimolar amounts of iodine and peptide

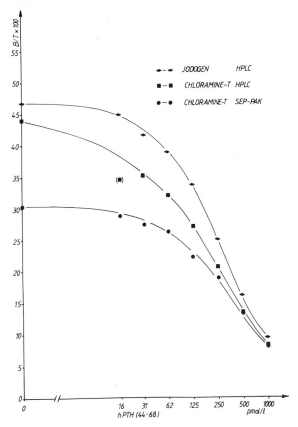

Fig. 3. MS6 assay: standard curves using Iodogen HPLC tracer, chloramine-T HPLC tracer, and chloramine-T Sep-Pak C_{18} tracer. We always used 0.5 mCi ^{125}I for labeling

(323 pmol = 1 µg). Free ^{125}I was negligible (less than 1% of the initial quantity). The amount of higher iodinated compounds (presumably diiodinated) increased (fractions 46 and 47). The radioactivity of all fractions amounted to 576 µCi (304 pmol iodine); the total amount of peptide (unlabeled and iodinated) was about 339 pmol, assuming that fractions 46 and 47 consisted of diiodinated Tyr^{43}-hPTH(44-68). When labeling 1 µg peptide with 0.7 mCi ^{125}I we hardly found any unlabeled peptide in the radiochromatogram (less than 1%; data not shown).

The absence of unlabeled peptide in the radiochromatogram is in favor of a simplified purification: employing Iodogen Tyr^{43}-hPTH(44-68) was iodinated with an excess amount of ^{125}I (0.7 mCi) and separated with a Sep-Pak C_{18} cartridge. The resulting tracer provided similar binding quality (45% B/T) as the monoiodinated Iodogen and chloramine-T tracers, both purified on HPLC.

Storing tracer at 4 °C (diluted in assay buffer with 20 g/liter BSA), the one purified on Sep-Pak C_{18} was found to be just as stable as the one processed on

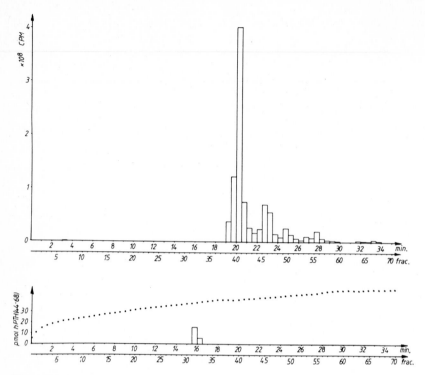

Fig. 4. *Upper*, reverse-phase C_{18}-HPLC radiochromatogram: 1 µg Tyr[43]-hPTH(44-68) was iodinated with 0.6 mCi ^{125}I using the Iodogen method. (For conditions see Fig. 1, *upper*.) *Lower*, nonlabeled Tyr[43]-hPTH(44-68) during the same chromatography. (For conditions see Fig. 1, *lower*

Table 2. Comparison of the stability of the labeled peptides: Iodogen HPLC, chloramine-T HPLC, and Iodogen Sep-Pak C_{18}

	Iodogen HPLC tracer			Chloramine-T HPLC tracer			Iodogen Sep-Pak tracer (0.7 mCi)		
Time (days)	0	14	28	0	14	28	0	14	28
B_{80}[a]	85	77	72	105	72	66	55	50	60
B_{50}[a]	290	290	260	300	270	250	226	205	233
B_{20}[a]	1000	1100	1100	1050	1000	960	893	828	896
B/T × 100 (%)	46.9	40.5	26.0	44.4	39.0	27.8	55.8	61.4	49.9

[a] 80%, 50%, and 20% B/B_0 in pmol/liter

HPLC. Table 2 demonstrates that Iodogen HPLC tracer, chloramine-T HPLC tracer, and Iodogen Sep-Pak tracer (labeled with 0.7 mCi ^{125}I) resulted in similar standard curves after 0, 14, and 28 days.

Figure 5 compares the standard curves of Iodogen HPLC tracer to those of our routine tracer (0.5 mCi ^{125}I, chloramine-T, Sep-Pak). The Iodogen HPLC tracer caused a shift of the standard curve to the left and resulted in a more sensitive assay. Thus a better discrimination of PTH levels within the normal range was achieved. The detection limits of assays using the different tracers are

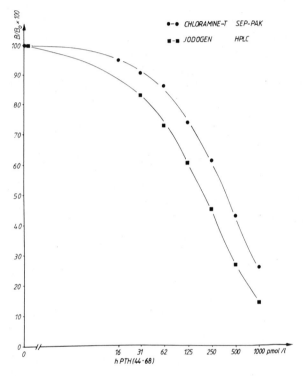

Fig. 5. MS6 assay: standard curves comparing Iodogen HPLC tracer and chloramine-T Sep-Pak C_{18} tracer

Table 3. Detection limits (90% B/B_0) of assays using three different tracers

Oxidant	Chloramine-T	Chloramine-T	Iodogen	Iodogen
mCi ^{125}I	0.5	0.5	0.5	0.7
Separation	Sep-Pak	HPLC	HPLC	Sep-Pak
90% B/B_0 (pmol/liter)	35	25	25	12

listed in Table 3. Sensitivity increased from 35 pmol/liter (chloramine-T, 0.5 mCi ^{125}I, Sep-Pak) to 25 pmol/liter (chloramine-T or Iodogen, 0.5 mCi ^{125}I, HPLC) and 12 pmol/liter (Iodogen, 0.7 mCi ^{125}I, Sep-Pak).

Discussion

High-performance liquid chromatography makes it possible to detect minimal differences of peptide structures. Separation of tyrosylated and nontyrosylated hPTH fragments, for example, was achieved [10]. This paper demonstrated that after separating radiolabeled hPTH fragments on HPLC there was a complete recovery of the iodine and peptide we started with. This was shown by summing up the radioactivity and the PTH concentration of the different fractions. It is suggested that the peak eluting with fraction 46 represented diiodinated peptide. As described by Seidah et al. [13], hydrophobicity and retention time of peptide increase with the number of iodine atoms incorporated into the peptide.

Sep-Pak C_{18} cartridges were used for tracer purification [11, 19]. This method was less cumbersome than HPLC and less radioactive waste was produced. After labeling hPTH with the chloramine-T method, we compared purification of the tracer on Sep-Pak cartridges and on HPLC. Maximum tracer binding of antiserum MS6 in relation to total activity of the tracer (B/T) was 44% with HPLC and 30% with the Sep-Pak cartridges. The results show that Sep-Pak cartridges achieved a good purification from free iodine (98%) but separation from nonlabeled and nonimmunoreactive peptide was not possible. This resulted in a loss of sensitivity in the MS6 assay. Therefore labeling with the Iodogen method was preferred which revealed a slightly higher binding. It is suggested that additional damage by reducing agents may have been circumvented.

Modifying the Sep-Pak C_{18} method we tried to compensate the disadvantage it has compared with the HPLC method. Using an excess amount of iodine for the labeling process with Iodogen (0.7 mCi), a significant reduction of the fraction representing nonlabeled peptide was achieved. Thus a separation of nonlabeled peptide was unnecessary. Assays using tracer purified on Sep-Pak cartridges and on HPLC revealed that the sensitivity and clinical usefulness were comparable. The use of more iodine than peptide increased the fraction of diiodinated peptide in the radiochromatogram. This led to increased radiolysis of the tracer which was compensated by labeling the peptides every 4 weeks.

We suggest that tracer purification on Sep-Pak C_{18} cartridges is sufficient for the routine assay of PTH, provided that the labeling process is performed with a slight excess of iodine. Routine purification by HPLC is too cumbersome and associated with exposure to radiation, but it is a suitable tool for optimizing labeling and purification techniques. Using the optimized tracer we were able to increase the sensitivity of our midregion assay. The detection limit (90% B/B_0) changed from 35 pmol/liter to 12 pmol/liter and discrimination of PTH levels within the normal range improved.

   In conclusion, we describe a monoiodinated tracer for the radioimmuno-logical assessment of midregion hPTH(44-68) fragment. [125]Iodine-labeled tyrosylated fragment ([^{125}I]Tyr[43]-hPTH44-68) is separated by reverse-phase C_{18} HPLC after iodination with either Iodogen or chloramine-T. The quality of the tracer purified on HPLC is compared with tracer purified on Sep-Pak C_{18} cartridges. Using the HPLC we obtained a fraction with monoiodinated tracer. This fraction did not contain any nonlabeled or nonimmunoreactive peptide and revealed a tracer binding of 47% B/T in contrast to the binding of 30% B/T achieved by the previous routine method (chloramine-T, Sep-Pak C_{18} car-tridges). The sensitivity of hPTH(44-68)RIA was increased by the use of the new Iodogen-labeled and HPLC-purified tracer, thus permitting a better discrimina-tion of PTH levels in the low normal range.

References

1. Butler SH, Lam RW, Fisher DA (1984) Iodination of thyroliberin by use of Iodogen. Clin Chem 30:547–548
2. Christie DL, Barling PM (1978) Isolation of iodinated bovine parathyroid hormone using ion exchange: demonstration of its immunological characteristics and biological activity. Endocrinology 103:204–211
3. Englebienne P, Doyen G (1982) Radioiodinated hormones purified by hydrophobic interaction chromatography. Clin Chem 28:2189–2190
4. Hitzler W, Schmidt-Gayk H, Spiropoulos P, Raue F, Hüfner M (1982) Homologous radioimmunoassay for human parathyrin (residues 53–84). Clin Chem 28:1749–1753
5. Hunter WM, Greenwood FC (1962) Preparation of the iodine-131 labelled human growth hormone of high specific activity. Nature 194:495–496
6. Janaky T, Toth G, Penke B, Kovacs K, Laslo FA (1982) Iodination of peptide hormones and purification of iodinated peptides by HPLC. Liquid Chromatography 5:1499–1507
7. Kao PC, Jiang NS, Klee GG, Purnell DC (1982) Development and validation of a new radioimmunoassay for parathyrin (PTH). Clin Chem 28:69–74
8. Mallette LE, Tuma SN, Berger RE, Kirkland JL (1982) Radioimmunoassay for the middle region of human parathyroid hormone using an homologous antiserum with carboxy-terminal fragment of bovine parathyroid hormone as radioligand. J Clin Endocrinol Metab 54:1017–1024
9. Marx SJ, Sharp ME, Krudy A, Rosenblatt M, Mallette LE (1981) Radioimmuno-assay for the middle region of human parathyroid hormone: studies with a radio-iodinated synthetic peptide. J Clin Endocrinol Metab 53:76–84
10. Schettler T, Aufm'Kolk B, Atkinson MJ, Radeke H, Enters C, Hesch RD (1984) Analysis of immunoreactive and biologically active human parathyroid hormone-peptides by high-performance liquid chromatography. Acta Endocrinol 107:60–69
11. Schmidt-Gayk H, Schmitt-Fiebig M, Hitzler W, Armbruster FP, Mayer E (1986) Two homologous radioimmunoassays for parathyrin compared and applied to disorders of calcium metabolism. Clin Chem 57:57–62
12. Schöneshöfer M, Kage A, Kage R, Fenner A (1982) A convenient technique for the specific isolation of ^{125}I-labelled peptide molecules. Fresenius Z Anal Chem 311:429–430

13. Seidah NG, Dennis M, Corvol P, Rochemont J, Chretien M (1980) A rapid high-performance liquid chromatography purification method of iodinated polypeptide hormones. Anal Biochem 109:185–191
14. Sharp ME, Marx SJ (1985) Radioimmunoassay for the middle region of human parathyroid hormone: comparison of two radioiodinated synthetic peptides. Clin Chim Acta 145:59–68
15. Stuart MC, Boscato LM, Underwood PA (1983) Use of immunoaffinity chromatography for purification of ^{125}I-labeled human prolactin. Clin Chem 29:241–245
16. Visser TJ, Buurman CJ, Birkenhäger JC (1979) Production and characterization of antisera to synthetic 1–34 human parathyroid hormone fragments: possible implications for the correctness of proposed structures. Acta Endocrinol (Copenh) 90:90–102
17. Wood WG, Butz R, Casaretto M et al. (1980) Preliminary results on the use of an antiserum to human parathyrin in a homologous radioimmunoassay. J Clin Chem Clin Biochem 18:789–795
18. Wood WG, Wachter C, Scriba PC (1981) Experiences using chloramine-T and 1,3,4,6-tetrachloro-3α,6α-diphenylglycoluril (Iodogen[R]) for radioiodination of materials for radioimmunoassay. J Clin Chem Clin Biochem 19:1051–1056
19. Zillikens D, Armbruster FP, Hitzler W, Horn J, Schmidt-Gayk H (1985) Schneller homologer Radioimmunoassay für human-Parathormon (hPTH) zur Differenzierung der hyperkalzämischen Krise. Ärztl Lab 31:151–156

Chapter 2.6

Homologous Radioimmunoassay for Human Parathyroid Hormone (Residues 28-48) with Tyrosylated Peptide as Tracer

I. AKER

Introduction

Berson and Yalow were the first to describe the heterogeneity of human parathyroid hormone (hPTH) in plasma [1]. Besides the intact hormone, fragments can be found of the C- and N-terminal and also of the midregional part of the hormone, of which the greatest part is biologically inactive [2, 3]. The fragments which appear result from proteolytic cleavage after their biosynthesis. They appear both intra- and extraglandularly [4]. Since the points of cleavage of the intact hormone are located between the amino acids 33/34 and 36/37 [5], it is assumed that detection of the intact hormone [6, 7, 8] is achieved by the radioimmunological detection of the sequence (28-48). So far only a few studies on this subject matter have been reported. For this reason a radioimmunoassay (RIA) for the measurement of hPTH(28-48) was developed and is described here.

Materials and Methods

Antibodies

The first antibody was produced by immunizing rabbits with synthetic hPTH(28-48) following the methods used by Sofroniew [9], i.e. conjugation of the peptide to bovine thyroglobulin, and Vaitukaitis [10]. To dilute the antibody assay buffer is used [phosphate buffer pH 7.4 from 800 ml Na_2HPO_4 67 mmol/liter and 200 ml KH_2PO_4 67 mmol/liter (Merck AG, Darmstadt, FRG), 1 g sodium azide (Merck AG), 400 mg ethlyenediaminetetraacetic acid (EDTA), and 1 g human serum albumin (Behringwerke AG, Marburg, FRG)]. To obtain a titer of 1:1000, 100 µl antiserum was added to 99.5 ml assay buffer and 400 µl normal rabbit serum. The affinity constant was calculated according to Scatchard's mathematical model [11]. The second antibody anti-rabbit IgG (donkey) was bought from Wellcome GmbH (Burgwedel, FRG) and diluted 1:21 in assay buffer.

Standards

Standard solutions were produced by diluting synthetic hPTH fragments in assay buffer with human serum albumin (HSA) (10 g human albumin/liter). (1-34), (28-48), (1-44), (44-68), and (53-84) hPTH were bought from Bachem, Bubendorf, Switzerland, (1-84) from Peptide Institute Inc., Osaka, Japan.

Tracer

Tracer was produced by radioactive labeling of the synthetic fragment Tyr^{27}-hPTH(28-48) (Bachem) with $Na^{125}I$ (Amersham Buchler, Frankfurt, FRG) using the chloramine-T or Iodogen methods. The chloramine-T labeling was carried out in modification of the method described by Hunter and Greenwood [12]: 5 mg chloramine-T and 12.5 mg sodium metabisulfite (both from Merck) are each dissolved in 50 ml aqua dest. To 1 µg Tyr^{27}-hPTH(28-48) is added: 2.5 µl $Na^{125}I$ solution (0.25 mCi) and 10 µl (1 µg) of chloramine-T. After 60 s at room temperature, the reaction is stopped by adding 10 µl sodium metabisulfite. With the Iodogen method [13] Eppendorf vials (Eppendorf Gerätebau, Fa. Netheler und Hinz, Hamburg, FRG) are initially coated with 50 µl Iodogen solution (1 mg in 25 ml dichloromethane, Iodogen from Pierce Chemical Company, Rockford, United States). This coating is stable at $-20\,^{\circ}C$ for about 3 months. For labeling, 2.5-3 µl $Na^{125}I$ and 1 µg peptide are put into the vial and incubated for 4 min during which time it is shaken; oxidation is stopped by transferring the mixture to another vial. To purify the tracer on Sep-Pak C_{18} cartridges (Waters Associates, Eschborn, FRG), the labeling mixture is applied to the cartridge together with 1 ml 0.05 M trifluoroacetic acid (TFA, Merck). The unbound ^{125}I is eluted with 2 ml 0.05 M TFA, the labeled peptide with 2 ml TFA/acetonitrile (60/40 v/v). Two milliliters assay buffer with 2% bovine serum albumin (BSA) is again pressed through the cartridge to increase the recovery of the tracer and to ensure protein protection of the tracer. To purify the tracer by high-performance liquid chromatography (HPLC), a Rad-Pak C_{18} column (Waters GmbH) is used. The mobile phase is composed of 100% acetonitrile and 0.05 M TFA (the composition alters within 30 min from 5/95 acetonitrile/TFA to 50/50 v/v), the flow rate is 1 ml/min, and the collection time per fraction is 1 min. The detection of unbound iodine and of tracer is carried out by measuring 10 µl of every fraction in the gamma counter. The tracer is diluted in assay buffer with 2% BSA (Serva Feinbiochemica, Heidelberg, FRG) to a total activity of approx. 30 000 cpm/100 µl (1000 Bq/100 µl).

Radioimmunoassay

The assay is carried out by sequential saturation: 100 µl first antibody 1:1000 and 100 µl standards (0.2–1000 pmol/liter) or samples from patients are incubated for 5 days in immunoassay vials (Chap. 1.4, Sarstedt, Nümbrecht, FRG) at $4\,^{\circ}C$. On the 6th day 100 µl tracer $[^{125}I]Tyr^{27}hPTH(28-48)$ is added.

After two further days of incubation at 4°C, the reaction is stopped by adding 100 μi of the second antibody and additionally 50 μl of normal human serum to the standards. After 2 h the tubes are centrifuged for 10 min at 3000 rpm and the supernatant fluid is aspirated. To reduce nonspecific binding the sediment is rinsed with 500 μl NaCl 0.9% and again centrifuged for 10 min at 3000 rpm. After the supernatant fluid has been aspirated, the sediment is measured in the gamma counter (Searle 1285, Zinsser, Frankfurt, FRG) for 1 min. All measurements are carried out in triplicate.

Results

By comparison of the 80%, 50%, and 20% intercept points of the antisera of different bleeding dates, "Ka Mi 4.5" was the most sensitive antiserum. With this antibody the assay was carried out at a dilution of 1:1000 (30% tracer binding). The affinity constant for the most sensitive population of antibodies was 1.56×10^{10} liter/mol. Twenty percent tracer displacement was found at

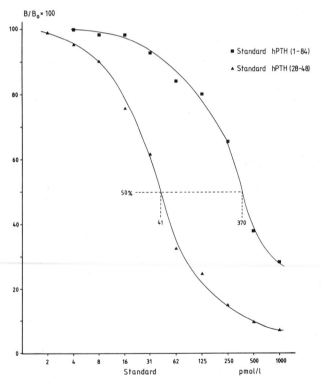

Fig. 1. Displacement of $[^{125}I]Tyr^{27}$-hPTH(28-48) by hPTH(28-48) and hPTH(1-84) standards. Comparison of standard curves (sequential saturation; total activity, 28 500 cpm)

14 pmol/liter, 50% at 41 pmol/liter, and 80% at 160 pmol/liter hPTH(28-48).
The fragments (1-44), (1-34), (44-68), and (53-84) caused no tracer displacement
[concentrations up to 1000 pmol/liter, (1–34) up to 8000 pmol/liter, were
tested]. The intact, synthetically manufactured hormone gave a weaker displacement of the tracer, about factor 9 on a molar basis, than the fragment (28-
48) (Fig. 1). The assay was optimized to obtain the highest possible sensitivity.

Sequential saturation with a cold preincubation of 5 days at 4 °C proved to
be favorable. When the incubation was carried out at room temperature, the
reactions reached equilibrium within 72 h; however, the tracer binding was
about 30% less than with the incubation at 4 °C.

Compared with the equilibrium technique, the same tracer displacement was
reached by using sequential saturation with only one-third of the amount of
standard. Extending the incubation time with sequential saturation increased
the sensitivity (Fig. 2). In carrying out the assay a distinct matrix error became
noticeable. The tracer binding in buffer was considerably weaker than in serum.

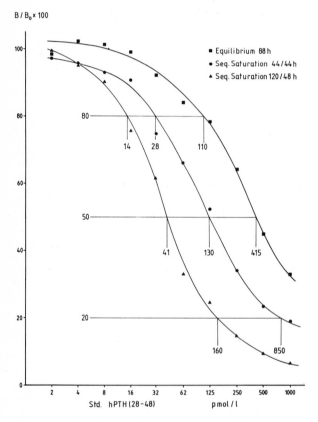

Fig. 2. Mode of saturation and assay sensitivity. Comparison of standard curves in
sequential saturation mode (44 h + 44 h, 120 h + 48 h) and in equilibrium mode

It proved impossible to compensate this by the addition of polyethylene glycol (PEG). Although PEG did increase precipitation in the buffer, it decreased binding in the serum at the same time, resulting in falsely high measurements. Aligning the protein concentration in the standards and samples by adding HSA the matrix error was compensated only incompletely. Diluting the standard solutions in charcoal-treated adenine-citrate-dextrose plasma (outdated blood bank plasma, charcoal-treated, "hormone-free" plasma) proved to be unsatisfactory as well since the binding was, to a high degree, non-specifically prevented (age of the plasmas, ACD and EDTA additive). The addition of 50 μl normal serum together with the second antibody to the buffer standards balanced the precipitation error satisfactorily (the effect was not reduced by freezing the serum up to four times; with more than 50 μl serum/tube the effect increased only negligibly). It was possible to measure dilution series of sera with increased PTH content accurately to scale (this was not the case with standard curves with HSA additive), as shown in Table 1.

Since $[^{125}I]Tyr^{27}hPTH(28-48)$ is degraded rapidly, experiments were carried out to reduce radiolysis (Table 2.). The labeling of the double quantity of peptide (2 μg) reduced the specific activity from 583 μCi/μg to 292 μCi/μg, but did not prevent disintegration of the tracer. Labeling with the Iodogen method

Table 1. Linearity of the measurements of different dilutions of a serum with high PTH content (C-high): undiluted, and diluted with assay buffer containing 10 g/liter HSA in the ratios 1:2, 1:4, and 1:8. In parallel, the addition of 50 μl serum/tube to the reaction mixture was tested. With added HSA, the count rates were partly higher than the count rate of the zero standard.

	HSA 8 μg/tube	HSA 13 μg/tube	Serum 50 μl/tube
C-high	45 pmol/liter	53 pmol/liter	53 pmol/liter
1:2	16.5	22.5	26
1:4	–	–	12.5
1:8	–	–	7.4

Table 2. Comparison of B_0/TA ratio (binding with zero standard/total activity) with increasing tracer age. HPLC and Sep-Pak purified tracer

	HPLC	Sep-Pak C_{18}
0 days	52.2	20.7
11 days	38.2	14.8
18 days	30.6	13.4
25 days	16.5	9.9

led likewise to a reduced specific activity (327 µCi/µg with the chloramine-T method, 107 µCi/µg with Iodogen using the same quantity of Na^{125}I); however, while the chloramine-T tracer showed a binding loss of 46% within 2 weeks, this loss amounted to merely 31% with the Iodogen tracer. When larger quantities of Na^{125}I were used for Iodogen labeling, the specific activity rose to 320 µCi/µg. Tests were then continued to see whether the quality and durability of the tracer would be increased by an improved method of separation. HPLC-purified tracer and Sep-Pak C_{18}-purified tracer were bound to 52% and to only 21%, respectively, with the same antibody dilution (Fig. 3). However, the length of life was not increased, the half-life of both tracers being about 18 days.

Before measuring the samples from patients, the influence of interfering factors on measurement was examined. Freezing of the samples and simple hemolysis did not alter the values. Heparin, citrate, EDTA and ACD, in that

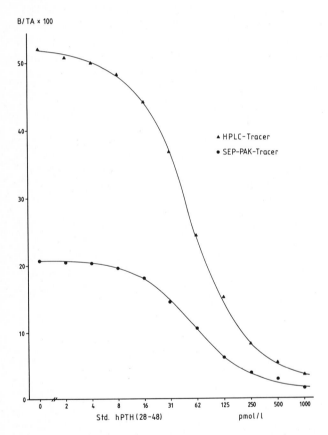

Fig. 3. Influence of tracer purification on tracer binding. Comparison of B/TA (bound/total activity) of Sep-Pak C_{18}- and HPLC-purified tracer

order, reduced the tracer binding in serum samples; the measurement was incorrectly high. Measurement was therefore only carried out in serum without any additives. The coefficient of variation was 1.1% when a sample was measured 12 times within one assay and 12.9% when measured on different days. The normal range was established by measuring 40 sera from normal persons by means of the mean value $\pm$ 2 standard deviations. The normal range is 3.6–16.4 pmol/liter (7.7–34.3 pg/ml). The lower detection limit is 3.3 pmol/liter (7.2 pg/ml).

Nineteen patients who were surgically proven to have primary hyperparathyroidism had values between 17.7 and 69 pmol/liter (37.7–148 pg/ml). One patient was within the normal range. The correlation between PTH and serum calcium in normal persons and patients with primary hyperparathyroidism was $r = 0.88$. Patients with secondary hyperparathyroidism could be distinguished by normal or lowered serum calcium. The values in the (28-48) assay were between 15.5 and 59 pmol/liter. One single value was at an excessively high level of 275 pmol/liter (Fig. 4). In the side localization of adenomas both the (44-68) and the (53-84) assays showed more distinct gradients than the (28-48) assay.

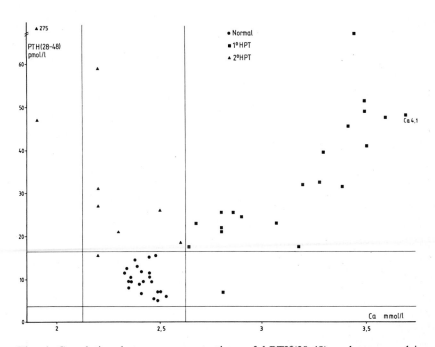

Fig. 4. Correlation between concentrations of hPTH(28-48) and serum calcium in normal persons and patients with primary and secondary hyperparathyroidism (primary HPT and secondary HPT). Lines indicate lower and upper limits of normal.

Discussion

The results of tracer-labeling with chloramine-T according to the methods of Hunter and Greenwood and with Iodogen [13] were compared. A higher specific activity was attained with chloramine-T than with Iodogen; the assay is therefore more sensitive. Tracer durability, however, is improved by the milder oxidation occurring in the Iodogen method. The separation of the reaction mixture both over Sep-Pak C_{18} cartridges and by HPLC has been described previously [14]. In the work presented here, purification of the tracer by HPLC resulted in considerably improved tracer quality. The same antibody dilution bound only one-fifth of the Sep-Pak-purified tracer but over one-half of the HPLC-purified tracer. While, therefore, a considerable quantity of immuno-reactive, nonlabeled peptide is present in the first tracer mentioned, mono-iodinated material can be extracted over HPLC. In this work, an RIA for hPTH(28-48) is described. $[^{125}I]Tyr^{27}hPTH(28-48)$ serves as tracer, hPTH(28-48) as standard, and a rabbit antiserum against hPTH(28-48) as binding protein.

The antibody has an affinity constant of 1.56×10^{10} liters/mol. The lower detection limit is 3.3 pmol/liter (7.2 pg/ml). The assay is therefore sufficiently sensitive to measure PTH in all normal persons. The assay was developed with the aim of measuring only intact PTH. The intact, synthetic hPTH(1-84) displaces the tracer at about factor 9 less than the fragment (28-48). The lower sensitivity for the sequence (1-84) than for fragments was also observed with other antisera [15]. It is probable that differences in conformation exist between the fragments and intact, synthetically manufactured peptide.

Since the tracer was not displaced by (1-34), (1-44), (44-48), or (53-84)hPTH, it can be assumed that the assay measures neither N- nor C-terminal fragments. Roos et al. [16] and Marx et al. [17] have described the appearance of midregional fragments (mol. wt. about 4400) in hypocalcemia and primary hyperparathyroidism. The results obtained from measuring selective blood samples from neck veins of hyperparathyroid patients showed sharper gradients in (44-68) and in (53-84) RIA than in (28-48) RIA. The first two RIAs might recognize sequences on PTH fragments secreted by the parathyroid glands, whereas the appearance of fragments with (28-48) immunoreactivity has not yet been described.

In contrast to other assays for the (28-48) region which have been described so far, the normal range of this assay corresponds to the PTH measurements of Goltzmann's cytochemical bioassay (1-30 pg/ml) and to those of Niepel's ad-enylate cyclase assay (19 pg/ml) [18, 19]. These assays measure biologically active PTH, i.e. the intact hormone and the N-terminal fragments, which likewise are present in very small concentrations. This relation supports the hypothesis that this assay does indeed mainly measure intact PTH.

For his assay of hPTH(28-48), Atkinson [6] has cited considerably higher measurements. His normal range is between 60 and 300 pg/ml. In her assay for hPTH(28-54), Gleed too [7] measured high concentrations of "intact" PTH. She has set 70 pg/ml as the upper limit of her normal range.

With one exception, the assay presented here distinguished well between normal persons and patients with primary hyperparathyroidism. No elevated values were measured in one case of primary hyperparathyroidism (adenoma confirmed by surgery, serum calcium 2.8 mmol/liter) in the assays for hPTH(28-48), (44-68) and (53-84). Long incubation periods and rapid tracer degradation are the main disadvantages of the hPTH(28-48) assay.

In conclusion a RIA for hPTH(28-48) was developed with the aim of measuring intact PTH. The antibody was produced by immunizing rabbits with synthetic hPTH(28-48) conjugated to bovine thyroglobulin. This antibody recognized only the intact hormone and the (28-48) fragment, but not the fragments (1-34), (1-44), (44-68), and (53-84). $[^{125}I]Tyr^{27}$-hPTH(28-48) served as the tracer, and hPTH(28-48) as the standard. The lower detection limit of the assay was 3.3 pmol/liter, the normal range 3.6–16.4 pmol/liter. With one exception, patients with primary hyperparathyroidism could be clearly distinguished from normal persons.

References

1. Berson SA, Yalow RS (1968) Immunochemical heterogeneity of parathyroid hormone in plasma. J Clin Endocrinol Metab 28:1037–1047
2. Potts JT Jr, Kronenberg HM, Rosenblatt M (1982) Parathyroid hormone: chemistry, biosynthesis, and mode of action. Adv Protein Chem 35:323–96
3. Slatopolsky E, Martin K, Morrissey J, Hruska K (1982) Current concepts of the metabolism and radioimmunoassay of parathyroid hormone. J Lab Clin Med 99:309–316
4. Armitage EK (1986) Parathyrin (parathyroid hormone): metabolism and methods for assay. Clin Chem 32:418–424
5. Segre GV, D'Amour P, Hultmann A, Potts JT Jr (1981) Effects of hepatectomy, nephrectomy/uremia on the metabolism of parathyroid hormone in the rat. J Clin Invest 67:439–448
6. Atkinson MJ, Wong CC, Jüppner H (1982) Intact human PTH (h1-84) radioimmunoassay using the h28-48 peptide. Acta Endocrinol (Copenh) Suppl 246:138
7. Gleed JH, Hendy GN, Nussbaum SR, Rosenblatt M, O'Riordan JLH (1986) Development and application of a mid-region specific assay for human parathyroid hormone. Clin Endocrinol 24:365–373
8. Mallette LE (1983) Immunoreactivity of human parathyroid hormone (28-48). Attempts to develop an assay for human parathyroid hormone. Metab Bone Dis Rel Res 4:329–332
9. Sofroniew MV, Madler M, Müller OA, Scriba PC (1978) A method for the consistent production of high quality antisera to small peptide hormones. Fresenius Z Anal Chem 290:163
10. Vaitukaitis J, Robbins JB, Nieschlag E, Ross GT (1971) A method for producing specific antisera with small doses of immunogen. J Clin Endocrinol 33:988–991
11. Scatchard G (1949) The attractions of proteins for small molecules and ions. Ann N Y Acad Sci 51:66

12. Hunter WM, Greenwood FC (1962) Preparation of iodine-131 labelled human growth hormone of high specific activity. Nature (London) 194:495–496
13. Wood WG, Wachter C, Scriba PC (1981) Experiences using Chloramin T and 1,3,4,6,-Tetrachloro-3,6-diphenylglycoluracil (Jodogen) for radioiodination of materials for radioimmunoassay. J Clin Chem Clin Biochem 19:1051–1056
14. Schöneshöfer M, Kage A, Kage R, Fenner A (1982) A convenient technique for the specific isolation of ^{125}I-labelled peptide molecules. Fresenius Z Anal Chem 311:429–430
15. Schmidt-Gayk H, Schmitt-Fiebig M, Hitzler W, Armbruster FP, Mayer E (1986) Two homologous radioimmunoassays for parathyrin compared and applied to disorders of calcium metabolism. Clin Chem 32:57–62
16. Roos BA, Lindall AW, Aron DC, Orf JW, Yoon M, Huber MB, Pensky J, Ells J, Lambert PW (1981) Detection and characterization of small midregion parathyroid hormone fragment(s) in normal and hyperparathyroid glands and sera by immunoextraction and region-specific radioimmunoassays. J Clin Endocrinol Metab 53:709–721
17. Marx SJ, Sharp ME, Krudy A, Rosenblatt M, Mallette LE (1981) Radioimmunoassay for the middle region of human parathyroid hormone: studies with a radioiodinated synthetic peptide. J Clin Endocrinol Metab 53:76–84
18. Goltzman D, Gomolin H, Wexler M, Meakins JL (1983) Cytochemical bioassay for parathyroid hormone: validation and clinical applications. In: Clinical disorders of bone and mineral metabolism, eds: Frame B, Potts JT Jr, Excerpta Medica, Amsterdam-Oxford-Princeton 1983:6–9
19. Niepel B, Radeke H (1982) Biologically active parathyroid hormone in serum: first results with a specially adapted adenylate cyclase assay. Acta Endocrinol 99 (Suppl 246):132–133

Chapter 2.7

Homologous Radioimmunoassay for Human Parathyroid Hormone (Residues 1-34) with Biotinylated Peptide as Tracer

A. STADLER

Introduction

Along with calcitonin and 1,25-dihydroxyvitamin D_3 the polypeptide parathyroid hormone (parathyrin) (PTH) is responsible for maintaining calcium and phosphorus homeostasis in vertebrates. Parathyrin is a polypeptide of 84 amino acids and produced by the parathyroid glands [1]. A change of 0.2 g/dl in the blood calcium concentration alters the secretory state of the parathyoid glands [2]. The cleavage of intact PTH into the amino-terminal, midregional, and carboxy-terminal fragments takes place in the liver and kidneys [3–5]. Besides the intact PTH only the amino-terminal part shows bioactivity. All other fragments are biologically inert [6]. PTH(1-34) interacts directly with bone and kidneys and—indirectly—with the intestine. This interaction increases the calcium level in human serum [1, 7, 8]. The diseases primary hyperparathyroidism (pHPT), secondary HPT, and hypoparathyroidism are closely connected with the PTH secretion of the parathyroid glands [8]. Detection of the PTH levels by radioimmunological procedures can provide the diagnosis for these diseases. Several homologous radioimmunoassays (RIAs) have been developed for the detection of the different PTH fragments [9–13]. To study the chronic secretory state of the parathyroid glands and to diagnose primary hyperparathyroidism the homologous RIA for the carboxy-terminal PTH is useful [13]. Human parathyrin hPTH (53-84) has a half-life of 1–2h [14]. It is possible to estimate the function of a transplanted kidney by measuring midregion PTH. The kidney eliminates the midregional part and the carboxy-terminal part from the circulation. This elimination depends on renal function [19]. Patients who have to undergo chronic hemodialysis show extremely high midregional PTH levels [12]. With the RIA for hPTH(28-48) intact PTH can be detected [11]. The development of a RIA for the detection of intact and amino-terminal PTH has proved to be extremely difficult because these two peptides have very short half-lives in the bloodstream (intact PTH, 10 min; hPTH(1-34), 1.5 min) [14]. Based on the short half-life of these peptides it is possible to evaluate the actual secretory state of the parathyroid glands with suitable RIAs. Furthermore the bioactivity of the secreted PTH can be detected in the blood stream [15]. Several homologous RIA systems have been developed to detect amino-terminal PTH (Table 1). They differ very much in their normal and abnormal ranges [10, 15–18].

Table 1. Levels of N-terminal parathyroid hormone in primary and secondary HPT

Authors	Normal range	Primary HPT	Secondary HPT
Papapoulos et al. (1980 [17]	0–120 pg/ml	100–1350 pg/ml	–
Gilberto et al. (1986) [10]	10–28 pmol/liter	10–519 pmol/liter	–
Desplan et al. (1977) [16]	70–450 pg/ml	50–3250 pg/ml	300–1750 pg/ml
Papapoulos et al. (1978) [18]	40–120 pg/ml	100–1650 pg/ml	45–4400 pg/ml
Segre (1983) [15]	11.9 ± 13.2 pg/ml	–	–

No author detected hPTH(1-34) in hypoparathyroid samples

We describe a homologous, sensitive RIA to detect aminoterminal PTH with an antibody raised in a goat against extracted PTH and another antibody raised in a rabbit against synthetic hPTH(1-34). Synthetic hPTH(1-34) is used as standard. The RIA is performed with $NLeu^8$-$NLeu^{18}$-Tyr^{34}-hPTH(1-34) and biotinylated hPTH(1-34)[^{125}I] streptavidin as tracer peptides. We describe a new RIA for the detection of amino-terminal PTH with good clinical utility. Furthermore we compare two antibodies and two tracers in the same RIA.

Materials and Methods

Production of assay buffers

One liter of assay buffer 1 was prepared by combining 800 ml of 67 mmol/liter Na_2HPO_4, 200 ml of 67 mmol/liter KH_2PO_4, 1 g sodium azide, 400 mg disodium ethylenediaminetetraacetic acid (EDTA), and 1 g human serum albumin (HSA) (Behringwerke AG, Marburg, FRG). All reagents were purchased from Merck, Darmstadt, FRG, in pro analysi quality, unless specified otherwise. In order to prepare 1 liter of assay buffer 2 we combined 900 ml assay buffer 1 and 100 ml of a hypoparathyroid serum which did not contain detectable levels of amino-terminal PTH, as proven by previous assay.

Production of 100 g/liter Polyethylene Glycol

Ten grams polyethylene glycol (PEG) was diluted in 100 ml assay buffer 1 and stored at 4 °C.

Standards

Standards were prepared by diluting the synthetic fragments hPTH(28-48), hPTH(44-68), and hPTH(53-84) in assay buffer 1. hPTH1(1-34) and hPTH(1-84)

standards were prepared with assay buffer 2 (all peptides were purchased from Peptide Institute Inc., Osaka, Japan).

Radioiodination Procedure

We radiolabeled 1.15 µg "NLeu^8-Nleu^{18}-Tyr^{34}-hPTH(1-34)" with 0.5 mCi Na^{125}I (Amersham Buchler, Braunschweig, FRG). The procedure was the chloramine-T method described by Hunter and Greenwood [20]. The peptide was diluted in 10 µl 67 mmol/liter phosphate buffer (pH 7.4). After adding 5 µl Na^{125}I solution the peptide was oxidized with aqueous chloramine-T (10 µl, 1 µg) at room temperature. After 60 s the oxidation was stopped with 10 µl 2.5 µg sodium metabisulfite. Then 200 µl assay buffer 1 + 20 g/liter HSA was added. The purification of the mixture of reactants was carried out by a Sep-Pak C$_{18}$ cartridge (Waters, Eschborn, FRG). Free ^{125}I was eluted with 2 ml of 0.05 M trifluoroacetic acid and discarded. Then the tracer was eluted with 2 ml of 0.05 M trifluoroacetic acid/acetonitrile (60:40, v/v). By adding 3 ml assay buffer 1 + 20 g/liter HSA the tracer was protected from radiolysis. Until use the tracer was stored at − 30 °C. For use the tracer was diluted in assay buffer 1 + 9 g/liter HSA to about 30 000 cpm/100 µl. For good assay performance the peptide NLeu^8-NLeu^{18}-Tyr^{34}-hPTH(1-34) was labeled monthly.

Preparing the Biotinylated hPTH(1–34) Tracer

[^{125}I] Streptavidin (purchased from Amersham Buchler, Braunschweig, FRG) was diluted in assay buffer 1 + 9 g/liter HSA to about 60 000 cpm/100 µl. One milliliter of a solution containing 1 µg biotinylated hPTH(1-34) (Bachem, Bubendorf, Switzerland) was diluted to 50 ml with assay buffer 1. For 100 tubes, 5 ml of this solution was preincubated with 10 ml of the [^{125}I] streptavidin solution at room temperature for 30 min.

Antisera

An antibody (G76/85.05.02; G76/84.09.12) against the N-terminal part of PTH was raised in a goat. Extracts from human adenomatous glands obtained during parathyroid surgery were used. They were purified by affinity chromatography (see Chap. 2.10). For use the antiserum was diluted in assay buffer 1 + 4 ml normal goat serum (NGS)/liter and stored at 4 °C (dilution: 1:1000). Another antibody (Rm/82.10.02) was raised in a rabbit against synthetic hPTH(1-34) which was conjugated to bovine thyroglobulin (Paesel KG, Frankfurt, FRG) [22]. The antiserum was diluted in assay buffer 1 + 4 ml normal rabbit serum (NRS)/liter (dilution: 1:50 000).

Second Antibody

Donkeys were immunized against goat IgG and rabbit IgG (Fa. Sigma, Deisenhofen, FRG). These second antibodies were diluted with assay buffer 1

Table 2. Flow diagram of the assay procedure

100 µl	Standard or sample
100 µl	First antibody (G76/85.05.02; dilution, 1:1000)
	48 h incubation at 4 °C
100 µl	Tracer
	48 h incubation at 4 °C
100 µl	Second antibody (goat IgG, 1:6)
	(rabbit IgG, 1:21)
100 µl	PEG solution
	1 h incubation at room temperature

- Centrifuge the tubes for 10 min at 1800 g
- Aspirate and discard the supernates
- Wash the sediments with 500 µl NaCl solution 0.85 g/liter
- Centrifuge the tubes for 10 min at 1800 g
- Aspirate and discard the supernates
- Count the radioactivity of the sediments in a gamma counter for 1 min
  (Searle 1285 gamma counter, Zinsser, Frankfurt/M., FRG)

(dilution of goat IgG, 1:6; rabbit IgG 1:21). The precipitation of the first antibodies was complete.

Samples

Coagulated blood was centrifuged for 10 min at 1800 g. The serum was stored at − 30 °C until use. The controls were obtained from apparently healthy donors. The controls were also prepared in EDTA plasma. The primary HPT samples were obtained from patients with diagnosed or surgically confirmed primary hyperparathyroidism. The secondary HPT samples were obtained from patients with chronic renal failure who had to undergo hemodialysis. The samples used for the RIA were fresh or thawed once.

Assay Procedure with the Labeled Peptide NLeu^8-NLeu^{18}-Tyr^{34}-hPTH(1-34)

The RIA was performed in immunoassay vials (Chap. 1.4) (Sarstedt, Nümbrecht, FRG).

Assay Procedure with the Biotinylated hPTH(1-34)[^{125}I] Streptavidin Tracer

The RIA was performed as described above. To each tube 150 µl biotinylated hPTH(1-34)[^{125}I] streptavidin preincubated tracer was added.

Serum Calcium Levels

Serum calcium levels were measured by calcein fluorometry.

Evaluation

To construct the standard curve the bound radioactivity in counts per minute
(y-axis) was plotted versus the concentration of the corresponding standards in
pmol/liter (x-axis) using half-logarithmic scales.

Results

Antibody Characteristics

To characterize the antibodies raised against the amino-terminal part of PTH,
the Rm/82.10.02 and G76/85.05.02 antisera were diluted 1:50 000 and 1:1000 in
assay buffer 1 + 4 ml NRS or NGS/liter. The displacement of labeled hPTH(1-
34) was tested with the peptides hPTH(1-34), hPTH(28-48), hPTH(44-68),
hPTH(53-84), and hPTH(1-84). For both antisera only hPTH(1-34) displaced
the labeled peptide within a PTH concentration from 0 to 64 pmol/liter. Ten
percent displacement was observed at a concentration of 1.4 pmol/liter
(Rm/82.10.02) and at a concentration of 2.4 pmol/liter PTH (G76/85.05.02). The
maximal binding of the tracer (B/T) was 18% (Rm/82.10.02) and 33%
(G76/85.05.02). The total activity of the tracer was about 30 000 cpm/100 μl.
hPTH(1-84) showed a displacement curve at higher concentrations. The displacement curve was parallel to the one with hPTH(1-34). No cross-reactivity
occurred with hPTH(28-48), hPTH(44-68), and hPTH(53-84) up to
2000 pmol/liter PTH.

Comparison of Tracers

Under routine conditions of the RIA, NLeu[8]-NLeu[18]-Tyr[34]-hPTH(1-34) and
biotinylated hPTH(1-34) [^{125}I] streptavidin tracer were added to the
G76/85.05.02 antiserum and incubated. The maximal binding of the NLeu[8]-
NLeu[18]-Tyr[34]-hPTH(1-34) tracer was 21% B/T and that of the biotinylated
hPTH(1-34) [^{125}I] streptavidin tracer was 30% B/T. 90% B/B$_0$ was observed at
a concentration of 2.4 pmol/liter PTH when the peptide NLeu[8]-NLeu[18]-Tyr[34]-
hPTH(1-34) tracer was used. When the biotinylated hPTH (1-34) [^{125}I] streptavidin tracer was used 90% binding was observed at a concentration of
1.4 pmol/liter PTH. Typical displacement curves are shown in Fig. 1.

Comparison of Antibodies

The Rm/82.10.02 antiserum showed a very high titer (dilution 1:50 000). Ninety
percent B/B$_0$ occurred at a concentration of 2.3 pmol/liter PTH. The

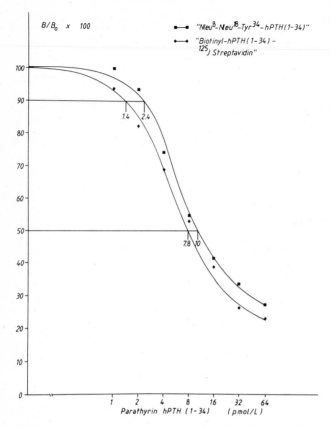

Fig. 1. Typical displacement curves with NLeu^8-NLeu^{18}-Tyr^{34}-hPTH(1-34) (■) and biotinylated hPTH(1-34) [^{125}I]-streptavidin (◆) as tracers

G76/84.09.12 antiserum showed a low titer (dilution 1:500) and 90% B/B_0 was observed at a concentration of 7 pmol/liter PTH (see Fig. 2 for results). In contrast to the goat antiserum the rabbit antiserum was of limited clinical usefulness. No distinction was possible between the PTH levels of the normals and the patients with primary hyperparathyroidism (see Fig. 3 for results).

Assay Developed with the G76/85.05.02 Antiserum and the Biotinylated hPTH(1-34) [^{125}I] Streptavidin Tracer

Further experiments demonstrated that the antigen-antibody reaction had reached equilibrium after 48 h at 4 °C. The lower detection limit (B_0–3 SD) dropped from 4.5 pmol/liter (equilibrium) to 0.5 pmol/liter PTH when the assay was performed in the sequential saturation mode. To find the best composition of the tracer, varied volumes of biotinylated hPTH(1-34) and [^{125}I] streptavidin were assayed. The combination of 100 µl [^{125}I] streptavidin with 50 µl bio-

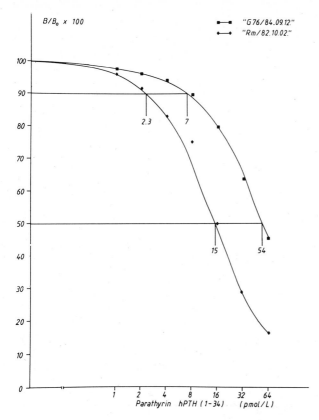

Fig. 2. Displacement curves of the G76/84.09.12 antiserum (■) and the Rm/82.10.02 antiserum (◆)

tinylated hPTH(1-34) per tube gave the best result. After 60 min the precipitation of the antigen-antibody complex was completed by adding 100 g/liter of polyethylene glycol (PEG 100 g/liter) to the second antibody.

Clinical Usefulness

To examine the clinical usefulness of the RIA, fresh serum samples or EDTA plasma samples were used. When the samples had been stored for a long time or thawed several times a significant degradation of amino-terminal PTH was observed.

Normal Range. Thirty-eight apparently healthy blood donors were assayed. PTH levels ranged from 1.3 to 6.8 pmol/liter (Fig. 4). The corresponding serum calcium levels ranged from 2.04 to 2.54 mmol/liter.

Hyperparathyroid Subjects. Forty-three patients with surgically confirmed or diagnosed primary hyperparathyroidism had values ranging from 4.5 to

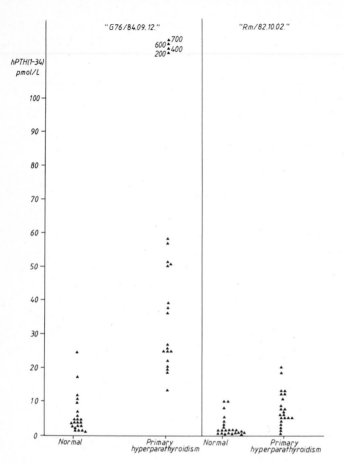

Fig. 3. Levels of hPTH(1-34) in 23 normals and 22 patients with primary hyper-parathyroidism assayed in the RIA with the G76/84.09.12 antiserum (*left*) and the Rm/82.10.02 antiserum (*right*)

52 pmol/liter PTH. Five patients had normal PTH values. The corresponding serum calcium levels ranged from 2.6 to 4.1 mmol/liter.

Patients with Chronic Renal Failure. Thirteen samples from patients with chronic renal failure who had to undergo hemodialysis were assayed before and after hemodialysis.

Ranges Before Hemodialysis. PTH: 6.8-15.5 pmol/liter
                                              Calcium: 1.89-2.53 mmol/liter

Ranges After Dialysis. PTH: 6.4–12.5 pmol/liter
                                       Calcium: 2.13–3.07 mmol/liter

(see Figs 4 and 5 for results)

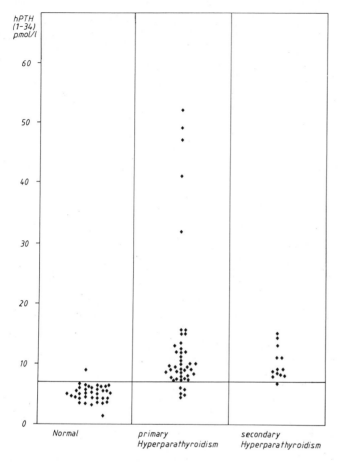

Fig. 4. Levels of hPTH (1–34) in 37 normals, 43 patients with primary hyperparathyroidism, and 13 patients with secondary hyperparathyroidism, assayed in the RIA
with the G76/85.05.02 antiserum. The *horizontal line* separates the normal range from the
hyperparathyroid range

The PTH ranges in serum samples did not differ from those in EDTA
samples.

Lower Detection Limit. The lower limit of detection was 0.5 pmol/liter PTH for
the described RIA. The "standard 0" sample was assayed 12 times ($\bar{x}$ B/B_0 − 3
SD).

Linearity

A hyperparathyroid sample was serially diluted with 0-standard medium.
Linearity was observed within the range from 1 to 64 pmol/liter PTH.

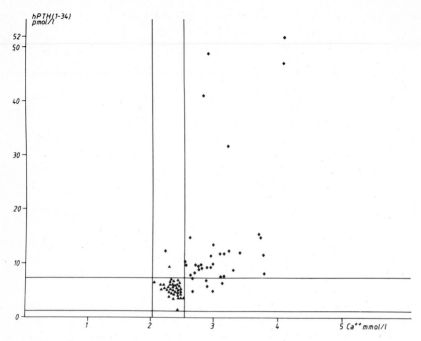

Fig. 5. Relationship between amino-terminal immunoreactive PTH and the serum calcium concentrations of 38 normals and 38 patients with primary hyperparathyroidism. The *horizontal lines* indicate the normal range of hPTH (1–34) and the *vertical line* indicates the normal range of the serum calcium levels. Normals (▲), primary HPT (◆)

Reproducibility

The intra- and interassay variations were estimated by repeatedly measuring a control serum from a normal and a hyperparathyroid subject. The results are shown in Tables 3 and 4.

Table 3. Estimation of intraassay variation by measurement of samples from a normal and a hyperparathyroid subject with one RIA

	Number of measurements	PTH(1-34) (pmol/liter)	CV %
Normal	32	4.9	8.3
Primary HPT serum	32	7.0	7.7

Table 4. Estimation of interassay variation by measurement of samples from a normal and a hyperparathyroid subject in eight different RIAs. The RIAs were performed within 5 weeks

	Number of measurements	hPTH(1-34) (pmol/liter)	$CV\%$
Normal	8	5.03	12.1
Primary HPT	8	16.3	17.1

Discussion

Very sensitive and specific RIAs are required to detect the amino-terminal part of PTH, which is very short-lived and which appears only in small amounts in human plasma [14, 23]. To achieve these conditions, suitable antibodies and tracers are necessary. When antibodies are raised against synthetic animo-terminal PTH a very sensitive RIA is available. Its clinical usefulness, however, is limited because the normal range overlaps the abnormal range. For antibodies raised against partially purified extracts from human adenomatous glands, the RIA is not so sensitive but there is only a slight overlap between the PTH levels of blood donors and hyperparathyroid patients [21]. A reason for this observation may be that the antibodies raised against human PTH are much more specific than the antibodies raised against synthetic hPTH(1-34). The high specificity is probably established in the tertiary structure of human PTH(1-34) used for immunization. To compensate for the lack of sensitivity of antibodies raised against human PTH a suitable tracer has to be applied. When the peptide NLeu[8]-NLeu[18]-Tyr[34]-hPTH(1-34) is labeled with [125]iodine, the peptide differs in three amino acids (Met[8]-Met[18]-Phe[34]) in its chemical structure and consequently in its immunological properties. During storage the peptide will undergo radiolysis, which also causes a change in chemical structure and in its immunological properties. The result is a tracer of limited specificity. By using the biotinylated hPTH(1-34) [^{125}I] streptavidin tracer these problems can be avoided. The biotin molecule is linked with the peptide at position one (manufactor's information). That is why the structure and the immunological properties of the peptide are not greatly altered. It is only during one incubation phase (48 h) that the tracer is in contact with the detector [^{125}I] streptavidin. Therefore, no major radiolysis of the peptide occurs. The result is a tracer with high affinity and the best immunological properties for the RIA.

The lower detection limit is 0.5 pmol/liter PTH. No other RIA described so far is adequate to detect 0.5 pmol/liter PTH [10, 15–18]. The levels of PTH detected by the cytochemical bioassay agree with measurements of the described assay [23]. Accurate measurement of the PTH levels within the normal range, however, is only possible when the RIA is performed in the more sensitive sequential saturation mode. With the development of an amino-terminal RIA

Segre has also achieved good results [15]. All the hitherto published RIAs for the amino-terminal PTH have much higher normal ranges which do not agree with those of the cytochemical bioassay. They also show an overlap between the normal and abnormal ranges. These facts are explainable by the reduced specificity and sensitivity of the published RIAs. The normal range and the range of primary HPT are discriminated nearly completely if the assay is performed with the biotinylated hPTH(1-34) [^{125}I] streptavidin tracer. Five hyperparathyroid samples had PTH levels within the normal range. This false measurement may have been due to the age of the samples and the degradation of hPTH(1-34) during storage. A good distinction between the PTH levels in normal and hyperparathyroid samples is achieved if the PTH and serum calcium levels are observed together. This explains why the diagnosis of the disease, primary hyperparathyroidism should only be established on the basis of the PTH levels and the corresponding serum calcium levels. Five patients with high PTH levels also had very high calcium levels. This demonstrates the positive correlation between the PTH and the calcium level in pHPT. All patients with chronic renal failure had increased hPTH(1-34) levels and low serum calcium levels before undergoing hemodialysis. The increased PTH(1-34) level might be a direct parameter for the degree of the renal osteopathy in patients with renal failure, because the elimination of biologically active amino-terminal PTH is thought to be independent from renal function. All other fragments of PTH are inert and their elimination is influenced by renal function [4, 5]. The PTH levels of all patients decreased after hemodialysis because the serum calcium levels increased during hemodialysis. The results demonstrate the rapid suppression of the parathyroid glands by increasing serum calcium levels. The extreme sensitivity and good clinical usefulness of the assay are due to the biotinylated hPTH(1-34) [^{125}I] streptavidin tracer and the antibody raised against the PTH of adenomatous glands. Based on the clinical use of the assay and the distinction of the normal range from hyperparathyroid PTH levels, acute and chronic alterations of the PTH levels connected with the bioactivity of PTH can be observed under physiological and abnormal conditions. For patients with chronic renal failure the RIA described has particular importance because the level of hPTH(1-34) may directly indicate the degree of renal osteopathy. In conclusion a RIA for the human amino-terminal hPTH(1-34) has been developed. One antibody raised in a rabbit against synthetic hPTH(1-34) is compared with another antibody raised in a goat against a partially purified extract from adenomatous glands. Furthermore the NLeu^8-NLeu^{18}-Tyr^{34}-hPTH(1-34) tracer is compared with the biotinylated hPTH(1-34) [^{125}I] strepavidin tracer. The RIA described detects hPTH(1-34) at a concentration of 0.5 pmol/liter. No cross-reactivity occurs with hPTH(28-48), hPTH(44-68), and hPTH(53-84). In normal subjects ($n = 38$) the concentrations range from 1.3 to 6.8 pmol/liter PTH. Patients with primary hyperparathyroidism have hPTH(1-34) levels from 4.5 to 52 pmol/liter ($n = 43$). Patients with chronic renal failure ($n = 13$) have hPTH(1-34) levels from 6.8 to 15.5 pmol/liter before undergoing hemodialysis.

References

1. Arnaud CD (1983) Hormonal regulation of calcium homeostasis. In: Bikle DD (ed) Assay of calcium regulating hormones. Springer, Berlin Heidelberg New York, pp 1–20
2. Brown EM (1982) PTH Secretion in vivo and in vitro. Miner Electrolyte Metab 8:130–150
3. Segre GV, Perkins AS, Wilkies LA, Potts JT Jr (1981) Metabolism of parathyroid hormone by isolated rat Kupffer cells and hepatocytes. J Clin Invest 67:449–457
4. Slatopolsky E, Martin K, Morrissey J, Hruska K (1982) Current concepts of the metabolism and radioimmunoassay of parathyroid hormone. J Lab Clin Med 99:309–316
5. D'Amour P, Segre GV, Robbs SJ, Potts JT Jr (1979) Analysis of parathyroid hormone and its fragments in rat tissue. J Clin Invest 63:89–98
6. Draper MW (1982) The structure of parathyroid hormone: its effects on biological action. Miner Electrolyte Metab 8:159–172
7. Nko M, Grisson M, Gueris J, Moukthar MS, Redel J (1982) Effects of vitamin D_3 dihydroxylated metabolites on parathyroid hormone in the rat. Miner Electrolyte Metab 7:67–75
8. Haas H (1979) Calziumhormone, Skelett-und Mineralstoffwechsel. In: Siegenthaler W (ed) Klinische Pathophysiologie. Thieme, Stuttgart, pp 335–359
9. Alexander LA, Famulare AJ, Worthy TE (1986) Evaluation of an assay for intact parathyroid hormone. Clin Chem 32:1152
10. Gilberto J, Vieira H, Oliviera AD, Maciel RMB, Mesquita CH, Russo EMK (1986) Development of an homologous radioimmunoassay for the synthetic amino-terminal (1-34) fragment of human parathyroid hormone using egg yolk-obtained antibodies. J Immunoassay 7:57–72
11. Mallette LE, Renfro M, Lemoncelli J, Rosenblatt M (1981) Radioimmunoassays for the 28-48 region of parathyroid hormone detect intact hormone but not hormone fragments. Calcif Tissue Int 33:375–380
12. Mallette LE, Tuma SN, Berger RE, Kirkland JL (1982) Radioimmunoassay for the middle region of human parathyroid hormone using a homologous antiserum with a carboxy-terminal fragment of bovine parathyroid hormone as radioligand. J Clin Endocrinol Metab 54:1017–1023
13. Hitzler W, Schmidt-Gayk H, Spiropoulos P, Raue F, Hüfner M (1982) Homologous radioimmunoassay for human parathyrin (residues 53–84). Clin Chem 28:49–53
14. Manning RM, Adami S, Papapoulos SE, Gleed JH, Hendy GN, Rosenblatt M, O'Riordan JLH (1981) A carboxy-terminal specific assay for human parathyroid hormone. Clin Endocrinol (Oxf) 15:439–449
15. Segre GV (1983) Amino-terminal radioimmunoassay for human parathyroid hormone. In: Frame B, Potts JS (eds) Clinical disorders of bone and mineral metabolism. Excerpta Medica Amsterdam, pp 14–17
16. Desplan C, Jullienne A, Moukthar MS, Milhaud G (1977) Sensitive assay for biological active fragment of human parathyroid hormone. Lancet ii:198–199
17. Papapoulos SE, Manning RM, Hendy GN, Lewin IG, O'Riordan JLH (1980) Studies of circulating parathyroid hormone in man using a homologous amino-terminal specific immunoradiometric assay. Clin Endocrinol (Oxf) 13:57–67
18. Papapoulos SE, Manning RM, Hendy GN, Lewin IG, O'Riordan JLH

(1978) Amino-terminal labeled antibody assay for human parathyroid hormone. J Endocrinol 19:33–39

19. Hehrmann R, Tidow J, Offner G, Hesch HP, Pichelmayer R (1980) Plasma Parathormon nach Nierentransplantation. Klin Wochenschr 58:249–258
20. Hunter WM, Greenwood FC (1962) Preparation of iodine-131-labeled human growth hormone of high specific activity. Nature 194:495–496
21. Fischer JA, Binswanger U, Dietrich FM (1974) Immunological characterization of antibodies against a glandular extract and the synthetic amino-terminal fragments 1-12 and 1-34 and their use in the determinaton of immunoreactive hormone in human sera. J Clin Invest 54:1382–1394
22. Sofroniew MV, Madler M, Müller OA, Scriba PC (1978) A method for the consistent production of high quality antisera to small peptide hormones. Fresenius Z Anal Chem 290:163
23. Goltzman D, Henderson B, Loveridge N (1980) Cytochemical bioassay of parathyroid hormone. Characteristics of the assay and analysis of circulating hormonal forms. J Clin Invest 65:1309–1317
24. Papapoulos SE (1977) Clearance of exogenous parathyroid hormone in normal and uraemic man. Clin Endocrinol (Oxf) 7:211–225

Chapter 2.8

Measurement of Intact Parathyroid Hormone by an Extracting Two-Site Immunoradiometric Assay*

E. Blind

Measuring intact human parathyroid hormone (hPTH) still presents many problems. Owing to the rapid uptake and cleavage of hPTH(1-84) by the liver, intact PTH is removed from the circulation within minutes [17]. As a consequence, plasma concentrations are very low. RIAs directed against the primary cleavage region of PTH (residues 28-48) appeared to be specific for intact PTH but were usually not sensitive enough to detect intact PTH in all healthy persons [15]. To obtain the necessary assay sensitivity, Lindall et al. [14] used an extraction step: columns with solid-phase-bound anti-N-terminal antibodies were used to extract and concentrate N-terminal fragments and intact PTH from samples. The intact hormone was finally detected in a subsequent RIA of midregion fragments.

Another way of improving assay sensitivity is to use the immunoradiometric assay (IRMA) technique first described by Miles and Hales [19]. The usually low nonspecific radioactive uptake makes it possible to detect very small changes in the specific uptake of the label [27]. Other advantages include a decrease in the time required for reactants to reach equilibrium, owing to a surplus of antibodies. Measuring the bioactive sequence hPTH(1-34) in a homologous IRMA of the classical one-site type was first reported by Papapoulos et al. [21], but even this sophisticated assay detected PTH in only 32% of healthy persons.

We have developed a new type of two-site assay for hPTH(1-84). We use two antisera, directed against the N-terminal and the C-terminal part of the hormone, to ensure the detection of only the intact (or essentially intact) hormone and to avoid any competition between these two antibodies (Fig. 1). The extraction of intact PTH and N-terminal fragments in a first step allowed us to eliminate all other components of serum, including the midregional and C-terminal fragments of the hormone. Immunoextraction and concentration further enhanced the sensitivity of this assay. In addition, we describe a method for labeling antibodies indirectly without previous purification.

* This work was supported by the Deutsche Forschungsgemeinschaft (Schm 400/7-1). Parts of this article have been published in *Clinical Chemistry*.

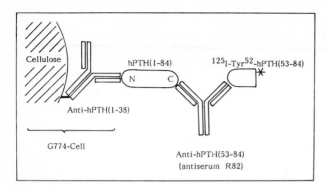

Fig. 1. Representation of the complex formed in the two-site assay procedure

Materials and Methods

Reagents

Most chemicals were from Merck AG, Darmstadt, Federal Republic of Germany. We prepared 1 liter *buffer A* (pH 7.4) by combining 800 ml 67 mmol/ liter Na_2HPO_4 solution, 200 ml 67 mmol/liter KH_2PO_4, 1 g sodium azide, 400 mg ethylenediaminetetraacetic acid (EDTA), and 1 g human serum albumin (Behringwerke AG, Marburg, FRG). To prepare 1 liter *buffer B*, we combined 900 ml buffer A and 100 ml hypoparathyroid serum previously determined to contain no detectable amounts of intact PTH. *Buffer C* was prepared by use of outdated blood-bank plasma: To remove intact PTH by adsorption, we added 80 g kaolin (Merck) to 1 liter plasma, and mixed and centrifuged the mixture (1800 *g*, 10 min). The supernatant was filtered twice through paper filters and then diluted tenfold in buffer A.

Standards and Samples

We prepared 10 nmol/liter stock solutions of the synthetic fragments hPTH(1-34), hPTH(1-44), hPTH(28-48), hPTH(39-84), hPTH(44-68), hPTH(53-84), and hPTH(69-84) in buffer A and of hPTH(1-84) in buffer B or buffer C. Standards were prepared by further diluting these solutions in the corresponding buffer. For the assay procedure, we prepared six concentrations of standard hPTH(1-84), ranging from 0 to 64 pmol/liter, and stored 0.5-ml aliquots at − 30°C. The PTH fragments were from Bachem Co., Bubendorf, Switzerland, except for hPTH(1-84), hPTH(39-84), and hPTH(69-84), which were from the Peptide Institute Inc., Osaka, Japan.

Serum or EDTA-treated plasma samples were separated from cells within 2 h, and stored at − 30 °C until assay.

Antisera

We raised, in goats, an antiserum (G774) against the N-terminal part of the hormone. We immunized the goats with extracts from human adenomatous glands obtained during parathyroid surgery. These glands were homogenized in 100 mmol/liter glycine HC1 (pH 3.0) at 0 °C. The homogenate was ultra-centrifuged and the supernate was then centrifuged in Centricon 30 cartridges (Amicon, Witten, FRG). The filtrate, which contained hPTH and other mole-cules smaller than mol. wt. 30 000, was generally emulsified with equal volumes of Freund's incomplete adjuvant (Sigma, Deisenhofen, FRG) and then injected subcutaneously at various sites, at 2-month intervals. The quantity of hormone injected ranged between 30 and 280 µg/application. The goats were bled 10–14 days after each booster. We incubated these antisera with four radioiodinated hPTH fragments to determine the titer and specificity of each antiserum. Bound tracer was determined by precipitation with antiserum against goat IgG in a conventional double-antibody assay system. The finally selected antiserum G774 was analyzed more precisely by simultaneous incubation with tracer and various concentrations of unlabeled fragments.

We obtained the antiserum (R82) against the C-terminal part of the hormone by immunizing rabbits with synthetic hPTH(53-84). This peptide had been conjugated to bovine thyroglobulin (Paesel KG, Frankfurt, FRG) in accordance with the method reported by Sofroniew et al. [25].

Preparation of Anti-hPTH(1-38)-Cellulose

The N-terminal antiserum G774 was fractionated. We followed a procedure described by Hebert et al. [11] and carried out repeated precipitations with solutions of ammonium sulfate (Merck AG). The precipitate was dialyzed against isotonic saline (NaCl, 0.85 g/liter) and finally against barbital buffer (50 mmol/liter, pH 8.0).

The covalent linkage of the IgG solution to cellulose particles was performed according to the method of Chapman and Ratcliffe [4] and Chapman et al. [5] and is described in detail here:

1. Prepare activated cellulose by dissolving 0.61 g 1,1'-carbonyldiimidazole (Sigma GmbH) in 25 ml acetone and add 5 g microcrystalline cellulose (Sigma GmbH). Incubate for 60 min (all incubations at 20 °C and rotated end over end). Wash the cellulose particles three times with 50 ml acetone by repeatedly mixing, centrifuging (1200 g, 5 min), and aspirating and discarding the supernatant. Let the activated cellulose air-dry on a filter paper.
2. Link the IgG as follows: Combine 2 g of the dried activated cellulose with 10 ml of the IgG solution (protein concentration 5 g/liter) and incubate overnight.
3. Wash the cellulose particles as described above with the following solutions: Incubate twice with bicarbonate buffer (0.5 mol/liter, pH 8.0) for 20 min,

acetate buffer (0.1 mol/liter, pH 4.0) for 60 min, acetate buffer overnight after sonicating for 30 s, and twice with the selected assay buffer for 20 min.
4. Dilute the cellulose particles with the assay buffer, store at 4°C, and mix on a magnetic stirring device just before use. Our assay uses a cellulose concentration of 8 g/liter in buffer A. The suspension was stable for at least 4 months.

Radioiodination Procedure

We radiolabeled 1 µg Nle[8,18],Tyr[34]-hPTH(1-34), Tyr[27]-hPTH(28-48), Tyr[43]-hPTH(44-68), and Tyr[52]-hPTH(53-84) with 0.5 mCi Na[125]I (Amersham Buchler, Braunschweig, FRG) as described previously [23]. The procedure is essentially the chloramine-T method described by Hunter and Greenwood [12], followed by a purification as reported by Schöneshöfer et al. [24]. Nle[8,18],Tyr[34]-hPTH(1-34) was supplied by Peptide Institute Inc.; the other tracer peptides were from Bachem Co. For routine assay performance we labeled the peptide Tyr[52]-hPTH(53-84) monthly; its specific activity was approximately 600 Ci/g. The tracer was further diluted to about 50 000 Bq/ml in buffer A to which human serum albumin was added to give a total albumin concentration of 10 g/liter.

Assay Procedure

1. Pipette 200 µl hPTH(1-84) standard, control sera (Table 1) or patients' samples into immunoassay vials (Chap. 1.4, 0.6 ml volume, Sarstedt, Nümbrecht, FRG) [22] in duplicate. Pipette 100 µl of the anti-hPTH(1-38)-cellulose into each vial. Close the vials with self-adhesive film and rotate end over end at 4 °C for 24 h.

Table 1. Accuracy and reproducibility

	Intraassay (n = 24)		Interassay (n = 9)[a]	
	Mean ± SD (pmol/liter)	CV (%)	Mean ± SD (pmol/liter)	CV (%)
Control sera				
Hypoparathyroid control	< 0.6[b]	–	< 0.6[b]	–
Normal control 1			2.6 ± 0.25	9.8
Normal control 2	3.9 ± 0.30	7.6		
High control	6.4 ± 0.58	9.0		
Hyperparathyroid control	26.3 ± 2.7	10.4	28.4 ± 3.9	13.7

[a] Determined in nine independent assays (different cellulose particle preparations, different standard preparations, different tracer preparations, etc.)
[b] For the hypoparathyroid control, values were constantly below the limit of detection

2. Centrifuge the samples (1800 g, 5 min), then aspirate and discard the supernates. Wash the vials by adding 400 μl isotonic saline, mix, recentrifuge, and again aspirate and discard the supernates. Add 20 μl of the C-terminal antiserum R82, diluted 100-fold in buffer A. Mix to produce a homogeneous suspension, then incubate, without shaking, at 4 °C overnight.
3. Wash the vials again as just described to remove unbound antibodies. Add 20 μl ^{125}I-labeled Tyr^{52}-hPTH(53-84) containing about 1000 Bq (30 000 cpm). Mix the contents of the vials and incubate at 4 °C for another 24 h.
4. Perform the same washing procedure twice more to remove unbound tracer. Count the radioactivity of the sediment in a gamma counter for 5 min (we used a Searle 1285 gamma counter from Zinsser, Frankfurt/M., FRG). Plot the bound radioactivity (y-axis) versus the concentration of the corresponding standard (in pmol/liter, x-axis), using linear scales. Samples with values > 30 pmol/liter should be diluted tenfold in buffer B and reassayed.

Results

Antibody Characteristics

N-Terminal Antiserum. The finally selected goat antiserum G774 bound Nle^{8,18},Tyr^{34}-hPTH(1-34) and Tyr^{27}-hPTH(28-48) but did not recognize Tyr^{43}-hPTH(44-68) or Tyr^{52}-hPTH(53-84). Displacement tests showed that the N-terminal tracer Nle^{8,18},Tyr^{34}-hPTH(1-34) was completely displaced by the peptides hPTH(1-34), hPTH(1-44), and hPTH(1-84). The fragment hPTH(28-48), however, failed to displace the tracer. When the N-terminal tracer was used, half-maximal competition for binding was observed at a concentration of 2.0 nmol/liter hPTH(1-34), 2.3 nmol/liter hPTH(1-84), and 2.7 nmol/liter hPTH(1-44).

Human parathyroid hormone (1-44), hPTH(28-48), and hPTH(1-84) were able to displace the tracer Tyr^{27}-hPTH(28-48) from the antibody, whereas hPTH(1-34) and hPTH(39-84) were ineffective. Hence, antiserum G774 consists of at least two large antibody populations which recognize hPTH within the sequence 1-38 at two distinct sites of the molecule.

C-Terminal Antiserum. The antiserum R82 bound Tyr^{43}-hPTH(44-68) and Tyr^{52}-hPTH(53-84) but failed to recognize Nle^{8,18}, Tyr^{34}-hPTH(1-34) or Tyr^{27}-hPTH(28-48). When the tracer Tyr^{43}-hPTH(44-68) was used, half-maximal displacement occurred at 1070 pmol/liter for hPTH(44-68) and at 520 pmol/liter for fragment hPTH(53-84). The tracer Tyr^{52}-hPTH(53-84) was displaced by 50% at 630 pmol/liter hPTH(53-84), whereas hPTH(69-84) did not influence the binding of the tracer. However, as shown in Chap. 2.11, the antibody does recognize sequences up to amino acid 76 of the hPTH (53-84) peptide.

Assay Development

We optimized several variables. We chose 4 °C as our assay incubation condition for all steps because under these conditions the standard curves were steeper and the count rates were higher compared with room temperature. Incubation for 24 h for the first phase of the assay, 14 h for the second, and 20 h for the third proved to be long enough for the reactants to reach equilibrium. A further prolongation of these incubation times did not increase the bound radioactivity of the highest standard (64 pmol/liter).

The C-terminal antiserum R82 and the ^{125}I-labeled Tyr^{52}-hPTH(53-84) were added in excess. For economic reasons, however, only 0.8 mg anti-hPTH(1-38)-cellulose was used per vial, thus resulting in a lower calibration curve for high standards (Fig. 2).

We observed no "hook" effect: with concentrations of hPTH(1-84) up to 4000 pmol/liter, bound activity increased steadily.

If the vial contents were not mixed during the first phase of incubation, bound activity fell by 30% for the whole range of standard concentrations.

The volume of incubation mixture chosen proved to be a determining factor in carrying out the assay. Owing to the low concentrations of hPTH(1-84) it was necessary to shift the equilibrium of the reactions toward the products. Figure 3

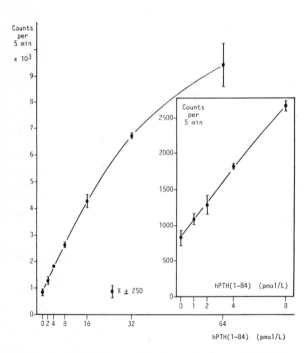

Fig. 2. Typical IRMA standard curve for intact PTH. *Vertical bars* indicate $\pm$ 2 SD. The *inset* shows the beginning of the curve at a larger scale

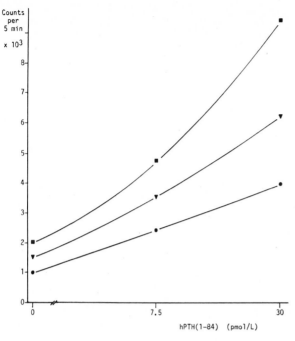

Fig. 3. Effect of volume on the IRMA for hPTH(1-84). Identical quantities of tracer (1000 Bq) dissolved in 20 µl (■), 50 µl (▼), or 100 µl (●) buffer were added to the sediment before the last incubation step

shows the increase in bound activity when the same quantity of tracer is dissolved in 20 µl buffer rather than in 100 µl.

Assay Characteristics

Detection Limit. The nonspecific uptake of the label was lower than 0.5% of the total activity added and reached values between 100 and 150 cpm (B_0). The lowest detectable concentration was defined as the point lying 3 SD above the B_0, as measured and calculated based on 32 samples of the zero standard. The lower limit of detection was 0.6 pmol/liter, which is equal to 1.2×10^{-16} mol or 1.1 pg hPTH(1-84)/tube.

Cross-Reactivity. Several synthetic hormone fragments did not cross-react. We tested the peptides hPTH(1-34), hPTH(1-44), hPTH(28-48), hPTH(39-84), hPTH(44-68), hPTH(53-84), and hPTH(1-84) at different concentrations ranging from 25 to 6400 pmol/liter. Only the intact hormone hPTH(1-84) showed an increase in bound activity.

Interference with C-Terminal Fragments. We tested what influence C-terminal fragments had on measuring hPTH(1-84). Various quantities of hPTH(39-84) were added to a serum sample enriched with 20 pmol synthetic hPTH(1-84)/

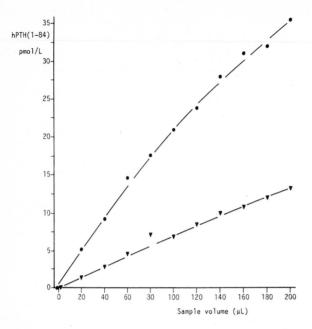

Fig. 4. Concentrations of intact hPTH(1-84) in serial dilutions of two hyperparathyroid plasma samples

liter. Detection of intact PTH was not influenced by concentrations of hPTH(39-84) up to 8000 pmol/liter.

Linearity and Recovery. Plasma samples of two patients with primary hyperparathyroidism were serially diluted with the zero-standard medium (buffer B). The results are shown in Fig. 4. The sample containing 36 pmol/liter at 200 μl showed slight nonlinearity; the slope at the beginning of the dilution curve indicates a concentration of about 50 pmol hPTH(1-84)/liter. From these data we concluded that we should reassay samples with concentrations exceeding 30 pmol/liter, using a tenfold dilution in buffer B.

We enriched a serum sample containing 2.1 (SD 0.22) pmol/liter hPTH(1-84) per liter with 2.0 and 20 pmol synthetic hPTH(1-84)/liter. The observed concentrations were 3.9 (SD 0.30) pmol/liter and 23.4 (SD 2.6) pmol/liter, the corresponding recoveries 95% and 106%.

Precision and Reproducibility. Intra- and interassay variations were estimated by repeatedly measuring three control sera from a healthy, a hyperparathyroid and a hypoparathyroid individual (Table 1).

Medium for the Preparation of Standards

Initial experiments with buffer A as a diluent for the standards showed flat standard curves (Fig. 5). Therefore we investigated degradation and adsorption of intact PTH in several media.

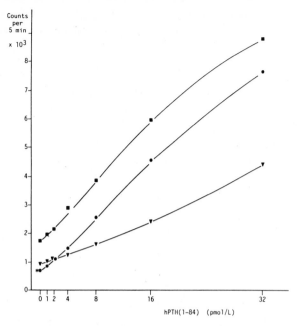

Fig. 5. Immunoradiometric standard curves with different standard media. Solutions used for the dilution of hPTH(1-84): pooled serum of normal persons (■), buffer C (●), buffer A (▼). One control from a patient with hypoparathyroidism is also shown (∗)

We added identical quantities of synthetic hPTH(1-84) to several solutions (serum, buffer A, buffer B, isotonic saline). After gentle mixing the solutions were stored in polypropylene tubes at room temperature for 3 h. One portion of these solutions was transferred five times into new vials during the incubation period in order to enhance adsorptive losses. To exclude any differences during assay performance the samples were diluted twofold in hypoparathyroid serum before assaying, except for the serum samples diluted with buffer A. The serum sample revealed a concentration of 14 pmol hPTH(1-84)/liter, without being influenced by repeated transfer into new vials. The sample in buffer A contained 13 pmol/liter. The value dropped by repeated transfer to 9.8 pmol/liter, an effect that was even stronger in the protein-free solution.

Addition of 100 ml hypoparathyroid serum to 900 ml buffer A, however, proved to be sufficient to obviate any adsorptive loss. That was why we chose this solution, referred to as buffer B, as the diluent for standards. We developed another medium based on treated blood-bank plasma (referred to as buffer C), which proved to be also suitable for the preparation of standards. Standards prepared with this buffer showed both a good parallel with standards prepared in pooled normal serum and a count rate of the zero standard which was identical to that of serum from patients with hypoparathyroidism (Fig. 5).

We observed no change in the PTH content of these standards when they were stored at 4 °C for 2 days or after three freeze-thaw cycles. To detect nonspecific adsorption of hPTH(1-84) onto the large surface of the cellulose particles, we performed the assay with cellulose that had been covalently coated with another protein. No standard curve was obtained.

Stability of Intact PTH in Samples

We examined the stability of intact PTH in 20 samples of EDTA-treated plasma, heparinized plasma, and serum from healthy and hyperparathyroid persons while the samples were stored at 4 °C for 2 days. We observed no decrease in the concentrations measured in the plasma samples, whereas one normal serum specimen showed a slight decrease and a renal-dialysis specimen a substantial decrease in the concentrations measured. Adding 2 mg EDTA to 1 ml of the latter sample lessened the loss. The concentration of intact PTH fell from 210 to 77 pmol/liter within 2 days. When EDTA was added it fell from 210 to only 160 pmol/liter.

Concentrations of intact hPTH(1-84) in serum differed slightly from values in plasma as determined in quadruplicate in simultaneously obtained blood specimens from one normal subject. The mean values were: EDTA plasma, 3.7 (SD 0.4); heparinized plasma, 3.5 (SD 0.8); plasma treated with kaolin-coated beads, 2.5 (SD 0.5); and serum (collected in plastic tubes), 3.1 (SD 0.4) pmol/liter. No significant differences of serum intact PTH concentrations were found in 11 patients with primary hyperparathyroidism from whom EDTA plasma and serum (in tubes with kaolin-coated beads) were obtained simultaneously. We therefore prefer EDTA plasma for sampling, but serum should also be suitable. Both serum and plasma samples are accepted for measurement of intact PTH if the specimens were assayed soon after the plasma or serum was separated from blood or was stored at − 30 °C until assay.

The concentrations of intact PTH did not change in several samples stored at − 30 °C for 3 months.

Clinical Use

Normal Range. Sixty apparently healthy blood donors were assayed. In all samples, intact PTH was detectable. The concentrations ranged from 1.9 to 6.8 pmol/liter (mean 3.7 pmol/liter, SD 1.3; median 3.3 pmol/liter). As the PTH values were not normally distributed on a linear scale, we obtained a 95% confidence interval by excluding the highest and lowest value and declaring the highest and lowest values of the remaining 58 patients as the limits of the normal range. The normal range established by this method was 2.0 to 6.3 pmol/liter.

Clinical Results. Thirty-two patients with surgically confirmed or diagnosed primary hyperparathyroidism and an average preoperative total calcium concentration of 3.03 mmol/liter (range 2.64–4.1 mmol/liter) in serum showed PTH values ranging from 7.0 to 80 pmol/liter (mean 19.4 pmol/liter, median 12.0). Four patients with hypoparathyroidism had no detectable amounts of intact

PTH(< 0.6 pmol/liter). Further clinical results with this assay are presented in Chap. 1.1.

Discussion

Conventional Methods of Measuring Intact PTH

Classical radioimmunoassay (RIA) methods have usually not been specific enough to detect only intact PTH and, at the same time, not sensitive enough to measure the rather low amounts of intact PTH in healthy persons [15, 16].

Region-specific RIAs combined with pre-assay extraction steps improved the sensitivity. The use of columns for immunoextraction was, however, a laborious procedure and required a large sample volume [10, 14]. These assays were not sensitive enough to detect intact PTH in all normal subjects. Characteristics of these assays are shown in Table 2 (assays 1, 2).

Techniques and Antibodies Used for the Assay

Sensitivity and Interference. By using the two-site method [19, 27] we obtained a lower limit of detection, 0.6 pmol/liter, which is sensitive enough to detect intact PTH in all healthy persons, thus permitting the distinction of hypoparathyroid patients from normal persons. Although our antibodies did not have a particularly high affinity, we achieved this sensitivity by adding reagents in excess and by working with small incubation volumes of about 25 µl, except for the extraction step.

To extract and concentrate intact PTH and N-terminal fragments, we used prior incubation of the samples with anti-hPTH(1-38)-cellulose. This step required additional time compared to the simultaneous addition of all assay components. On the other hand, it allowed us to reduce the volume of the subsequent incubations. In particular, this step removed circulating substances which might have interfered nonspecifically during the subsequent assay procedure and ensured that all C-terminal and midregional fragments were eliminated. As high concentrations of these fragments can accumulate in patients suffering from renal failure [17] it was important to exclude any interference with them.

Antibodies and Labeling. We did not label the C-terminal antibody directly because the C-terminal antiserum was of low titer and the necessary purification would have caused heavy losses. To circumvent this problem we labeled the antibodies indirectly. Oxidative damage to the C-terminal antibody was thus avoided, and the antiserum was used economically. This method was initially intended to screen several different C-terminal antisera for their suitability for this assay, but it also proved to be satisfactory even for routine assay purposes. The tracer peptide Tyr^{52}-hPTH(53-84) is commercially available, can be radioiodinated by a simple and reliable method [23], and is stable over a period of

Table 2. Assays of intact hPTH

No.	Solid-phase antibody	Labeled antibody	Label	Assay standard	Sample volume (ml)	Normal range (pmol/liter)	Mean of normal ± SD (pmol/liter)	Detection limit (pmol/liter)	Reference
Extraction assays based on RIA									
1.	Chicken anti-hPTH(1-34)	(midregion RIA)	^{125}I	Tyr^{43}-hPTH(44-68)	2.5		4.8 ± 0.3 4.8 ± 2.4	2.1^a	Lindall et al. [14] Supplier's information[b]
2.	Goat anti-hPTH (1-34)	(midregion RIA As Giselle 3)	^{125}I	hPTH(1-84)	1.8	1.0–10.6	4.4 ± 2.3		Hackeng et al. [10]
Two-site immunoradiometric assays									
3.	Goat anti-hPTH(1-34)	Rabbit anti-hPTH(53-84)	^{125}I	hPTH(1-84)	0.2	2.0–6.3	3.7	0.6	Blind et al. (cited in Chap. 1.1)
4.	Goat anti-hPTH(53-84)	Goat anti-hPTH(1-34)	^{125}I	hPTH(1-84)	0.2	1.3–6.9^a 1.1–5.8^a	3.0^a	0.1^a	Nussbaum et al. [20] Supplier's information[c]
Two-site chemiluminometric assays									
5.	Mouse monoclonal anti-hPTH(44-68)	Sheep anti-hPTH(1-34)	Acridinium ester	hPTH(1-84)	0.1		3.4	0.8	Brown et al. [2]
6.	Goat anti-hPTH(1-34)	Rabbit anti-hPTH(53-84)	Isoluminol derivative	hPTH(1-84)	0.2	1.8–5.9	3.8	0.5	Böhler (Chap. 2.9)

[a] Original values were in nanograms per liter and were converted to picomoles per liter by division by 9.43

[b] Supplier's information, Immuno Nuclear Corporation, Stillwater, MI, United States

[c] Supplier's information, Nichols Institute Diagnostics, San Juan Capistrano, CA, United States

at least 6 weeks. Indirect labeling of antibodies might be applied to other peptide hormone assays if it is intended to set up a two-site system on the basis of an established RIA procedure.

The slight nonlinearity of samples containing large amounts of PTH required a reassay of these samples in tenfold dilution. This effect may be provoked by circulating N-terminal fragments which reduce the number of binding sites of the cellulose particles in the case of high plasma PTH concentrations. One might overcome this insufficiency by purifying the N-terminal antiserum using affinity chromatography. This method has the disadvantage of a considerable antibody consumption but ought to achieve a higher density of antibodies on the cellulose particles. The use of affinity chromatography seems to be the method of choice to obtain pure high-affinity antibodies [2] because monoclonal antibodies against PTH were inferior to polyclonal antibodies so far: Monoclonal antibodies against hPTH(44-68) showed only medium affinity and had to be used in large excess for use in a two-site assay [2]. Monoclonal antibodies against hPTH(1-34) have also been investigated for use in a two-site assay but were inferior to purified polyclonal antibodies [3].

Specificity of the Assay

The use of two antibodies against two distinct sites of the peptide (sequences 1-38 and 53-76) prevented any steric inhibition of antibody binding and assured measurement of only intact PTH, thus resulting in increased specificity compared with one-site methods.

Because this method is an immunochemical one, the term "intact PTH" used in this chapter refers not only to intact hPTH(1-84) in a narrow sense but also to smaller peptides containing the regions 1-38 and 53-76. Detection is, however, restricted to intact PTH in a physiological sense, i.e. PTH prior to cleavage in the region 34-37, which is thought to be the first important step in PTH metabolism [17]. The mean concentration of PTH in plasma of normal individuals, as detected by cytochemical bioassay [9], is 11.3 ng/liter (1.2 pmol/liter), which is lower than concentrations detected by the two-site immunoradiometric assay. This may be caused by alterations of the intact peptide in circulation, e.g. removal of only a few amino acids from the N-terminal end, that alter its bioactivity but might not influence its detection in our assay. Concentrations of PTH as measured by cytochemical bioassay can vary more than 20-fold within minutes [8]. We found no comparable pulsatility of intact PTH release with our intact PTH assay. The concentrations of intact PTH in plasma correlate closely, however, with values for circulating PTH bioactivity [14].

Stability of Intact PTH in Samples

Intact PTH as measured in EDTA-treated plasma samples with our assay was stable at 4 °C for days. Occasionally, this was not the case with some serum samples. Values were marginally lower when the samples were obtained by using kaolin-coated beads, probably due to adsorption of intact PTH onto the surface of the beads. EDTA plasma was recommended for assay 1 of Table 2 because intact PTH degraded rapidly in serum at room temperature with this assay (Immuno Nuclear Corporation, supplier's product information). In contrast, intact PTH was more labile in plasma than in serum as measured with a new two-site IRMA of intact PTH tested by Chu and Chu [7]. The kind of sample was less critical with our assay. We prefer EDTA plasma for sampling but accept all specimens which are assayed soon after the plasma or serum was separated from blood or were stored at $-30\,°C$ until assay. The preferable kind of sample seems to be method-related and should be selected for each assay individually.

Assay Standard Medium

Intact PTH in solutions is easily adsorbed onto glass and plastic surfaces [1], an effect which can be reduced by the presence of albumin or plasma and which is less distinct for the fragments hPTH(1-34) or hPTH(53-84) [13]. Albumin, even in high concentrations, was not sufficient to prevent losses of intact PTH in our assay. We therefore developed a medium (buffer C) based on plasma which was freed from intact PTH by adsorption in a way described similarly by Christensen [6]. The medium met all needs for the preparation of intact PTH assay standards: In contrast to hypoparathyroid serum it was available in large quantities, could be prepared easily, did not contain detectable quantities of intact PTH, and showed good parallelism with standards of full serum.

Normal Range of Intact PTH

The normal range and the mean value of intact PTH in healthy persons was very similar to the values reported by others (Table 2). This applies especially to the new two-site assays of intact PTH (assays 3–6 in Table 2), which do consistently use synthetic hPTH(1-84) as standard. Measurement of intact PTH in such assays leads to more standardized results when the detection of PTH is restricted to the intact, or essentially intact, hormone. By contrast, assays directed against the midregional or C-terminal part of the hormone often give very different values because the various forms of inactive degradation products as well as the intact hormone are detected to different degrees, depending on the antisera used [18, 23]. Sokoll et al. [26] measured intact PTH in healthy postmenopausal women with a two-site IRMA (assay 4 of Table 2). The normal range from 1.5 to 6.4 pmol/liter (mean 3.4 pmol/liter) was slightly higher than the originally reported values for this assay ([20], Table 2). There was a positive but not significant correlation between age and intact PTH.

References

1. Barrett PQ, Neuman WF (1978) The cleavage and adsorption of parathyroid hormone at high dilution—implications for receptor binding studies. Biochim Biophys Acta 541:223–233
2. Brown RC, Aston JP, Weeks I, Woodhead JS (1987) Circulating intact parathyroid hormone measured by a two-site immunochemiluminometric assay. J Clin Endocrinol Metab 65:407–414
3. Brown RC, Aston JP, John AS, Woodhead JS (1988) Comparison of poly- and monoclonal antibodies as labels in a two-site immunochemiluminometric assay for intact parathyroid hormone. J Immunol Methods 109:139–144
4. Chapman RS, Ratcliffe JG (1982) Covalent linkage of antisera to microparticulate cellulose using 1,1'-carbonyldiimidazole: a rapid, practical method with potential use in solid-phase immunoassay. Clin Chim Acta 118:129–134
5. Chapman RS, Sutherland RM, Ratcliffe JG (1983) Application of 1,1'-carbonyldiimidazole as a rapid, practical method for the production of solid-phase immunoassay reagents. In: Hunter WM, Corrie JET (eds) Immunoassays for clinical chemistry, 2nd edn. Churchill Livingstone, Edinburgh, pp 178–190
6. Christensen MS (1976) A sensitive radioimmunoassay of parathyroid hormone in human serum using a specific extraction procedure. Scand J Clin Lab Invest 36:313–322
7. Chu SY, Chu AK (1988) Assessment of INCSTAR's two-site immunoradiometric assay (IRMA) of intact parathyrin. Clin Chem 34:989–990
8. Dixit M, Moniz C, Cundy T (1987) Pulsatile secretion of parathyroid hormone in normal subjects. Ann Clin Biochem [Suppl 1] 24:143–144
9. Goltzman D, Henderson B, Loveridge N (1980) Cytochemical bioassay of parathyroid hormone. Characteristics of the assay and analysis of circulating hormonal forms. J Clin Invest 65:1309–1317
10. Hackeng WHL, Lips P, Netelenbos JC, Lips CJM (1986) Clinical implications of estimation of intact parathyroid hormone (PTH) versus total immunoreactive PTH in normal subjects and hyperparathyroid patients. J Clin Endocrinol Metab 63:447–453
11. Hebert GA, Pelham PL, Pittman B (1972) Determination of the optimal ammonium sulfate concentration for the fractionation of rabbit, sheep, horse, and goat antisera. Appl Microbiol 25:26–36
12. Hunter WM, Greenwood FC (1963) Preparation of iodine-131 labeled human growth hormone of high specific activity. Nature 194:495–496
13. Jüppner H, Mohr H, Hesch RD (1980) Adsorption of parathyrin: pitfall for solid phase assays using radiolabelled antibodies? J Clin Chem Clin Biochem 18:585–590
14. Lindall AW, Elting J, Ells J, Roos BA (1983) Estimation of biologically active intact parathyroid hormone in normal and hyperparathyroid sera by sequential N-terminal immunoextraction and midregion radioimmunoassay. J Clin Endocrinol Metab 57:1007–1014
15. Mallette LE (1983) Immunoreactivity of human parathyroid hormone (28-48): attempt to develop an assay for intact human parathyroid hormone. Metab Bone Dis Rel Res 4:329–332
16. Mallette LE, Renfro M, Lemoncelli J, Rosenblatt M (1981) Radioimmunoassays for

the 28-48 region of parathyroid hormone detect intact PTH but not hormone fragments. Calcif Tissue Int 33:375–380

17. Martin KJ, Hruska KA, Freitag JJ, Klahr S, Slatopolsky E (1979) The peripheral metabolism of parathyroid hormone. N Engl J Med 301:1092–1098

18. Marx SJ, Sharp ME, Krudy A, Rosenblatt M, Mallette LE (1981) Radioimmunoassay for the middle region of human parathyroid hormone: studies with a radio-iodinated synthetic peptide. J Clin Endocrinol Metab 53:76–84

19. Miles LEM, Hales CN (1968) Labelled antibodies and immunological assay systems. Nature 219:186–189

20. Nussbaum SR, Zahradnik RJ, Lavigne JR, Brennan GL, Nozawa-Ung K, Kim LY, Keutmann HT, Wang C, Potts JT Jr, Segre GV (1987) Highly sensitive two-site immunoradiometric assay of parathyrin, and its clinical utility in evaluating patients with hypercalcemia. Clin Chem 33:1364–1367

21. Papapoulos SE, Manning RM, Hendy GN, Lewin IG, O'Riordan JLH (1980) Studies of circulating parathyroid hormone in man using a homologous amino-terminal specific immunoradiometric assay. Clin Endocrinol (Oxf) 13:57–67

22. Schmidt-Gayk H, Wahl HM, Limbach HJ, Walch S (1979) Ein spezielles Gefäß zur Durchführung des Radioimmunoassay (RIA). Medizintechnik 99:103–104

23. Schmidt-Gayk H, Schmitt-Fiebig M, Hitzler W, Armbruster FP, Mayer E (1986) Two homologous radioimmunoassays for parathyrin compared and applied to disorders of calcium metabolism. Clin Chem 32:57–62

24. Schöneshöfer M, Kage A, Kage R, Fenner A (1982) A convenient technique for the specific isolation of ^{125}I-labelled peptide molecules. Fresenius Z Anal Chem 311:429–430

25. Sofroniew MV, Madler M, Müller OA, Scriba PC (1978) A method for the consistent production of high quality antisera to small peptide hormones. Fresenius Z Anal Chem 290:163

26. Sokoll LJ, Morrow FD, Quirbach DM, Dawson-Hughes B (1988) Intact parathyrin in postmenopausal women. Clin Chem 34:407–410

27. Woodhead JS, Addison GM, Hales CN (1974) The immunoradiometric assay and related techniques. Br Med Bull 30:44–49

Chapter 2.9

Measurement of Intact Parathyroid Hormone by a Two-Site Immunochemiluminometric Assay*

U. BÖHLER

Introduction

Using the advantages of two-site immunoradiometric assays (IRMAs), especially in terms of short incubation time, high specificity, and high sensitivity [27], it has recently become possible to measure intact human parathyroid hormone (hPTH) both sensitively and specifically [2, 3, 15]. These assays have allowed a more direct estimation of the secretory activity of the parathyroid gland compared with conventional PTH assays and, among other advantages, have been able to separate normal from subnormal PTH levels reliably. In this chapter we describe the development and clinical utility of a two-site immunochemiluminometric assay (ILMA) of intact hPTH that combines the advantages of a nonisotopic tracer peptide with the convenience of a simplified separation procedure based on the use of the "coated-tube" technique [4]. Additionally, this ILMA makes use of a highly purified label peptide.

The isoluminol derivative 6-[N-(4-aminobutyl-N-ethyl)-2,3-dihydrophthalazine-1,4-dione] hemisuccinimide (ABEI-H) coupled via succinimide ester was used to label synthetic hPTH(53-84). Reverse-phase high-performance liquid chromatography (HPLC) was used to purify the ABEI-H-labeled hPTH(53-84). Thus, ABEI-H-labeled was not only separated from unlabeled peptide and from free ABEI-H, but also the ABEI-H-labeled hPTH(53-84) conjugate with the highest incorporation ratio was selected.

The two-site ILMA design is based on the method of "indirect antibody labeling" as developed with an IRMA of intact hPTH in our clinical laboratory [2]: the immune complex formed in this assay consists of an immobilized antibody against the N-terminal part of hPTH, intact hPTH, and an antibody against the C-terminal part of hPTH whose second free binding site has been labeled in a final step with ABEI-H-labeled hPTH(53-84).

Finally, we report the application of the present ILMA to the measurement of intact hPTH in specimens from healthy subjects and patients with disorders of calcium metabolism.

*This chapter has partly been published in Clinical Chemistry (1989) 35:215–222.

Materials and Methods

Reagents

Intact PTH and hPTH(39-84) were purchased from Peptide Institute Inc., Osaka, Japan; the other fragments hPTH(1-34), hPTH(1-44), hPTH(28-48), hPTH(44-68), and hPTH(53-84) were from Bachem Co., Bubendorf, Switzerland. 6-[N-4-Aminobutyl-N-ethyl)-2,3-dihydrophthalazine-1,4-dione] hemisuccinimide (ABEI-H) was purchased from LKB-Wallac, Turku, Finland. Microperoxidase (MP11, sodium salt, from equine heart cytochrome c was purchased from Sigma Chemical Co., St. Louis, MO, United States; human and bovine serum albumin were from Behringwerke AG, Marburg, Federal Republic of Germany. Water and acetonitrile used for the HPLC were from Baker Co., Deventer, The Netherlands; trifluoroacetic acid, dimethylformamide, and reagents used for preparation of buffer and the alkaline peroxide solution were from Merck, Darmstadt, Federal Republic of Germany, and N-hydroxysuccinimide and dicyclohexylcarbodiimide were from Serva Feinbiochemica, Heidelberg, Federal Republic of Germany. Aqua pro injectione was obtained from Braun-Melsungen AG, Melsungen, Federal Republic of Germany. Protein A-agarose gel was from Bio-Rad Laboratories, Richmond, CA, United States.

Assay Buffer. This was phosphate buffer (67 mmol/liter, pH 7.4) containing 1 g sodium azide, 400 mg ethylenediaminetetraacetic acid (EDTA), and 1 g human serum albumin/liter.

Reagents for the Luminescent Reaction. The microperoxidase working solution was 5 µmol/liter microperoxidase in phosphate buffer (50 mmol/liter, pH 8.0), containing 400 mg bovine serum albumin, 5.84 g sodium chloride, and 1 g sodium azide/liter.

Alkaline Peroxide Solution. The final version contained 2 mol/liter sodium hydroxide and 625 µl/liter hydrogen peroxide. We freshly prepared this working solution by adding 100 µl of the 300 ml/liter hydrogen peroxide stock solution to 48 ml of the 2 mol/liter sodium hydroxide stock solution. The first version contained 330 mmol/liter sodium hydroxide with 10 ml/liter hydrogen peroxide and 0.1 mol/liter sodium chloride. We incubated the alkaline peroxide working solution for 30 min at room temperature.

Reagents for the Reverse-Phase HPLC. Eluant A was a 50-mmol/liter trifluoroacetic acid solution in HPLC-grade water; eluant B was acetonitrile.

Antisera

C-Terminal Antiserum. The antiserum R12 against the C-terminal part of PTH was obtained by immunizing rabbits with synthetic hPTH(53-84), which was covalently linked to bovine thyroglobulin. This antiserum bound specifically to the sequence 53-68 [2] and was diluted 150-fold in the assay buffer.

N-Terminal Antiserum. The antiserum Rm against the N-terminal part of the hormone was raised in rabbits using synthetic hPTH(1-34). This antiserum recognized the hPTH(1-34) fragment and did not recognize the fragments hPTH(28-48), hPTH(44-68), and hPTH(53-84).

Standards and Specimens

The standards were prepared by diluting the synthetic fragments hPTH(1-34), hPTH(1-44), hPTH(28-48), hPTH(44-68), hPTH(39-84), hPTH(53-84), and the intact hPTH in assay buffer containing 100 ml/liter hypoparathyroid serum. The hypoparathyroid serum was assayed in advance and contained no detectable amounts of intact hPTH. For the routine assay we prepared standards with concentrations of 0, 1, 4, 16, 32, 64, and 125 pmol/liter intact hPTH. All standards and sera and the EDTA-treated plasma samples were divided into 0.5-ml aliquots and stored at $-30\,°C$ until use.

Instrumentation

The light-generating reaction was carried out in the automatic luminescence analyzer LB 950 (Laboratorium Berthold, Wildbad, FRG). This computer-assisted analyzer allows fully automated measurement of up to 400 samples. Reverse-phase HPLC was performed using a radial pak liquid chromatography cartridge C_{18}, 5 μm, 8 mm ID. The column, radial compression separation system Model RCM-100, gradient controller Model 680, injection system Model U6K, and solvent delivery system Model 6000A were all purchased from Waters Associates, Milford, MA, United States.

Preparation of ABEI-H-Labeled hPTH(53-84)

To couple the label ABEI-H (molecular mass, 512.4) with hPTH(53-84), we first synthesized its succinimide ester by the method reported by Gadow et al. [7]. We dissolved 10 mg (27 μmol) ABEI-H in 800 μl dry dimethylformamide under slight warming. As soon as the solution had cooled down to room temperature, 3.1 mg (27 μmol) *N*-hydroxysuccinimide was added while stirring the mixture. Subsequently we added 16.7 mg (81 μmol) dicyclohexylcarbodiimide dissolved in 200 μl dry dimethylformamide and incubated the reaction mixture under light exclusion for 20 h at room temperature. This solution contained 27 μmol/ml activated ABEI-H.

   To couple hPTH(53-84), a molar ratio hPTH(53-84): ABEI-H active ester of 2:1 was chosen. A 14.23-mmol/liter hPTH(53-84) solution was prepared by dissolving 0.25 mg synthetic hPTH(53-84) in 0.5 ml of 67 mmol/liter phosphate buffer pH 7.4. To this solution (containing 71.1 nmol hPTH(53-84) we added 5.35 μl of the ABEI-H-active ester solution (containing 142.3 nmol activated ABEI-H) and incubated the reaction mixture for 24 h under light exclusion at

4°C. Subsequently, 250 µl of the reaction mixture was filled into a gas-tight syringe and subjected to HPLC.

Purification of Conjugates

Separation of unreacted components and different ABEI-H-labeled hPTH(53-84) conjugates was carried out by reverse-phase HPLC. We used a reverse-phase (radial pak cartridge C_{18}) concavely gradient chromatography of 5%–50% eluant B over 30 min at a flow rate of 1 ml/min. Seventy 0.5-ml fractions were mechanically collected in polypropylene tubes containing 1 ml assay buffer.

Firstly 70 µl phosphate buffer (67 mmol/liter, pH 7.4) containing 54 pmol ABEI-H-active ester was chromatographed. We pipetted 20 µl of each fraction in immunoassay vials (see Chapter 1.4, polystyrene type, volume 600 µl; Sarstedt, Nümbrecht, FRG) [17], and performed the light measurement as described below.

Subsequently, 250 µl of the coupling mixture was chromatographed and 10 µl of each fraction diluted in 10 ml phosphate buffer (67 mmol/liter, pH 7.4) for further investigation. We tested 50 µl of each diluted fraction for its luminescence activity as described below. The amount of immunoactive hPTH(53-84) of each fraction was determined with a radioimmunoassay (RIA) for hPTH(53-84). This assay was performed as described previously [18]. We performed three HPLC runs as described above. To prevent unsatisfactory separation of the ABEI-H-labeled hPTH(53-84) conjugates, which might be caused by overloading the used column, we did not subject more than 125 µg hPTH(53-84) to a single HPLC run.

Anti-hPTH(1-34) Solid Phase

The anti-hPTH(1-34) solid phase consisted of the N-terminal antibody coated to the polystyrene surface of the immunoassay vials.

Purification of Antibody. We first purified 40 ml of the antiserum Rm by affinity chromatography on protein A-agarose as described by Goding [8]. The antiserum was passed over a column of 50 ml protein A-agarose gel containing 2 mg protein A/ml wet gel (Fig. 1).

After washing the column with phosphate-buffered saline (PBS; 20 mmol/liter, pH 7.4) containing 7.59 g sodium chloride and 0.05 g merthiolate (thimerosal)/liter, the bound material was eluted with 0.58% (v:v) glacial acetic acid containing 8.76 g sodium chloride/liter (Fig. 2).

Subsequently the eluate was dialyzed against 4 liter buffer pH 9.3 containing 17.3 g sodium hydrogen carbonate and 8.6 g sodium carbonate/liter. 108.5 ml IgG fraction with a concentration of 4.85 g/liter was obtained. This solution was finally diluted 100-fold in aqua pro injectione. The pH of this salt-free, non-buffered aqueous IgG solution was between 9.0 and 9.5.

Immobilization of the N-Terminal Antibody. We adsorptively coated the N-terminal antibody onto the polystyrene surface of the immunoassay vials by

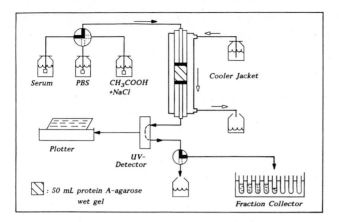

Fig. 1. One-step purification of IgG from whole rabbit serum. Rabbit serum (40 ml) against the N-terminal part of hPTH was passed over a column of protein A-agarose, washed with PBS and eluted with acetic acid. The protein A-agarose column was attached to an ultraviolet absorption detector and a fraction collector and was constantly cooled at 4 °C with cooling water

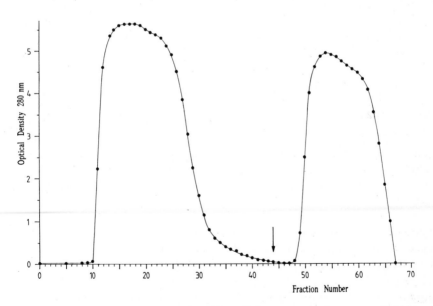

Fig. 2. Elution profile (OD_{280}) of rabbit IgG from protein A-agarose. Rabbit serum (40 ml) against the N-terminal part of hPTH was passed over a column of protein A-agarose and washed with PBS. The optical density at 280 nm (OD_{280}) of the effluent was continuously measured and fractions were collected every minute. After the plotter pen had returned to the baseline, the bound IgG was eluted with acetic acid (*arrow* marks start of elution). The flow rate was 6.2 ml/min

incubating 250-μl aliquots of the diluted IgG solution in each vial for 48 h at 4°C under slight shaking. The contents were aspirated and collected, and the vials were washed twice by adding 500 μl isotonic saline. Then 250 μl assay buffer was added containing 20 g/liter bovine serum albumin and incubation was performed for 2 h under the same conditions as described above. The vials were again washed twice and dried by centrifuging them upside down mounted on filter paper. Then the vials were closed with adhesive film and stored at − 20°C until use. Under these conditions the coated tubes were stable for at least 2 months.

Immunoluminometric Assay Procedure

Pipette 200-μl aliquots of the intact hPTH standards and samples in duplicate into the immunoassay vials coated with N-terminal antibody as described above, close the vials with adhesive film, and incubate for 24 h at 4°C. Aspirate the contents, wash the vials by adding 500 μl isotonic saline, mix, and again aspirate the content. Add 200 μl of the C-terminal antiserum, diluted 150-fold in assay buffer, close the vials, and incubate for 12 h at 4°C. Perform the same washing procedure and add 200 μl ABEI-H-labeled hPTH(53-84) stock solution, diluted 500-fold in assay buffer. This dilution contains approximately 1.35 nmol/liter ABEI-H-labeled hPTH(53-84). Incubate for 8 h at 4°C, wash three times as described to remove unbound ABEI-H-labeled hPTH(53-84), and perform the light measurement as described below.

For generation of the light output, add 200 μl of the microperoxidase working solution and fit the immunoassay vials into the 3.5-ml polystyrene tubes (No. 55 484, Sarstedt) of the sample chain of the luminescence analyzer. Initiate the light-producing reaction by automatic injection of 100 μl of the alkaline peroxide working solution (optimized version). Express the light emission as total photon counts and integrate over 24 s after initiation. At this time the reaction is at least 91% complete. Perform the light-measuring procedure at room temperature. To construct the assay standard curves, plot the concentration of the respective standard, in picomoles per liter, versus the mean photon counts over a 24-s integral, using linear scales.

Immunoradiometric Assay of Intact hPTH

We compared the results of the present assay by measuring the same samples with an IRMA of intact hPTH used for routine determination in our clinical laboratory, as described previously [2].

Results

Tracer Evaluation

Figure 3a shows the luminescence chromatogram of 0.2 μl ABEI-H activated ester solution, prepared as described above, consisting of at least six different

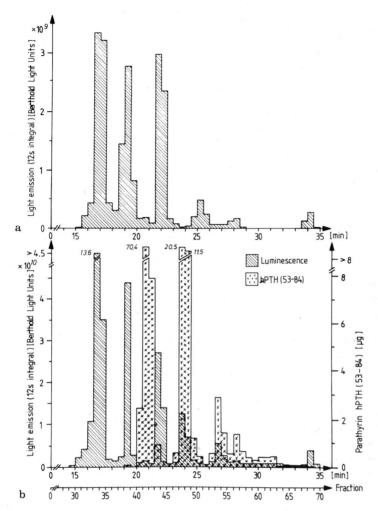

Fig. 3. a Luminescence chromatogram on a C_{18} reverse-phase HPLC of 5.3 nmol-activated ABEI-H. A concave gradient of 5%–50% acetonitrile in 50 mmol/liter tri-fluoroacetic acid solution in water was used with a flow rate of 1 ml/min over 30 min. **b** Luminescence chromatogram and immunoreactivity of hPTH(53-84) chromatogram. 250 μl coupling mixture containing 35.5 mmol hPTH(53-84) and 71.1 nmol activated ABEI-H in 67 mmol/liter phosphate buffer, pH 7.4, were used; performance in the same manner as in Fig. 1a. Fractions with luminescence above 4.5×10^{10} cps or with hPTH(53-84) amounts above 8 μg are indicated

luminescent compounds. The chromatogram of the immunoactivity for hPTH(53-84) and the luminescence of the reaction mixture are shown in Fig. 3b. Four peaks with immunoactive hPTH(53-84) were identified: the first (fractions 41-43) showed nearly no luminescence despite the high hPTH(53-84) level. The second (fractions 48, 49), third (fractions 54, 55) and fourth (fractions 57, 58) peaks showed good luminescence. Therefore we assumed the fractions 41-43 to

Table 1. Characteristics of the ABEI-H-labeled hPTH(53-84) conjugates

Fraction no.	R_f (min)	Incorporation molar ratio[a] (ABEI-H/hPTH(53-84)) Mean ± SD	Specific activity[b] (counts/mol label)
48 + 49	24.2	0.44 ± 0.007	2.06×10^{18}
54 + 55	27.2	1.63 ± 0.37	6.31×10^{18}
57	28·5	0.76 ± 0.10	3.17×10^{18}

[a] Calculated by two independent methods as described in the text
[b] Measured with the first version of the measuring procedure

consist of unlabeled hPTH(53-84), and the other three peaks to consist of differently labeled hPTH(53-84). We calculated the total amount of labeled hPTH(53-84) to be 36.0% by adding the measured amounts of fractions 45-64 and comparing them with the amount of hPTH(53-84) applied.

We estimated the incorporation of label into hPTH(53-84) for all three obtained peaks consisting of ABEI-H-labeled hPTH(53-84). The hPTH(53-84) content of each fraction was measured by RIA, and the ABEI-H contents of the respective fractions were calculated by comparing the light intensity of each single fraction with the total intensity of all fractions which represented the applied 71.1 nmol activated ABEI-H. To confirm this estimation, we again determined the ABEI-H concentration of each fraction containing labeled hPTH(53-84) by measuring the intensity of light emission, using different concentrations of activated ABEI-H as standards. Table 1 shows the incorporation ratios, defined as the molar ratio of ABEI-H to hPTH(53-84), as the mean ± SD of both calculations for each peak containing ABEI-H-labeled hPTH(53-84). Three different ABEI-H-labeled hPTH(53-84) conjugates were separated by HPLC.

The conjugates of fractions 54 and 55 appeared to have the highest incorporation ratio and were therefore used as the luminescent tracer for evaluation of the ILMA. We pooled fractions 54, 55, and the respective fractions of three additional HPLC runs performed in the same manner. The 9 ml stock solution obtained contained 675 nmol/liter ABEI-H-labeled hPTH(53-84) with an incorporation of 1.63 ± 0.37 mol ABEI-H/mol hPTH(53-84). Incorporation to this extent corresponded to a specific molar activity of 6.31×10^{18} counts /mol label, when measured with the first version of the measuring procedures described below. The ABEI-H-labeled hPTH(53-84) stock solution was stored at $-20\,°C$ for about 1 year without any significant loss of either immunological or luminescent activity.

Optimization of Light Measurement

We investigated several variables of the light-measuring procedure to obtain a wide dynamic range of the standard curve (i.e. difference between the response of

the 125 pmol/liter and the zero standard) and a maximum of sensitivity.
Increasing the sodium hydroxide concentration in the alkaline peroxide solution
up to 2 mol/liter led to a rise in light emission (Fig. 4).

To avoid any damage to the injection system by using higher sodium
hydroxide concentrations, 2 mol/liter was chosen as the working concentration.
Accordingly, the hydrogen peroxide was chosen as 625 µl/liter (Fig. 5).

We tested the light emission obtained by using different volume ratios of the
added microperoxidase solution and the injected alkaline peroxide solution.
Both volumes were varied from 50 to 350 µl, and the ratio found to generate the
highest dynamic range of the standard curve was 200 µl microperoxidase
solution : 100 µl alkaline solution (Fig. 6).

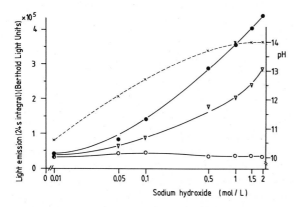

Fig. 4. Light emission of the standards 0(○———○), 64(▽———▽), and 125
(●———●) pmol/liter intact hPTH at different concentrations of sodium hydroxide in
the alkaline peroxide solution. The hydrogen peroxide concentration was constantly
625 µl/liter. The *dotted line* indicates the pH of the alkaline peroxide solutions

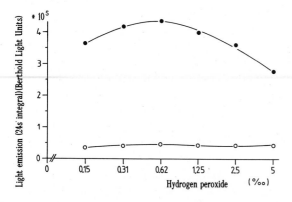

Fig. 5. Light emission of the standards 0 (○———○) and 125 (●———●) pmol/liter
intact hPTH at different concentrations of hydrogen peroxide in the alkaline peroxide
solution. The sodium hydroxide concentration was constantly 2 mol/liter

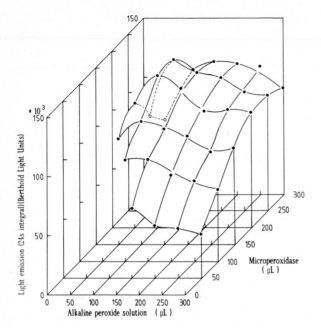

Fig. 6. Dynamic range of standard curve (difference between the light signal of the standards 125 and 0 pmol/liter intact hPTH) as a function of different volumes of the added microperoxidase solution and different volumes of the injected alkaline peroxide solution. The alkaline peroxide solution was 2 mol/liter sodium hydroxide containing 625 μl/liter hydrogen peroxide; the microperoxidase solution was 5 μmol/liter microperoxidase in phosphate buffer (50 mmol/liter, pH 8.0). Integration time was 12 s. Lines behind the perspective plane are indicated by *dotted lines*

Finally the integration time was chosen. The reaction kinetics of the 125 pmol/liter and of the zero standard showed that the maximum was reached at 1.33 s after injection of the alkaline peroxide solution with a half-maximum time of 5.33 s. The whole reaction was almost finished within 1 min. We chose to integrate the light signal from 0 to 24 s. This response represents 91% of the dynamic range obtained by integration from 0 to 60 s (Fig. 7).

These optimized measuring conditions were used for all light measurement, except for the evaluation of the luminescent tracer for which the nonoptimized measuring conditions were as follows: addition of 100 μl microperoxidase working solution diluted with 200 μl isotonic saline, injection of 350 μl alkaline peroxide working solution (first version) and integration of the light signal over 12 s.

This optimized measuring procedure led to a 37.7-fold increase of the specific molar activity of the tracer which was now 2.38×10^{20} counts/mol ABEI-H-labeled hPTH(53-84) over a 24-s integral. The background count rate was defined as the response obtained by performing the entire light-measuring procedure (including the addition of microperoxidase solution) with a plain

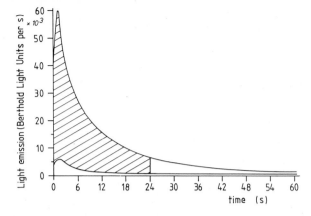

Fig. 7. Time course of the light signal obtained upon oxidation of the 125-pmol/liter standard (*upper curve*) and the zero standard (*lower curve*). The dynamic range of the standard curve obtained with integration over 24 s is represented by the *hatched area*

tube and usually ranged between 15 000 and 30 000 counts/24-s integral. The background was markedly dependent on the quality of the microperoxidase solution, which was stable for at least 1 month when stored at 4 °C.

Assay Development

We chose 4 °C as the incubation temperature for the coating of the N-terminal antibody and for all incubation steps of the assay procedure, except for the light measuring which was performed at room temperature. The influence of different incubation times of each assay phase on the standard curve is shown in Fig. 8.

Incubation or coating at room temperature led neither to a wider dynamic range of the standard curve nor to better sensitivity. Incubation of the vials with assay buffer containing 20 g/liter bovine serum albumin after coating decreased the nonspecific uptake of the label. Dose-response curves were generated using various concentrations of IgG solution of the N-terminal antiserum, C-terminal antiserum, and the ABEI-H-labeled-hPTH(53–84). All final conditions were chosen to obtain maximum sensitivity and steepness of standard curve.

Characteristics of ILMA for Intact hPTH

Immunoluminometric Assay Standard Curve. A typical standard curve for intact hPTH is shown in Fig. 9.

The nonspecific uptake of the label, defined as the difference between the response of the zero standard and the background count rate, was lower than 2% of the range of the standard curve and about 0.1% of the total activity added. Neither a "hook" effect nor a saturation of the anti-hPTH(1–34) solid phase was observed up to concentrations of 8000 pmol/liter intact hPTH.

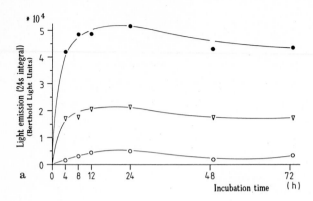

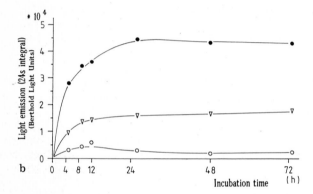

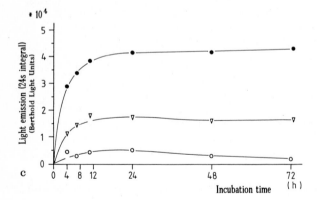

Fig. 8a–c. Kinetics of the ILMA: effect of different incubation times of the first **a**, second **b**, and third **c** assay phase on the light emission of the standards 0 (O———O), 32 (▽———▽), and 125 (●———●) pmol/liter intact hPTH. The incubation time of each assay phase was varied from 4 to 72 h while the incubation time of the other two phases was kept at 48 h. The incubation temperature was 4 °C

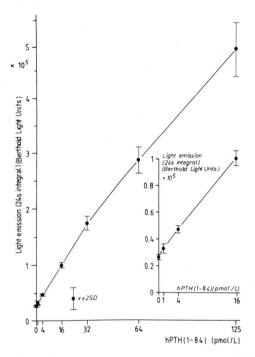

Fig. 9. Typical standard curve for intact hPTH obtained after subtraction of the background signal of 17 752 counts over a 24-s integral. Each point of the standard curve is the mean of six duplicate determinations. The zero standard gave a mean of 26 482 counts over a 24-s integral

Sensitivity. The lower limit of detection was defined as the minimal concentration of intact hPTH which could be distinguished from a sample containing no intact hPTH. Distinction was based on the confidence limits of the estimate of the zero standard. We calculated the 99.7% confidence limits of the zero estimate on the basis of 12 replicate determinations and ascertained the point where these confidence limits intersected the standard curve. The minimal detection limit determined in this manner was 0.5 pmol/liter (= 4.75 ng/liter).

Precision. We examined variance throughout the ILMA standard curve by assaying each standard sixfold in duplicate and calculating the coefficient of variation (*CV*) and the standard deviation (SD) for each standard. Figure 10 depicts the assay SD, which declines to approximately 0.2 pmol/liter at low concentrations of intact hPTH. The total measurement *CV*s are 15.3% or less for intact hPTH concentrations of 1 pmol/liter or greater. The intraassay variance was assessed by performing 22 replicate determinations of 2 sera from healthy persons, 2 sera from patients with primary hyperparathyroidism, and 1 serum from a patient with hypoparathyroidism. The interassay variance was assessed by analyzing aliquots of three sera from a healthy person, a patient with

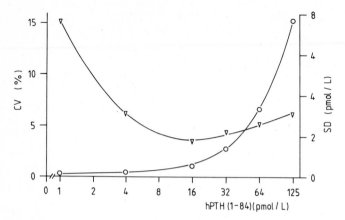

Fig. 10. Precision profile of the ILMA. Each standard was assayed six times in duplicate. The SD of the ILMA (○———○) declined to 0.2 pmol/liter at low concentrations of hPTH(1-84). Total measurement *CV*s (▽———▽) were also calculated

Table 2. Assay precision

Sample	Intact hPTH(pmol) Mean ± SD		CV(%)
Interassay (n = 7)			
Hypoparathyroid serum	< 0.5ᵃ		–
Normal serum	3.5 ± 0.41		11.5
Hyperparathyroid serum	33.1 ± 3.70		11.1
Intraassay (n = 22)			
Hypoparathyroid serum	< 0.5ᵇ		–
Normal serum 1	3.4 ± 0.39		11.4
Normal serum 2	3.1 ± 0.43		13.8
Hyperparathyroid serum 1	27.6 ± 1.60		5.7
Hyperparathyroid serum 2	11.9 ± 1.76		14.7

ᵃ For hypoparathyroid serum, three determinations were below the limit of detection and four determinations ranged from 0.7 to 1.2 pmol/liter with a mean of 0.8 pmol/liter
ᵇ For the hypoparathyroid serum all values were below the limit of detection, except one, which was 0.9 pmol/liter

hypoparathyroidism, and a patient with primary hyperparathyroidism in duplicate in seven consecutive assays. Intra- and interassay variations are shown in Table 2.

Specificity. To prove that only the intact hormone was measured we examined the ILMA for its cross-reactivity with several synthetic hPTH fragments. We assayed different concentrations of hPTH(1-44), hPTH(44-68), hPTH(39-84), and hPTH(53-84), ranging from 64 to 8000 pmol/liter. None of these fragments showed an increase in bound activity.

Interference with hPTH Fragments. Since circulating hPTH fragments are present in specimens we investigated the influence of diverse synthetic hPTH fragments on the detection of intact hPTH. We added different amounts of hPTH(1-44), hPTH(44-68), hPTH(39-84), and hPTH(53-84) to a standard containing 32 pmol/liter intact hPTH. No influence on the detection of intact hPTH was observed by the C-terminal and the midregional fragments at concentrations up to 4000 pmol/liter, and by the N-terminal fragment at concentrations up to 250 pmol/liter.

Linearity. We serially diluted two sera of patients with primary hyperparathyroidism with the zero standard medium (assay buffer containing 100 ml/liter hypoparathyroid serum). The intact PTH concentrations of the undiluted sera were 14.4 and 100.5 pmol/liter. We used linear regression analysis to establish correlations (Fig. 11). Both dilution experiments gave a linear response up to 14.4 and 100.5 pmol/liter, respectively.

Analytical Recovery. We added different known amounts of synthetic intact hPTH to a serum and an EDTA-treated plasma sample, both from patients with surgically proven primary hyperparathyroidism. Subsequently we measured the

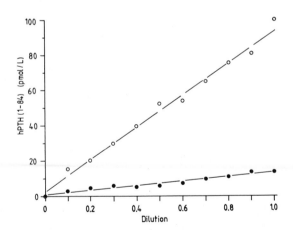

Fig. 11. Dilution of two hyperparathyroid sera containing 100.5 pmol/liter ($\bigcirc$—$\bigcirc$) and 14.4 pmol/liter ($\bullet$——$\bullet$) intact hPTH, each serially diluted in zero standard medium and then assayed. Regression of the dilution versus the measured intact hPTH concentration yielded the regression equations $y = 2.14$ pmol/liter $+ 92.34 x$ ($n = 11$, $r = 0.995$) for the serum containing 100.5 pmol/liter intact hPTH and $y = 0.85$ pmol/liter $+ 12.96x$ ($n = 11$, $r = 0.970$) for the serum containing 14.4 pmol/liter intact hPTH

total amount of intact hPTH in duplicate to assess the analytical recovery. Percentage recovery was calculated by subtracting the endogenous intact hPTH from the measured total amount, divided by the amount added and multiplied by 100. The mean recovery was 100.8% ($n = 11$; SD 25.2%) (Fig. 12).

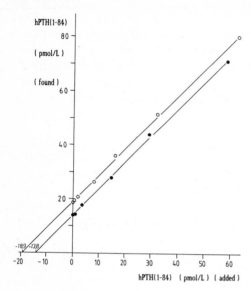

Fig. 12. Analytical recovery. Different known amounts of synthetic intact hPTH were added to a serum sample (○——○) and an EDTA-treated plasma sample (●——●), both from patients with primary hyperparathyroidism. The added and the found amounts of intact hPTH are shown

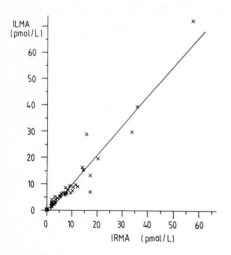

Fig. 13. Correlation between intact hPTH concentrations in human serum as measured by the present ILMA and an immunoradiometric assay (IRMA). ILMA = − 1.36 pmol/liter + 1.12 IRMA, $r = 0.96$, $n = 42$, $P < 0.001$

Correlation with IRMA. We measured intact hPTH concentrations in 42 samples by the present ILMA (y) and by an immunoradiometric assay method (x) (Fig. 13). The relationship was calculated by linear regression analysis and described by the equation:

$$y = -1.36 \text{ pmol/liter} + 1.12x \ (n = 42, r = 0.96, P < 0.001)$$

The intact hPTH values ranged from 0 to 72 pmol/liter ILMA. For samples with intact hPTH values below 5.9 pmol/liter (representing the normal range) the regression equation was:

$$y = -1.79 \text{ pmol/liter} + 0.98x \ (n = 20, r = 0.91, P < 0.001).$$

Clinical Results

All concentrations of intact hPTH measured in specimens from normal subjects and patients are shown in Fig. 14.

Normal Range. The intact hPTH concentration was determined in samples from 37 healthy adults. Intact hPTH was detectable in all samples, with a mean of 3.87 pmol/liter and a median of 3.8 pmol/liter. Omitting the highest and lowest detected values we defined the normal interval as 1.8 to 5.9 pmol/liter intact hPTH.

Hyperparathyroid Subjects. Fifty-six patients with surgically proven primary hyperparathyroidism had elevated serum levels of intact hPTH, except one patient, whose intact hPTH value of 5.9 pmol/liter was at the upper limit of the normal interval. The intact hPTH values of this group ranged from 5.9 to 113 pmol/liter, with a mean of 22.0 pmol/liter and a median of 16.1 pmol/liter.

Eight patients with presumed primary hyperparathyroidism (not surgically proven) had elevated serum levels of intact hPTH, ranging from 6.0 to 48.4 pmol/liter (mean 16.6; median 11.6). Additionally we tested 22 patients with primary hyperparathyroidism after they had undergone surgical exploration. Parathyroid adenoma or hyperplasia was found in all cases, and all specimens were collected at least 2 days after surgical exploration. Nine patients of this group had intact hPTH levels within the normal range, eight had levels below the normal range, and five showed remarkably elevated intact hPTH levels.

Hypoparathyroid Subjects. We assayed serum samples from six patients with idiopathic hypoparathyroidism. All measured intact hPTH levels were below the lower limit of the normal interval. Two patients had values of 0.6 and 0.7 pmol/liter, and four patients had no detectable amount of intact hPTH.

Patients with Transplanted Kidneys. Twenty-nine serum samples from patients with kidney transplants, none of them receiving hemodialysis, were studied. The intact hPTH values obtained were widely spread from 2.9 to 98 pmol/liter

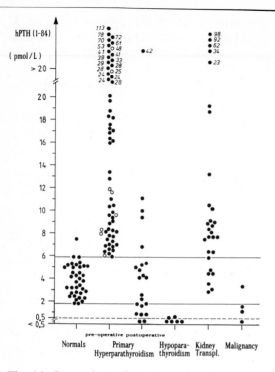

Fig. 14. Comparison of the intact hPTH concentrations measured in samples of 37 healthy volunteers, 64 patients with primary hyperparathyroidism [56 surgically proven (●); 8 presumed (○)], 22 patients with surgically proven primary hyperparathyroidism but measured 2 days after successful surgical exploration, 6 patients with idiopathic hypoparathyroidism, 29 patients with transplanted kidneys, and 4 patients with malignancy-associated hypercalcemia. The minimal detection limit is indicated by the *dotted line*. The normal interval from 1.8 to 5.9 pmol/liter is marked off by the *continuous lines*. Points indicating values above 20 pmol/liter are shown with their respective concentration

(mean 17.5; median 8.1). Only seven patients of this group had intact hPTH values within the normal interval whereas 22 patients showed elevated levels.

Patients with Malignancy-Associated Hypercalcemia. Four patients with malignancy-associated hypercalcemia had mostly intact hPTH levels below the normal interval except for one value of 3.4 pmol/liter.

Rapid Calcium Infusion Test. We performed a calcium infusion test in a patient with surgically proven hyperparathyroidism. The serum intact hPTH concentration was measured before and every 2.5 min after intravenous infusion of 10 ml calcium 10%. The result is shown in Fig. 15.

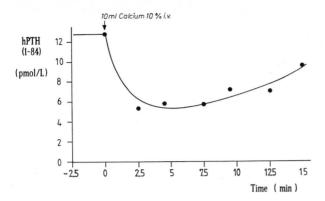

Fig. 15. Rapid calcium infusion test in a patient with primary hyperparathyroidism (surgically proven). The calcium infusion test was performed only in patients with serum calcium levels below 3.0 mmol/liter

Discussion

Radioimmunoassays are widely used for measuring circulating fragments of PTH [1] but except for one two-site ILMA using an acridinium ester-labeled antibody [3], all assays of intact hPTH make use of ^{125}I-labeled proteins as tracer [2, 9, 11, 15].

These assays all suffer from the well-known disadvantages of ^{125}I-labeled tracers: contact with radioactive material, short tracer half-life, and instability due to radiolytic damage of the labeled protein. Furthermore, long counting times are required to achieve sufficient sensitivity. For these reasons, many nonisotopic labels have been developed and investigated for their use in immunoassays, but most of them have failed to yield assays with the sensitivity attainable by the use of ^{125}I [26].

Luminescent labels have proved to be efficient in terms of both specificity and sensitivity and are therefore suitable for replacing radioisotopes as labels [22]. Many chemiluminescent labels and their use in labeling proteins have been described in the literature [7, 13, 20], but only few reports describe the preparation of tracer peptides of low molecular weight [25]. We used ABEI-H because it is commercially available, shows good luminescence, and also because its active ester can be synthesized without requiring much expertise [7]. For the synthesis of ABEI-H-labeled hPTH(53-84), N-hydroxysuccinimide was used. This method has proven to be far superior to alternative coupling reagents because the succinimide ester reacts with the amino moieties of the peptide under nonoxidative conditions and therefore the immunoreactivity of the tracer is mostly retained [7, 25].

The succinimide ester of ABEI-H binds to the lysine amino groups of the polypeptidic chain. The hPTH(53-84) molecule, however, has only six lysine amino groups, thus limiting the number of possibly incorporated luminescent labels. Furthermore, the small size of hPTH(53-84) increases the possibility that incorporation of the luminescent label will affect the immunoreactivity of the PTH fragment. Therefore we chose a molar ratio of hPTH(53-84) to ABEI-H active ester that was half as much as the corrected substitution ratio recommended by Gadow et al. [7]. Different techniques for the purification of ^{125}I-labeled hPTH fragments and other ^{125}I-labeled peptide hormones have been described, but none of them has been investigated for its practicability for purifying luminescent-labeled hPTH fragments [5, 6, 10, 19, 21, 24]. An easily performed method is reverse-phase chromatography using Sep-Pak C_{18} cartridges, but even this method does not remove the unlabeled peptide. Reverse-phase HPLC has been recommended because it gives the best purification of the tracer by separating labeled from unlabeled peptide [19].

In our experience this method has proved to be an excellent one for purifying ABEI-H-labeled hPTH(53-84): reverse-phase HPLC not only separated free ABEI-H-active ester from ABEI-H-labeled hPTH(53-84) but also ABEI-H-labeled hPTH(53-84) from native hPTH(53-84). Moreover, different ABEI-H-labeled hPTH(53-84) conjugates with differing molar incorporation of luminescent label were isolated without any overlap. Thus we obtained a highly purified tracer peptide with a high specific activity.

The amount of purified ABEI-H-labeled hPTH(53-84) obtained by four HPLC runs was sufficient to perform about 22 500 single determinations of intact hPTH. HPLC is therefore also an economical method for producing large amounts of luminescent tracer. So far it has not been possible to purify labeled antibodies directly in a manner comparable to that achieved with the hPTH(53-84) label because of its low molecular weight (3512 vs approximately 150 000). We even succeeded in separating tracer fractions with different molar label incorporations, thus increasing the assay sensitivity. In contrast, directly labeled antibodies are a mixture of proteins with various label incorporation ratios, and our antiserum would have required affinity chromatography purification before being labeled because it had a low titer.

Compared to other published assays of intact PTH [2, 3, 15], the performance of this assay was simplified by coating the N-terminal antibody at the surface of the immunoassay vials. This method was suitable after purification of the N-terminal antiserum by affinity chromatography on protein A-agarose. Thus centrifugation steps were replaced by more rapid and cost-effective washing, aspiration or decantation steps. We used isotonic saline as washing solution, and no nonionic detergents, to avoid removal of the adsorbed antibody from the surface of the polystyrene vial. The small nonspecific uptake of the tracer proved that isotonic saline was a satisfactory washing solution. Chemiluminescent reaction conditions were optimized to promote maximum total light output, resulting in increased sensitivity. For this benefit we accepted slower light reaction kinetics.

Due to the specific architecture of the present ILMA, the term "intact hPTH" refers to all PTH molecules that possess both the N-terminal and the C-terminal part of the hPTH, i.e. only hPTH molecules prior to cleavage in region 34-37 [12] will be recognized by the present ILMA. Accordingly, no cross-reaction was found with synthetic hPTH(1-44), hPTH(44-68), hPTH(39-84), and hPTH (53-84) fragments in concentrations of up to 8000 pmol/liter.

The first step of the present ILMA extracts intact hPTH and N-terminal hPTH fragments. All other circulating substances, including C-terminal and midregional fragments, are eliminated. Therefore no interference was observed when synthetic hPTH(44-68), hPTH(39-84), and hPTH(53-84) up to 4000 pmol/liter were added. No interference was found by adding synthetic hPTH(1-44) up to 250 pmol/liter; at higher concentrations, however, the N-terminal antibody of the solid phase became increasingly saturated. Neverthe-less it is unlikely that the measurement of intact hPTH by the present ILMA will be interfered with by circulating N-terminal fragments since it was shown that these fragments reach only low circulating levels [14, 16].

The use of highly purified ABEI-H-labeled hPTH(53-84) as tracer led to a high signal-to-noise ratio which resulted in a high sensitivity and a high precision of the ILMA. Another benefit of this tracer was the faster kinetics of the indirect labeling of the C-terminal antibody, which shortened the total incubation time to 48 h, two-thirds of the total incubation time required if ^{125}I-labeled Tyr^{52}-hPTH(53-84) is used as tracer [2]. Because of the linearity of samples containing up to 100 pmol/liter intact hPTH and the absence of a high-dose-hook effect it was not necessary to repeat measurements of diluted samples containing large amounts of intact hPTH.

The levels of intact hPTH in normal subjects, as measured by different assays, are remarkably similar. On the other hand, reference intervals differ slightly in different laboratories, even with the same assay; the commercially available Allegro Intact hPTH kit (Nichols Institute Diagnostics, San Juan Capistrano, CA, United States) suggests a normal range from 1.1 to 5.8 pmol/liter, whereas Nussbaum et al. [15] have defined a normal range from 1.3 to 6.9 pmol/liter in 72 healthy subjects with the same assay, and Sokoll et al. [23] have determined a normal range from 1.5 to 6.8 pmol/liter based on 245 healthy postmenopausal women. The reference interval of the commercially available IRMA of intact hPTH (Immundiagnostik GmbH, Bensheim, FRG) developed in our clinical laboratory [2] ranged from 1.9 to 6.8 pmol/liter in 60 healthy persons, with a normal interval of 2.0 to 6.3 pmol/liter. Thus the normal range of the present ILMA (1.8–5.9 pmol/liter) is similar to those described above, and the mean of the normal range (3.8 pmol/liter) is similar to the values reported by Lindall et al. [11] (4.8 pmol/liter) and Brown et al. [3] (3.4 pmol/liter).

The intact hPTH values of patients with surgically proven primary hyper-parathyroidism were above the normal range and completely different from those of normal subjects, patients with idiopathic hypoparathyroidism, and patients with malignancy-associated hypercalcemia. The elevated intact hPTH levels of 20% of the patients after successful surgical exploration might have been due to the immense deficiency of calcium in bone, especially if their primary hyperparathyroidism had been of long standing.

In conclusion, a two-site immunochemiluminometric assay for intact hPTH is described. A solid-phase antibody directed against the N-terminal part of hPTH was adsorptively immobilized onto the polystyrene surface of the assay vial and extracted the intact hPTH and N-terminal fragments. Another antibody against synthetic hPTH(53-84) bound to the C-terminal part of intact hPTH and was indirectly labeled at its second free binding site with luminescent hPTH(53-84). This was synthetic hPTH(53-84) conjugated via succinimide linkage to ABEI-H. Purification of the labeled hPTH(53-84) by reverse-phase HPLC allowed the isolation of the conjugate with the highest incorporation ratio of 1.6 mol ABEI-H/mol hPTH(53-84). The assay has a detection limit of 0.5 pmol/liter, is accurate, precise and reliable and shows linearity for samples containing up to 100 pmol/liter. The normal interval ranged from 1.8 to 5.9 pmol/liter; 56 patients with surgically proven primary hyperparathyroidism presented levels ranging from 5.9 to 113 pmol/liter. The levels detected in patients with idiopathic hypoparathyroidism or malignancy-associated hypercalcemia were below the normal range.

References

1. Armitage EK (1986) Parathyrin (parathyroid hormone): metabolism and methods for assay [review]. Clin Chem 32:418–424
2. Blind E, Schmidt-Gayk H, Armburster FP, Stadler A (1987) Measurement of intact human parathyrin by an extracting two-site immunoradiometric assay. Clin Chem 33:1376–1381
3. Brown RC, Aston JP, Weeks I, Woodhead JS (1987) Circulating intact parathyroid hormone measured by a two-site immunochemiluminometric assay. J Clin Endocrinol Metab 65:407–414
4. Catt KJ, Tregear GW (1967) Solid phase radioimmunoassay in antibody coated tubes. Science 158:1570–1571
5. Christie DL, Barling PM (1978) Isolation of iodinated bovine parathyroid hormone using ion exchange: demonstration of its immunological characteristics and biological activity. Endocrinology 103:204–211
6. Englebienne P, Doyen G (1982) Radioiodinated hormones purified by hydrophobic interaction chromatography. Clin Chem 28:2189–2190
7. Gadow A, Fricke H, Strasburger CJ, Wood WG (1984) Synthesis and evaluation of luminescent tracers and hapten-protein conjugates for use in luminescence immunoassays with immobilized antibodies and antigens. J Clin Chem Clin Biochem 22:337–347
8. Goding JW (1976) Conjugation of antibodies with fluorochromes: modifications to the standard methods. J Immunol Methods 13:215–226
9. Hackeng WHL, Lips P, Netelenbos JC, Lips CJM (1986) Clinical implications of estimation of intact parathyroid hormone (PTH) versus total immunoreactive PTH

in normal subjects and hyperparathyroid patients. J Clin Endocrinol Metab 63:447–453

10. Janaky T, Toth G, Penke B, Kovacs K, Laszlo FA (1982) Iodination of peptide hormones and purification of iodinated peptides by HPLC. J Liquid Chromatogr 5:1499–1507

11. Lindall AW, Elting J, Ells J, Roos BA (1983) Estimation of biologically active intact parathyroid hormone in normal and hyperparathyroid sera by sequential N-terminal immunoextraction and midregion radioimmunoassay. J Clin Endocrinol Metab 57:1007–1014

12. Martin KJ, Hruska KA, Freitag JJ, Klahr S, Slatopolsky E (1979) The peripheral metabolism of parathyroid hormone. N Engl J Med 301:1092–1098

13. Messeri G, Schroeder HR, Caldini AL, Orlando C (1986) Synthesis of cheminolumic conjugates with dimethyladipimidate for sensitive immunoassays. Methods Enzymol 133:557–568

14. Newman DJ, Thakkar H, Ashby JP (1987) Clinical utility of region-specific parathyroid hormone assays in the investigation of hypercalcemia. Ann Clin Biochem 24 [Suppl 1]: 150–151

15. Nussbaum SR, Zahradnik RJ, Lavigne JR, Brennan GL, Nozawa-Ung K, Kim LY, Keutmann HT, Wang C, Potts JT Jr, Segre GV (1987) Highly sensititive two-site immunoradiometric assay of parathyrin, and its clinical utility in evaluating patients with hypercalcemia. Clin Chem 33:1364–1367

16. Papapoulos SE, Manning RM, Hendy GN, Lewin IG, O'Riordan JLH (1980) Studies of circulating parathyroid hormone in man using a homologous amino-terminal specific immunoradiometric assay. Clin Endocrinol (Oxf) 13:57–67

17. Schmidt-Gayk, Wahl HM, Limbach HJ, Walch S (1979) Ein spezielles Gefäß zur Durchführung des Radioimmunoassay (RIA). Medizintechnik 99:103–104

18. Schmidt-Gayk H, Schmitt-Fiebig M, Hitzler W, Armbruster FP, Mayer E (1986) Two-homologous radioimmunoassays for parathyrin compared and applied to disorders of calcium metabolism. Clin Chem 32:57–62

19. Schöneshöfer M, Kage A, Kage R, Fenner A (1982) A convenient technique for specific isolation of ^{125}I-labeled peptide molecules. Fresenius Z Anal Chem 311:429–40

20. Schroeder HR, Boguslaski RC, Carrico RJ, Buckler RT (1978) Monitoring specific protein binding reactions with chemiluminescence. In: De Luca MA (ed) Bioluminescence and Chemiluminescence. Methods Enzymol 57:424–445

21. Seidah NG, Dennis M, Corvol P, Rochemont J, Chretien M (1984) A rapid high-performance-liquid-chromatography purification method of iodinated polypetide hormones. Acta Endocrinol (copenh) 107:60–69

22. Seitz WR (1984) Immunoassay labels based on chemiluminescence and biolumin-escence. Clin Biochem 17:120–124

23. Sokoll LJ, Morrow FD, Quirbach DM, Dawson-Hughes B (1988) Intact parathyrin in postmenopausal women. Clin Chem 34:407–410

24. Stuart MC, Boscato LM, Underwood PA (1983) Use of immunoaffinity chromato-graphy for purification of ^{125}I-labeled human prolactin. Clin Chem 29:241–245

25. Tode B, Messeri G, Bassi F, Pazzagli M, Serio M (1987) Chemiluminescence immunoassay for somatomedin C in serum. Clin Chem 33:1989–1993

26. Weeks I, Sturgess ML, Woodhead JS (1986) Chemiluminescence immunoassay: an overview [review]. Clin Sci 70:403–408

27. Woodhead JS, Addison GM, Hales CN (1974) The immunoradiometric assay and related techniques. Br Med Bull 30:44–49

Chapter 2.10

A Sensitive Adenylate Cyclase Bioassay for Parathyroid Hormone

H. Scharfenstein

Adenylate Cyclase System

A large number of substances such as dopamine, secretin, prostaglandin E_2, β-adrenergic catecholamines, and parathyroid hormone (PTH) activate adenylate cyclase by interacting with appropriate endogenous ligands on the cell surface. These interactions ultimately result in stimulation of adenylate cyclase activity and thus in an increase of cAMP production. Prostaglandin F_2 and α_2-adrenergic substances, however, lower the cAMP level by inhibiting adenylate cyclase.

Mechanism of Adenylate Cyclase Regulation

All hormone-sensitive adenylate cyclases are complex systems with multiple functions and several sites of regulation. The system consists of three main components (see Fig. 1).

- The hormone receptor (R), which binds the hormone.
- The guanine-nucleotide-binding regulatory proteins (G_s and G_i), which combine the receptor with the catalytic unit.
- The catalytic unit (C) or adenylate cyclase in the narrow sense, which catalyzes ATP to cAMP in the presence of Mg^{2+}.

There are stimulatory and inhibitory receptors. The stimulatory receptors include those for β-adrenergic agonists, adrenocorticotropic hormone (ACTH), gonadotropins, PTH and many others, while inhibitory control is exerted by such agents as α_2-adrenergic and muscarinic agonists, and opioids [1].

Each receptor has a G-protein which either has stimulatory (G_s) or inhibitory (G_i) functions. The G-proteins control the activity of the actual catalyst, the catalytic unit. G_s and G_i consist of nonidentical subunits (α, β, δ). G_s and G_i have the same β- and δ-subunits with molecular weights of 45 000 and 10 000, respectively. The α-subunits with the guanine nucleotide-binding sites, however, are different. The whole G_s-protein has a molecular weight of about 45 000, while that of the G_i-protein is 41 000. The activation of G_s, caused by hormone

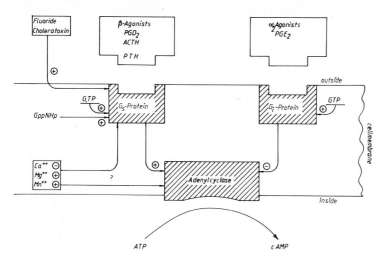

Fig. 1. Adenylate cyclase model. Part of the plasma membrane is shown, in which the adenylate cyclase is localized. (According to Gilman and Auf'mkolk [28])

binding at the stimulatory receptor is followed by the release of an α-subunit. The α-subunit probably activates the catalytic unit. The mechanism for the inhibition of the system by G_i has not yet been elucidated. There is no doubt that guanosine triphosphate (GTP) plays an important role in this process. GTP and its nonhydrolysable analogue guanylimidodiphosphate (GppNHp) probably adheres to the α-subunit of the G-protein and activates it. Because GppNHp is resistant to hydrolysis it can permanently activate the catalytic unit [1, 2]. The same result can be achieved by cholera toxin which decreases GTPase activity [3]. The third component, the catalytic unit, has not been selectively isolated as yet. But it can be separated from the G-proteins without loss of function [4].

Cyclic AMP: Mode of Action

Cyclic AMP mediates its effect inside the cell by activating protein kinases which in turn phosphorylate a large number of substances. The activation mechanism results from the adhesion of cAMP to regulatory subunits with the consequent release of catalytic subunits.

Cyclic AMP: Metabolism

Intracellular cAMP is quickly hydrolyzed to 5'AMP and phosphate by phosphodiesterases. These enzymes have been detected in the cytoplasm as well as in the membrane fractions. The phosphodiesterases are controlled by calmodulin and calcium [5].

Adenylate Cyclase Assay for Human Parathyroid Hormone

Human serum contains different fragments of human parathyroid hormone (hPTH). Because, in a radioimmunological assay, antisera for hPTH may react even with fragments, the specificity of the measurement might be lowered [6]. In addition, the detection of a fragment in a radioimmunoassay (RIA) does not give any information about the biological activity of this fragment. The RIA is not suitable for distinguishing between biologically active and inactive hPTH. In 1967 Chase and Aurbach discovered that adenylate cyclase in the renal cortex can be stimulated by hPTH [7]. Marcus and Aurbach later succeeded in performing an in vitro bioassay for hPTH [8]:

- Isolation of adenylate cyclase from the cell membranes of the renal cortex
- Incubation of the membranes with substrate (ATP) and hPTH, in which ATP is converted into cAMP
- Measurement of the cAMP produced

The first isolation of adenylate cyclase from rat kidneys was described by Marcus and Aurbach [9]. This was followed by publications about the isolation of the enzyme from bovine [10–12], chicken [13–15], canine [16], rabbit [17], and porcine [18] tissues.

The PTH-responsible adenylate cyclase is localized in the cortical nephron [19] and probably in the glomerulus [20]. The adenylate cyclase of the cortical membranes is highly specific for PTH. To achieve the same stimulation effect of PTH with other stimulatory agonists, the concentration of this agent must be much higher than the concentration of hPTH: 5000 times higher for vasopressin, calcitonin, and glucagon, and even 500 000 times higher for epinephrine than the concentration of hPTH [2].

The aim of this study was to develop a highly sensitive adenylate cyclase assay for hPTH and to monitor the isolation of hPTH from human adenomas.

Incubation

Apart from adenylate cyclase, ATP and hPTH, the incubation systems include the following reagents:

An ATP-regenerating system consisting of creatine phosphate and creatine kinase. Although ATP is added in surplus, a cumulation of AMP is avoided. 3-Isobutyl-1-methylxanthine (Mix) inhibits the phosphodiesterase which reduces cAMP to AMP. Magnesium is an important cation in the process of activating phosphohydrolases such as adenylate cyclase. Mg^{2+} is a component of the $MgATP^{2-}$ complex and thus a necessary cofactor for PTH-sensitive adenylate cyclase [8]. While Mg^{2+} stimulates the adenylate cyclase system [21], Ca^{2+} is an inhibitor [22]. To avoid the negative influence of calcium, ethylene glycol tetraacetic acid (EGTA) is added. Hunt et al. have shown that the K_m for PTH was decreased eight times by the addition of GppNHp, the nonhydrolysable analogue of GTP [24]. After incubation the amount of cAMP produced is related to the concentration of PTH added to the incubation. cAMP can be measured by cAMP-binding assay.

Materials

The following materials were used: a Beckman L 2-65 B centrifuge with a JA 20 rotor; a Beckman L 5-65 centrifuge with a Ti 60 Beckman rotor; a Beta-counter (Liquid Scintillation Systems LS, Beckman 8000 Munich, FRG); a Biofuge B centrifuge (Heraeus-Christ); filters, size 0.45 μm and 0.2 μm (Schleicher & Schüll, Dassel, FRG); a Hamilton repeating dispenser (Deutsche Hamilton, Darmstadt, FRG); a C12927 homogenizer (Thomas, Philadelphia, United States); Pharmacia columns K9/30 and K26/40 (Pharmacia, Uppsala, Sweden); a Sorvall RC 2B centrifuge with SS 24 and SS 34 rotors; and an Ultra-Turrax homogenizer (Janke & Kunkel, Staufen, FRG).

Reagents

The following reagents were used: Affi-Gel (cat. No. 153–6046 Bio-Rad, Munich, FRG); cAMP (Amersham, Braunschweig, cat. No. 102300 Boehringer, Mannheim, FRG); [³H]cAMP; ATP (cat. No. 126888, Boehringer, Mannheim, FRG); creatine kinase (cat. No. 127566, Boehringer, Mannheim, FRG); creatine phosphate (cat. No. 126977, Boehringer, Mannheim, FRG); EGTA (Merck, Darmstadt, FRG); GTP (cat. No. 106372, Boehringer, Mannheim, FRG); GppNHp (cat. No. 106402, Boehringer, Mannheim, FRG); Mix (cat. No. 26445, Serva, Heidelberg, FRG); Percoll (Pharmacia, Uppsala, Sweden); hPTH(1-34) (Bachem, Bubendorf, Switzerland); and Sephadex-G 15 (Pharmacia, Uppsala, Sweden).

Preparation of Membranes

Buffer A contained 50 mM Tris/HCl, 1 mM EDTA, and 0.25 M sucrose, at pH 7.4. Buffer B contained 50% Percoll, 50 mM Tris/HCl, 1 mM EDTA, and 0.25 M sucrose, at pH 7.4. Percoll is a medium for density gradient centrifugation of cells and subcellular particles being composed of colloidal silica coated with polyvinylpyrrolidone (PVP). The centrifugation of Percoll results in the spontaneous formation of a density gradient due to the heterogeneity of the particle sizes in the medium.

Fresh bovine renal cortex was prepared as described by Marx et al. and Mohr and Hesch [25, 11]. All solutions were kept at 4 °C. The bovine kidneys were obtained from a local slaughterhouse and deep frozen during transport. Cortex slides were cut off from the organs and suspended in the same amount of buffer A. The tissue was minced by a short burst with the Ultra Turrax homogenizer. The suspension was further homogenized in a homogenizer until no solid particles could be seen. The homogenate was diluted in the same amount of buffer A. This crude homogenate was placed in the SS 34 rotor of a Sorvall RC-2B centrifuge at 4 °C. As soon as the motor reached 4500 rpm it was turned off. The supernatant fluid was decanted and the pellet, containing unhomogenized tissue, red blood cells, and nuclei, was discarded. This centrifugation was repeated twice more. The supernatant fluid was then centrifuged at 4500 rpm for 15 min. The supernant fluid, now containing mitochondria, microsomes, and lipid, was discarded and the upper portion of the resulting double-layered pellet was resuspended in chilled buffer A by gentle swirling. This suspension was rehomogenized and again centrifuged at 4500 rpm for 15 min. The resulting pellet was suspended in 30 ml buffer A and then mixed with 20 ml buffer B. This suspension was centrifuged at 15 000 rpm in the Beckman L2-65 B centrifuge with a JA 20 rotor. The membrane fraction appeared as a fluffy band near the top of the resulting gradient and was isolated with the aid of a Pasteur pipette. The membranes were diluted in 50 ml buffer A and centrifuged for 10 min at 10 000 rpm., thereby rinsing out the percoll. This centrifugation was repeated. The resulting pellet was diluted with buffer A so that a final concentration of 2 mg protein/ml was obtained. (The yield of membranes was about 1% of the wet cortex tissue.) The solution was homogenized and stored in 500-µl portions at − 70 °C.

Incubation System of the Adenylate Cyclase Assay

The incubation system consisted of ATP (1.8 mM), MgCl$_2$ (5 mM) Mix (1 mM), EGTA (1.25 mM), GppNHp (100 nM or 1 µM), creatine kinase (0.1 mg), creatine phosphate (0.5 mg), and bovine serum albumin (BSA) (0.2 mg).

Cyclase buffer was 50 mM Tris/HCl, pH 7.4.

The incubation system plus the PTH standards were prepared at 4 °C. The actual incubation was started by the addition of the membranes and the transfer of the tubes from 4 °C to 30 °C and was stopped after 30 min by protein denaturation at 85 °C for 5 min. (Blank values were provided by three tubes without PTH addition.) The suspension was centrifuged for 3 min at 12 000 rpm and 100 µl supernatant fluid was added to the cAMP-competitive binding assay.

Results

Adenylate Cyclase Activity

The possible loss of adenylate cyclase activity was proved in a pilot test in which the enzyme was stimulated by sodium fluoride. Sodium fluoride stimulates the adenylate cyclase system unspecifically by binding to the G$_s$-protein (Fig. 1). The

Table 1. Pipetting scheme

Reagent	Original concentration	Final concentration	Volume per tube
ATP	36 mM	1.8 mM	10 µl
MgCl$_2$	100 mM	5 mM	10 µl
Mix	10 mM	1 mM	20 µl
EGTA	10 mM	1 mM	20 µl
GppNHp	1 µM	100 nM	20 µl
Creatine kinase			0.1 mg
Creatine phosphate			0.5 mg
BSA			0.2 mg
Buffer			15 µl
		Total	100 µl
Incubation system	100 µl		
PTH standard or sample	50 µl		
Membranes (adenylate cyclase)	50 µl	(= 25 µg)	
Final volume	200 µl		

maximum cAMP production rate thus achieved by this was 200 pmol cAMP/mg membranes × min.

The same effect could be achieved with a GppNHp concentration of 100 nM. Therefore an assay concentration of 100 nM or 1 µM GppNHp was chosen.

Standard Curve for Biologically Active hPTH

An intraassay comparison of two standard curves gave the following results. The first curve was obtained with 100 nM GppNHp, the second with 10 µM GTP. Figure 2 shows that with GppNHp there was a rise in stimulation at a hPTH concentration of 100 pM while GTP could not increase the cAMP production until a hPTH concentration of 1nM was reached. Thus GppNHp made the system ten times more sensitive than GTP.

Improvement of Incubation Conditions

The aim was to find the GppNHp concentration which would show the best difference between the blank value and the lowest standard. Therefore hPTH(1-34) concentrations between 10 pM and 1 nM were compared with GppNHp concentrations from 100 nM to 10 µM. The results are shown in Fig. 3. In the following assays a concentration of 1 µM GppNHp was preferred because it showed a good difference and, with higher concentrations, sometimes the blank value already had such a high level due to GppNHp that a difference from the blank value was not visible.

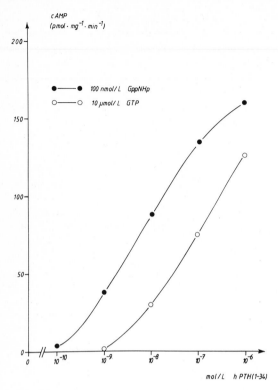

Fig. 2. Standard curves of biologically active hPTH(1-34) with 100 nM GppNHp and 10 μM GTP

Gel Filtration of Human Parathyroid Adenoma Extract

In order to separate the strong KCl and urea solutions from the protein (see Table 2) a gel filtration was performed. The column was Pharmacia K 26/40, gel Sephadex G 15 by Pharmacia. Buffer was 0.1 M glycine/HCl, pH 3.0. Figure 4 shows that a total separation of the protein peak from the salt peak was achieved. A measurement of all fractions in the bioassay as well as in the RIA(44-68) confirmed that hPTH eluted in the protein peak only (Fig. 5).

Affinity Chromatography

For further separation of hPTH fragments, affinity chromatography was performed. The method for fractionating rabbit antisera against hPTH(1-34) was cold precipitation with half-saturated ammonium sulfate as described by Hebert et al. [26]. These antisera were linked to Affi-Gel 10, an agarose gel.

Buffer A was 0.1 M NaHCO$_3$, pH 8.0; buffer B was 0.1 M glycine/HCl, pH 2.2.

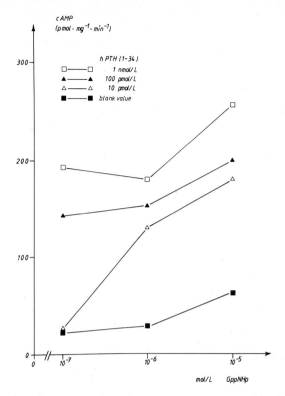

Fig. 3. Stimulation of adenylate cyclase with hPTH(1-34) concentrations from 10 pmol/liter to 1 nmol/liter and a blank value at GppNHp concentrations from 100 nM to 10 µmol/liter

Figure 6 shows that all N-terminal fragments were linked to the antibodies on the gel matrix. No fragments with biological activity were eluted in the 1–20 fractions which included all non-N-terminal fragments.

Discussion

Despite the development of different RIAs for hPTH there is obviously a need for a sensitive bioassay. A large number of adenylate cyclase assays have been described in the past few years [2, 24, 27, 28]. Only the bioassay gives some information about the bioactivity of the fragments obtained while the RIAs can only give information about the immunoreactivity.

The plasma membranes were prepared as described by Mohr and Hesch [11]. Because the self-performing Percoll gradient was used instead of a sucrose gradient, the preparation took only 4 h and was easy to perform. The yield of membrane protein was 1% of the wet cortex tissue, higher than the 0.3% as

Table 2. Extraction of hPTH from human
parathyroid adenoma: Extraction scheme

Mincing the adenomas

Homogenization

Centrifugation

60 min at 9500 rpm

Centrifugation
12 h at 40 000 rpm

Filtration
Filter size 0.45 μm and 0.2 μm

Gel filtration
Sephadex G 15

Lyophilization

Affinity chromatography
Affi-Gel 10

Reverse-phase chromatography
Extraction buffer was: 0.1 M glycine/HCl
$\qquad\qquad\qquad$ 3 M KCl
$\qquad\qquad\qquad$ 8 M Urea
$\qquad\qquad\qquad$ pH 3.0

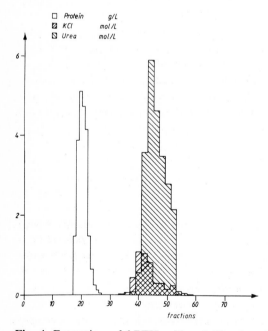

Fig. 4. Extraction of hPTH with gel filtration (Sephadex G15). Separation of the
protein peak containing biologically active hPTH and hPTH(44-68) from KCl and urea

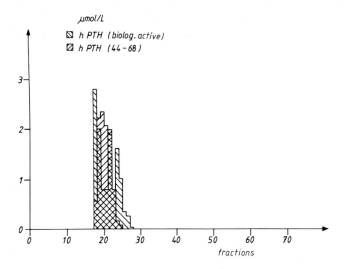

Fig. 5. Extraction of hPTH with gel filtration (Sephadex G15). Measurement of the biologically active hPTH and hPTH(44-68).

reported by Niepel et al. [2]. The maximum stimulation of 250 pmol cAMP/mg per minute ranged between the published data from 160 to 450 pmol/mg per minute [2, 24]. With the addition of 100 nM GppNHp, adenylate cyclase stimulation was ten times higher than with 10 μM GTP. Various optimal GppNHp concentrations have been published. While Niepel et al. [2] added 10 μM, Nissenson et al. [24] had the best results with 100 μM, and Seshadri et al. [15] even found 1 mM to be optimal. In our experiments a concentration of 1 μM was the most suitable. With higher levels the blank values were already stimulated so much that the lowest PTH standards could not be differentiated. Numerous variables make it difficult to compare the described adenylate cyclase assays, for instance the difference in species from which the cortical tissue is obtained, and the specific activity of the enzyme which is easily altered by the length of time spent in situ, transport, and preparation. Our detection range of 10 pmol/liter hPTH(1-34) is comparable to published data of 3–5 pmol/liter.

Different teams have tried to lower the detectable value of hPTH below 1 pM. That has not yet been achieved. Therefore and because of the quite difficult handling of the assay, a fresh incubation system must be produced for each assay; it does not seem reasonable to use this assay as a daily routine diagnostic procedure. An advantage of the bioassay is the possibility of obtaining the results very quickly. In connection with the cAMP-protein-binding assay, results can be obtained within 10 h, while RIAs usually take 2–5 days. Another advantage of this assay is its usefulness for research purposes, especially for the extraction of biologically active hPTH. As shown in Figs. 4–6 the assay is suitable for the examination of fractions after chromatography procedures. As the concentration of hPTH in these fractions was much higher than the serum

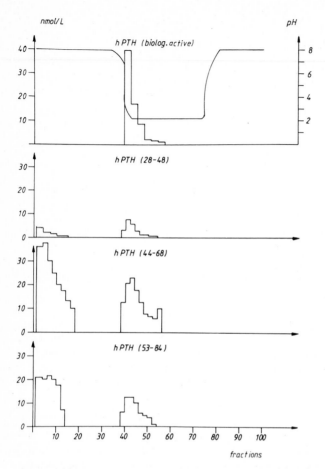

Fig. 6. Affinity chromatography (Affi Gel 10). The diagrams give the concentration of the eluted hPTH in the bioassay and the RIAs(28-48), (44-68), and (53-84). The *upper part of the figure* also shows the pH gradient during chromatography

levels, there was no difficulty in detecting the fractions which were of interest.

Affinity chromatography seemed to be an appropriate method for separating N-terminal fragments from mid- and C-regional fragments. The limiting factor, however, was the volume of antisera, so that only a column with a bed volume of 20 ml could be installed. This problem was overcome by the immunization of goats instead of rabbits which yield higher amounts of antisera.

In conclusion, a sensitive assay for biologically active hPTH is presented. This assay is based upon the stimulation of adenylate cyclase in the renal cortex by hPTH. The result is an increase in intracellular cAMP production. cAMP was measured with the cAMP-protein-binding assay as described in Chap. 3.1. Adenylate cyclase was prepared from bovine renal cortical plasma membranes by different centrifugation steps and with the help of Percoll, a self-performing gradient. The plasma membrane yield was 1% of the wet kidney tissue.

The following incubation system was used for the adenylate cyclase assay: ATP, 1.8 mM; MgCl$_2$, 5 mM; EGTA, 1.25 mM; 3-isobutyl-1-methyl-xanthine (Mix), 1 mM; creatine kinase, 0.1 mg; creatine phosphate; 0.5 mg; BSA, 0.2 mg; adenylate cyclase, 25 µg in 50 mM Tris/HCl, pH 7.4. By the addition of the GTP analogue guanylimidodiphosphate (GppNHp) in a concentration of 1 µM the sensitivity of the assay was 10 pmol/liter hPTH(1-34). The bioassay was used to examine the biological activity of hPTH extracted from the parathyroid glands of patients with confirmed primary hyperparathyroidism. The hormone extraction was performed by centrifugation, gel filtration (Sephadex G 15), and affinity chromatography (Affi Gel 10). The affinity chromatography with antibodies against the N-terminal fragment (1-34) coupled with the Affi Gel showed good separation of the biologically active N-terminal fragments from mid- and C-regional fragments.

References

1. Gilman AG (1984) G proteins and dual control of adenylate cyclase. Cell 36:577–579
2. Niepel B, Radeke H, Atkinson MJ, Jueppner H, Hesch RD (1983) A homologous biological probe for parathyroid hormone in human serum. J Immunoassay 4:21–47
3. Katada T, Ui M (1982) ADP ribosylation of the specific membrane protein C 6 cells by islet activating protein associated with modification of adenylate cyclase activity. J Biol Chem; 257:7210–7216
4. Tomlinson S, Mac Neil S, Brown BL (1985) Calcium, cyclic AMP, and hormone action. Clin Endocrinol (Oxf) 23:595–610
5. Cohen P (1985) The role of protein phosphorylation in hormonal control of enzyme activity. Eur J Biochem 154:439–448
6. Chambers DJ, Dunham J, Zanelli JM, Parsons JA, Bitensky L, Chayen J (1978) A sensitive bioassay of parathyroid hormone in plasma. Clin Endocrinol (Oxf) 9:375–379
7. Chase LR, Aurbach GD (1967) Parathyroid function and the renal excretion of 3',5'-adenylic acid. Proc Natl Acad Sci USA 58:518–525
8. Marcus R, Aurbach GD (1971) Adenyl cyclase from renal cortex. Biochim Biophys Acta 242:410–421
9. Marcus R, Aurbach GD (1969) Bioassay of parathyroid hormone in vitro with a stable preparation of adenylate cyclase from rat kidney. Endocrinology 85:801–810
10. Di Bella FP, Dousa TP, Miller SS, Arnaud CD (1974) Parathyroid hormone receptors of renal cortex - specific binding of biologically active, [125]-I-labeled hormone and relationship to adenylate cyclase activation. Proc Natl Acad Sci USA 71:723–726
11. Mohr H, Hesch RD (1980) Different handling of parathyrin by basal-lateral and brush-border membrane of the bovine kidney cortex. Biochem J 188: 649–656
12. Zull JE, Chuang J (1985) Characterization of parathyroid hormone fragments produced by Cathepsin D. J Biol Chem 260:1608–1613
13. Martin TJ, Vakakis N, Eismann JA, Livesey SJ, Tregaer GW (1974). Chick kidney

adenylate cyclase: sensitivity of parathyroid hormone and synthetic human and bovine peptides. J Endocrinol 63:369–375

14. Nissenson RA, Nyiredy KO, Arnaud CD (1981) Guanyl nucleotide potentiation of parathyroid hormone stimulated adenylate cyclase in chicken renal plasma membranes: a receptor independent effect. Endocrinology 108:1949–1953

15. Seshsadri MS, Chan YL, Wilkinson MR, Mason RS, Posen S (1985) Some problems associated with adenylate cyclase bioassays for parathyroid hormone. Clin Sci 68:311–319

16. Segre GV, Rosenblatt M, Reiner BL, Mahaffey JE, Potts JT Jr (1981) Characterization of parathyroid hormone receptors in canine renal cortical plasma membranes using a radioiodinate sulfur-free hormone analogue. J Biol Chem 254:6980–6986

17. Liang CT, Sacktor B (1977) Preparation of renal cortex basal-lateral and brush border membranes—localization of adenylate cyclase and guanylate cyclase activities. Biochim Biophys Acta 466:474–487

18. Bader CA, Monet JD, Rivaille P, Gaubert CM, Moukhtar MS, Milhaud G, Funck-Brentano JL (1976) Comparative in vitro biological activity of 1-34 N-terminal synthetic fragments of human parathyroid hormone on bovine and porcine kidney membranes. Endocr Res Commun 3:167–186

19. Jackson BA, Hui YSF, Northrup TE, Dousa TP (1980) Differential responsiveness of adenylate cyclase from rat, dog, and rabbit kidney to parathyroid hormone, vasopressin and calcitonin. Miner Electrolyte Metab 3:136–145

20. Sraer J, Sraer JD, Chansel D, Jüppner H, Hesch RD, Ardaillou R (1978) Evidence for glomerular receptors for parathyroid hormone. Am J Physiol 235:F96-F103

21. Somkuti SG, Hildebrandt JD, Herberg JT, Iyengar R (1982) Divalent cation regulation of adenylate cyclase. J Biol Chem 257:6387–6393

22. Bellorin-Font E, Martin KJ (1981) Regulation of the PTH-receptor-cyclase system of canine kidney: effects of calcium, magnesium and guanine nucleotides. Am J Physiol 241:F364–F373

23. Hunt NH, Martin TJ, Michelangeli VP, Eismann JA (1976) Effect of guanyl nucleotides on parathyroid hormone-responsive adenylate cyclase in chick kidney. J Endocrinol 69:401–412

24. Nissenson RA, Abbott SR, Teilelbaum AP, Clark OH, Arnaud CD (1981) Endogenous biologically active human parathyroid hormone: measurement by a guanyl nucleotide amplified renal adenylate cyclase assay. J Clin Endocrinol Metab 52:840–846

25. Marx SJ, Fedak SA, Aurbach GS (1972) Preparation and characterization of a hormone-responsive renal plasma membrane fraction. J Biol Chem 247:6913–6918

26. Hebert GA, Pelham PL, Pittman B (1972) Determination of the optimal ammonium sulfate concentration for the fractionation of rabbit, sheep, horse, and goat antisera. Appl Microbiol 25:26–36

27. Di Bella FP, Arnaud CD, Brewer HB Jr (1976) Relative biologic activities of human and bovine parathyroid hormones and their synthetic NH_2-terminal (1-34) peptides, as evaluated in vitro with renal cortical adenylate cyclase obtained from three different species. Endocrinology 99:429–436

28. Londos C, Salomon Y, Lin MC, Harwood JP, Schramm M, Wolff J, Rodbell M (1974) 5'-Guanylimidodiphosphate, a potent activator of adenylate cyclase systems in eukaryotic cells. Proc Natl Acad Sci USA 71:3087–3090

29. Auf'mkolk B (1983) Untersuchungen zur Charakterisierung des biologisch aktiven Parathormons im Menschen mit einem optimierten Adenylatcyclase-Bioassay. Dissertation, University Hannover

Chapter 2.11

Immunological Properties of Asparagine versus Aspartic Acid at Residue 76 of Human Parathyroid Hormone (Residues 53-84)

K. HERFARTH, E. BLIND, H. SCHMIDT-GAYK, and F.P. ARMBRUSTER

The amino acid sequence of human PTH (hPTH) was found in 1978 by applying Edman degradation to the isolated peptide [1]. The structure of the peptide was confirmed by cDNA techniques in 1981, except for residue 76, which is asparagine and not aspartic acid [2] (Fig. 1). We tested the significance of this amino acid residue for raising antisera against this region and for using them together with commercially available synthetic peptides of both sequences in immunoassays.

Materials and Methods

Antisera were raised in different species and are in use for established immuno-assays. An antiserum was raised by injecting extracts of human parathyroid adenomas into a goat (antiserum Goat H4); the hormone had been partly purified by gel permeation chromatography. This antiserum is used for a rapid (Chap. 2.3) and a sensitive (Chap. 2.2) RIA of C-terminal PTH. We immunized a guinea pig with a similar extract (antiserum MS7, Chap. 2.1). Another guinea pig was initially immunized with an extract of bovine parathyroid glands (partly purified extract) and subsequently also with human parathyroid hormone (antiserum GPB). A rabbit antiserum was obtained by injecting synthetic Asp^{76}-hPTH(53-84) conjugated to bovine thyroglobulin (antiserum R82). This anti-serum is used in a two-site assay of intact PTH (Chap. 2.8).

These well characterized antisera recognize, at least in part, the sequence 53-84 of hPTH. The antisera were compared in a conventional double-antibody RIA system (equilibrium conditions) as described in detail in Chap. 2.4.

The synthetic carboxyterminal peptide with the correct structure, Asn^{76}-hPTH(53-84), was used as the standard and as ^{125}I-labeled Tyr^{52}-hPTH(52-84), and compared with its analogue Asp^{76}-hPTH(53-84). The peptides were from Bachem (Bubendorf, Switzerland). The procedure used for labeling peptides was essentially the chloramine T method and was performed as described in Chap. 2.8.

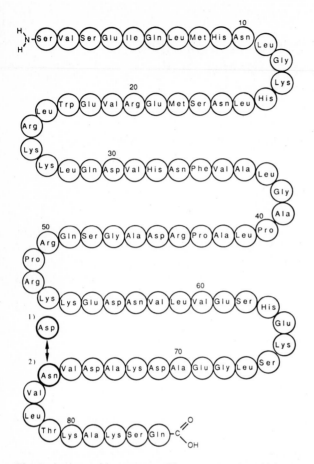

Fig. 1. Amino acid sequence of human parathyroid hormone. *1* Structure according to reference [1]; *2* structure according to reference [2].

Results

Antiserum MS7 (against hPTH) bound Tyr[52], Asn[76]-hPTH(52-84), and its Asp[76] analogue equally well. Both tracers were similarly displaced by Asn[76]-hPTH(53-84) and Asp[76]-hPTH(53-84), as shown in Fig. 2.

In the assay with the antiserum Goat H4 (against hPTH), the tracer with the correct human structure displayed a twofold better binding. Both tracers, however, were displaced by Asn[76]-hPTH(53-84), as shown in Fig. 3.

In contrast, antiserum GPB (against bovine PTH) exclusively bound the Asp[76] tracer. Asn[76]-hPTH(53-84) was not able to displace the tracer (Fig. 4). Antiserum GPB cross-reacts exclusively with Asp[76]-hPTH.

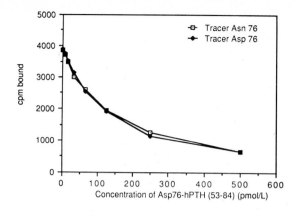

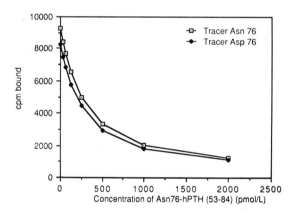

Fig. 2. Guinea pig antiserum MS7 against extracted hPTH. Displacement of different hPTH(53-84) tracers by their Asp[76] (*upper panel*) and Asn[76] (*lower panel*) analogues

The antiserum R82 raised against synthetic Asp[76]-hPTH(53-84) gave better binding to the corresponding tracer peptide than to ^{125}I-labeled Tyr[52]-Asn[76]-hPTH(52-84), as shown in Fig. 5.

The PTH content in sera from two hypoparathyroid patients, seven healthy controls, and 5, respectively 4 hyperparathyroid patients was determined with the antiserum MS7, Goat H4 (both against extracted hPTH), and R82. The displacement of the corresponding tracer peptide is shown in Fig. 6. Antiserum R82 against synthetic Asp[76]-hPTH(53-84), i.e. the "old" or wrong structure, was not able to discriminate patients with primary hyperparathyroidism from healthy controls (Fig. 6).

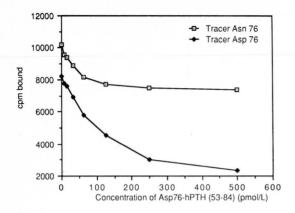

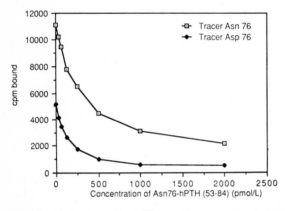

Fig. 3. Antiserum Goat H4 against extracted hPTH. Displacement of different hPTH(53-84) tracers by their Asp[76] (*upper panel*) and Asn[76] (*lower panel*) analogues

Discussion

The change of the amino acid residue at position 76 of the human structure (in material for immunization, standards, or tracer) had a strong influence on assay performance. Antisera against the "old" structure, i.e. Asp[76]-hPTH, seemed to be usually less suitable, especially when used together with "new" standard or tracer material (i.e. Asn[76]-hPTH). This was the case with antiserum R82 against synthetic Asp[76]-hPTH(53-84) which cross-reacts poorly with Asn[76]-hPTH. One fraction of antiserum R82 probably recognizes sections of PTH that do not contain amino acid 76 (Fig. 5). The antiserum was, however, still useful for the two-site assay with Asn[76]-hPTH as standard, as antibodies were added in large excess. A comparable antiserum raised against Asn[76]-hPTH(53-84) might improve assay performance.

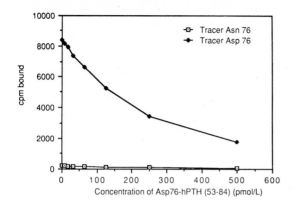

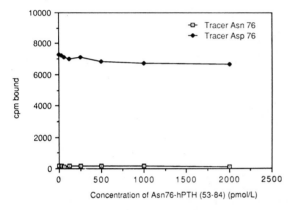

Fig. 4. Guinea pig antiserum GPB against extracted bovine and human PTH. Displacement of different hPTH (53–84) tracers by their Asp[76] (*upper panel*) *and* Asn[76] (*lower panel*) analogues

Gleed et al. [3] demonstrated that Asp[76]-hPTH(1-84) was markedly less reactive than Asn[76]-hPTH(1-84) in their C-terminal-specific assay for hPTH using labeled antibodies. In earlier studies they found synthetic Asp[76]-hPTH(1-84) to be 4–5-fold more reactive than hPTH(53-84) prepared from native hPTH with an anti-bovine PTH antiserum [3]. The immunological data supplement the results of cDNA studies that aspartic acid is the correct amino acid residue 76 in bovine PTH.

Extraction and purification of hPTH from gland tissue does not seem to result in spontaneous deamidation of asparagine at position 76, as demonstrated by cation-exchange high-performance liquid chromatography [4]. In agreement with our results, antisera raised against extracts of human parathyroid glands show full cross-reaction with the "correct" hPTH peptide sequence.

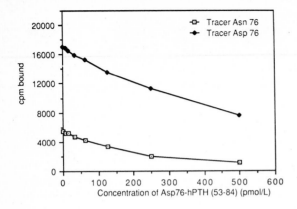

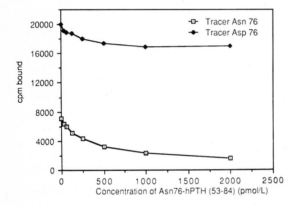

Fig. 5. Rabbit antiserum R82 against synthetic Asp[76]-hPTH(53–84). Displacement of different hPTH(53-84) tracers by their Asp[76] (*upper panel*) and Asn[76] (*lower panel*) analogues

Synthetic hPTH(53-84) with the "wrong" amino acid (Asp[76]) has been commercially distributed for years. In retrospect, this might explain in part the failure of several C-terminal assays of PTH to determine reliably the activity of the parathyroid gland [5].

In conclusion, the change of one single amino acid residue at position 76 of the human structure (in material for immunization, standards, or tracer) might have a strong influence on assay performance. Only our antisera against extracted and partly purified human parathyroid hormone (Goat H4 and MS7) were able to discriminate patients with primary hyperparathyroidism from healthy controls in C-terminal specific assays.

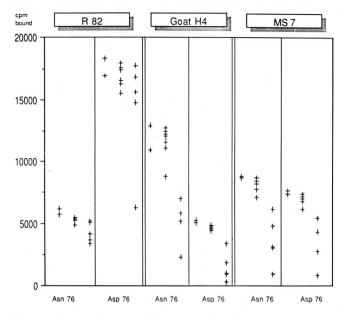

Fig. 6. Assay performance with antisera R82, Goat H4, and MS7 by using ^{125}I-labeled Tyr^{52}, Asn^{76}-hPTH(52-84), and Tyr^{52}, Asp^{76}-hPTH(52-84). The binding of the tracer is shown on the y-axis. In each panel, hypoparathyroid patients (*left column*), normal controls (*middle column*), and hyperparathyroid patients (*right column*) are shown

References

1. Keutmann HT, Sauer MM, Hendy GN, O'Riordan JLH, Potts JT Jr (1978) Complete amino acid sequence of human parathyroid hormone. Biochemistry 17:5723–5729
2. Hendy GH, Kronenberg HM, Potts JT Jr, Rich A (1981) Nucleotide sequence of cloned cDNAs encoding human preproparathyroid hormone. Proc Natl Acad Sci USA 78:7365–7369
3. Gleed JH, Hendy GN, Kimura T, Sakakibara S, O'Riordan JLH (1987) Immunological properties of synthetic human parathyroid hormone: effect of deamidation at position 76. Bone Min 2:375–382
4. Kumagaye KY, Takai M, Chino N, Kimura T, Sakakibara S (1985) Comparison of reversed-phase and cation-exchange high-performance liquid chromatography for separating closely related peptides: separation of Asp^{76}-human parathyroid hormone (1-84) from Asn^{76}-human parathyroid hormone (1-84). J Chromatogr 327:327–332
5. Gorog RH, Hakim MK, Thompson NW, Rigg GA, McCann DS (1982) Radioimmunoassay of serum parathyrin: comparison of five commercial kits. Clin Chem 28:87–91

3 Parathyroid Hormone-Related Protein

Chapter 3.1

Parathyroid Hormone-Related Protein

W.A. RATCLIFFE and J.G. RATCLIFFE

Introduction

Characterisation of PTH-rP

Parathyroid hormone-related protein (PTH-rP) is a protein with potent para-thyroid hormone (PTH)-like activity which acts on PTH receptors in bone and kidney with generation of cAMP. It was initially purified from the BEN lung tumour cell line and breast and renal carcinomas associated with hyper-calcaemia (Moseley et al. 1987; Burtis et al. 1987; Strewler et al. 1987). Com-plementary DNA (cDNA) cloned from the BEN cell line predicted a protein of 141 amino acids and molecular weight of 16 000 daltons (Suva et al. 1987). The amino-terminal region of the protein has a high degree of homology with PTH, with identity of eight of the first thirteen amino acids in both proteins (Table 1). This structural homology may explain common effects on bone resorption, adenylate cyclase stimulation and inhibition of renal phosphate reabsorption. Genomic DNA of PTH-rP was located on chromosome 12 (Mangin et al. 1988b).

Subsequently PTH-rP was shown to occur in tumours as a heterogeneous mixture of proteins arising from transcriptional, translational and/or post-translational processing. Northern analysis of mRNA from tumours and normal tissues has revealed several hybridising transcripts (Mangin et al. 1988a). Three of these mRNA species are thought to arise from alternative splicing and encode three proteins which differ at the carboxyl terminus (Table 1) and may be expressed to different extents in endocrine and non-endocrine tissues. Post-translational modification and proteolytic cleavage may also occur since species of molecular weights 7000–9000 and 17 000 daltons have been isolated from different tumours (Stewart et al. 1987) and multiple components with adenylate cyclase-stimulating activity demonstrated (Moseley et al. 1987; Docherty and Heath 1989). Lysine and arginine-rich regions (e.g. residues 88-91, 96-98, and 102-106) may be sites of post-translational cleavage. However, the final secreted forms of PTH-rP have yet to be identified.

Potential Role of PTH-rP in Hypercalcaemia of Malignancy

Malignancies most commonly associated with humoral hypercalcaemia of malignancy (HHM) include squamous carcinoma of lung and head and neck,

Table 1. Amino-acid sequence of PTH-related proteins predicted from the base sequence of cloned cDNA

A

[1]ALA *VAL SER GLU HIS GLN LEU LEU HIS* ASP LYS LYS *GLY LYS* SER ILE GLN ASP LEU ARG *ARG*[20]

[21]ARG PHE PHE *LEU* HIS HIS LEU ILE ALA GLU ILE *HIS* THR ALA GLU ILE ARG ALA THR SER[40]

[41]GLU VAL SER PRO ASN SER LYS PRO SER *PRO* ASN THR *LYS* ASN HIS PRO *VAL* ARG PHE GLY[60]

[61]*SER* ASP ASP GLU GLY ARG TYR LEU THR GLN GLU THR ASN LYS VAL GLU THR THR TYR *LYS* GLU[80]

[81]GLN PRO LEU LYS THR PRO GLY LYS LYS LYS LYS GLY LYS PRO GLY LYS ARG LYS GLU GLN[100]

[101]GLU LYS LYS LYS ARG ARG THR ARG SER ALA TRP LEU ASP SER GLY VAL THR GLY SER GLY[120]

[121]LEU GLU GLY ASP HIS LEU SER ASP THR SER THR THR SER LEU GLU LEU ASP SER ARG[139]

B

[140]ARG HIS[141]

C

[140]THR ALA LEU LEU TRP GLY LEU LYS LYS LYS LYS GLU ASN ASN ARG ARG THR HIS HIS MET[159]

[160]GLN LEU MET ILE SER LEU PHE LYS SER PRO LEU LEU LEU[173]

Cloning of cDNA from *A* renal carcinoma cell line 786-0 (Thiede et al. 1988), *B* BEN lung tumour cell line (Suva et al. 1987) and *C* human renal carcinoma SKRC-1 (Mangin et al. 1988a) has predicted three forms of PTH-rP consisting of 139, 141 and 173 amino acids respectively. Sequence 1–139 is common to the three forms of PTH-rP, which are thought to arise by alternative splicing of mRNA derived from a single copy of genomic DNA. Homology with the sequence of human PTH is indicated by underlining and carcinoma of ovary and kidney (Mundy et al. 1984). The secretion of PTH-rP from tumours associated with hypercalcaemia provides an attractive hypothesis to explain the clinical, biochemical and histological manifestations of HHM. Synthetic amino-terminal fragments of PTH-rP are hypercalcaemic in vivo and in vitro, resorb bone and inhibit phosphate transport, and stimulate cAMP production in osteoblast-like cells and renal membranes (Rabbani et al. 1988; Pizurki et al. 1988; Thompson et al. 1988).

The biological effects of the potential factor(s) involved in HHM resemble those of PTH in some respects (e.g. hypercalcaemia, increased phosphate excretion, increased nephrogenous cAMP, increased osteoclastic bone resorption), but other effects suggest that the factors differ from PTH (Burtis et al. 1988). Thus there is greater hypercalciuria for a given serum calcium level in HHM than in primary hyperparathyroidism, and decreased osteoblastic bone formation in HHM compared to primary hyperparathyroidism, while osteoclastic bone resorption is increased in both syndromes. Circulating 1,25 dihydroxy vitamin D levels are typically reduced in HHM, whereas they are increased in primary hyperparathyroidism due to PTH stimulation of renal 1-hydroxylation. Circulating PTH levels measured by specific two-site immunometric assays are low in HHM, but inappropriately increased in primary hyperparathyroidism. Finally, PTH mRNA has not been detected reliably in tumours associated with HHM.

PTH-rP may not, however, be the only humoral mediator of hypercalcaemia since other bone resorbing factors have been extracted from tumours or are present in conditioned media from tumour cell lines. These include, for example, transforming growth factors α and β (TGF α, β), cytokines (interleukin 1 and tumour necrosis factor) and prostaglandins (Martin et al. 1988).

Thus hypercalcaemia of malignancy may be multifactorial depending on tumour type and presence of skeletal metastases. Nevertheless, in solid tumours without metastases (e.g. squamous cell carcinoma of lung, skin, head and neck and carcinoma of kidney, pancreas and ovary) PTH-rP seems the likely major hypercalcaemic factor, though TGFs and cytokines may be synergistic. In haematological malignancies, local cytokines may be more important. In metastatic hypercalcaemia local osteolytic factors such as prostaglandins and tumour enzymes may be involved with an uncertain contribution by humoral factors. Overall, there is evidence of an underlying humoral mechanism in the majority of cases of hypercalcaemia of malignancy associated with unselected solid tumours.

Nevertheless, the importance of PTH-rP as a hypercalcaemic factor in malignancy has yet to be established by measurement of circulating concentrations of the protein by specific assays.

Distribution of PTH-rP

PTH-rP bioactivity has been extracted from many cell lines or tumours associated with hypercalcaemia, including lung, breast, kidney and T cell lymphoma (HTLV-1 infected) (Motokura et al. 1988). Immunohistochemical staining of tumours not associated with hypercalcaemia has identified PTH-rP commonly in squamous cell carcinoma from many sites, renal cell carcinoma, malignant melanoma and unexpectedly in small cell lung cancer, but rarely in adenocarcinoma (Danks et al. 1989). This suggests that PTH-rP may be a useful histogenetic marker.

There is as yet little information on the distribution of PTH-rP in normal tissues or its physiological role. A survey of localisation in the rat showed that PTH-rP mRNA was detected only in the lactating mammary gland, suggesting that the protein may be involved in mobilisation or transfer of calcium to the milk during lactation (Thiede and Rodan 1988). PTH-rP bioactivity is present in the placenta and foetal ovine parathyroid glands (Rodda et al. 1988), and experimental studies suggest that PTH-rP may be responsible for maintaining a higher serum calcium concentration in the foetus than in the mother, possibly by stimulating placental calcium transfer. PTH-rP is secreted by keratinocytes in culture (Merendino et al. 1986) and stimulates adenylate cyclase activity in human dermal fibroblasts, suggesting that it may have a role in skin physiology (Wu et al. 1987).

Assays for PTH-rP

In vitro bioassays have been used to monitor the purification and character-isation of PTH-rP from tissue extracts and culture supernatants and to examine the bioactivity of synthetic fragments of PTH-rP. The most widely used methods utilise osteosarcoma cells, renal cells or renal membranes, with quantitation of generated cAMP (Rabbani et al. 1988). PTH-rP has also been measured by highly sensitive cytochemical bioassays with quantitation of the glucose-6-phosphate dehydrogenase activity generated in renal tubules (Stewart et al. 1983). Since PTH-rP and PTH appear to interact with the same receptor (Juppner et al. 1988), PTH-rP specificity is achieved in these assays by blocking PTH activity with an antiserum to PTH.

The development of immunoassays, especially immunometric assays for PTH-rP with low PTH cross-reactivity, are anticipated to improve assay specificity and sensitivity. Furthermore, the use of region-specific antisera may help to elucidate the molecular forms present.

A commercial RIA kit for PTH-rP 1-34 is available from Peninsula Labor-atories Ltd. (St Helens, Cheshire, England). A 50% inhibition of tracer PTH-rP is given by 22.3 pg/tube, and cross-reaction with PTH 1-34 is less than 1%. The manufacturers also recommend a protocol for extracting PTH-rP from plasma (1 ml) which involves adsorption and subsequent elution of PTH-rP from a C_2 column. An independent validation of this procedure has yet to be published.

Most recently a RIA for PTH-rP 1-34 has been reported from this laboratory with a detection limit of 5 pg/tube and cross-reaction with PTH 1-34 of < 0.025% (Ratcliffe et al. 1988). This assay is based on the use of a polyclonal antiserum to PTH-rP 1-34 and immunoextraction of the protein from biological fluids or tissues with a monoclonal antibody to the same sequence. Experimental details of this assay and its applications are described in subsequent sections.

Radioimmunoassay of PTH-rP 1-34

This assay is based on that described by Ratcliffe et al. (1988).

Materials

Synthetic PTH-rP 1-34, and [Tyr^0]-PTH-rP 1-34 were obtained from Peninsula Laboratories Ltd. (St. Helens, Cheshire, England). [Tyr^{34}]-PTH-rP 1-34 was synthesized by Alta Bioscience (Birmingham, England). Bovine thyroglobulin, 1-ethyl-3-(3-dimethyl-amino-propyl)carbodiimide (EDC), chloramine-T, and Polypep (low viscosity) were from Sigma Chemical Co. (Poole, Dorset, England). Sheep anti-mouse immunoglobulin and donkey anti-rabbit immunoglobulin were from the Scottish Antibody Production Unit (Carluke, Lanarkshire, Scotland). Polyethylene glycol (PEG) 6000 was from Koch Light (Haverhill, Suffolk, England), foetal calf serum from Sera-lab (Crawley Down, Sussex, England), and hypoxanthine-aminopterin-thymidine (HAT) was from Flow Laboratories (Rickmansworth, Hertfordshire, England). Sac-Cel was from Immunodiagnostic Systems (Washington, Tyne and Wear, England), and protein A Sepharose CL-4B and cyanogen bromide (CNBr)-activated Sepharose 4B from Pharmacia (Milton Keynes, Buckinghamshire, England). Disposable polystyrene chromatography columns were from Pierce Warriner (Chester, Cheshire, England), C$_{18}$ Sep-Pak cartridges were from Waters Associates (Milford M. A., U.S.A.). [^{125}I]Sodium iodide (100 mCi/ml) was from Amersham International (Amersham, Buckinghamshire, England).

Preparation of Iodinated Tracer

To [Tyr^0]-PTH-rP 1-34 (2 μg) in 10 μl 0.05 M phosphate buffer pH 7.4 was added 10 μl 0.5 M phosphate buffer pH 7.4, 5 μl [^{125}I]sodium iodide (0.5 mCi) and 10 μl of chloramine-T (1 mg/ml) in 0.05 M phosphate buffer. After 20 s, 10 μl of sodium metabisulphite (2 mg/ml) in 0.05 M phosphate buffer pH 7.4 was added. The reaction mixture was diluted to 1.0 ml with 0.1% trifluoroacetic acid (TFA) and applied to a C$_{18}$ Sep-Pak cartridge, previously washed with 10 ml methanol and 10 ml water. Free iodide was eluted with 10 ml water; the iodinated peptide was eluted with 5 ml of 60% acetonitrile in 0.1% TFA and stored at 4 °C. The specific activity of ^{125}I-[Tyr^0]-PTH-rP 1-34 was in the range 150–200 μCi/ug.

Polyclonal Antisera

Synthetic PTH-rP 1-34, 400 μg, (Peninsula) was coupled to 2.5 mg bovine thyroglobulin at pH 7.0 in the presence of ^{125}I-[Tyr^0]-PTH-rP 1-34 (61 000 cpm) and 4.3 mg EDC, with stirring at room temperature overnight. A total of 67% of the radioactivity was recovered in the conjugate after dialysis against phosphate-buffered saline, yielding a conjugate of molar ratio 6.7:1 (PTH-rP 1-34:thyroglobulin). Six New Zealand White rabbits were injected s.c. and i.m. with 100 μg conjugate emulsified in complete Freunds adjuvant:saline (2:1 vol/vol) and boosts of 25 μg conjugate were given s.c. and i.m. at monthly intervals. Antibodies to PTH-rP were detected by binding to ^{125}I-[Tyr^0]-PTH-rP 1-34 (20 000 cpm) in assay diluent consisting of 0.25% Polypep, 0.1% Triton X-100, 0.01% sodium azide in phosphate buffered saline, pH 7.4. Precipitation of antibody-bound tracer was by the addition of donkey anti-rabbit immunoglobulin precipitating serum. After two boosts, two rabbits showed no response, whereas titres (defined as the dilution binding 50% of added tracer) in the remaining four rabbits ranged from 1:1000 to 1:500000. The highest titre antiserum (code R 4/2) was selected for further studies.

Monoclonal Antibodies

Balb/c mice were injected s.c. with 100 μg PTH-rP:thyroglobulin conjugate in complete Freunds adjuvant:saline (2:1 vol/vol), and were boosted s.c. or i.p. with 10–25 μg conjugate at monthly intervals. Approximately half the mice responded to the immunogen and those with highest antibody titres were selected as donors of spleen cells for fusion. Pre-fusion boosts were given by two regimes; either 25–75 μg conjugate was given i.v. and i.p. 3 days before fusion, or 50 μg conjugate and 200 μg [Tyr^{34}]-PTH-rP 1-34 were given i.p. and i.v. 4 and 3 days before fusion, followed by 25 μg conjugate i.p. 2 days before fusion. Spleen cells from the hyperimmunised mice were fused with NSO mouse myeloma cells (ratio of 10:1) using 50% PEG 6000. Hybrids were grown in medium containing 20% foetal calf serum and non-immune spleen feeder cells (1.5×10^6 cells/ml), and selection of hybrids was with HAT. Antibodies were detected by binding to ^{125}I-[Tyr^0]-PTH-rP 1-34, with precipitation of antibody bound tracer by addition of sheep anti-mouse immunoglobulin. Four out of six fusions yielded a total of 25 secreting hybrids; 18 hybrids were selected for cloning by limiting dilution and production of ascites in mice. These 18 monoclonal antibodies have been partially characterised in terms of titre in culture fluid, avidity and cross-reactivity with PTH 1-34 and PTH-rP from keratinocytes. Titres in culture fluid ranged from 1:10 to 1:6000, with ten and four having titres in excess of 1:100 and 1:1000, respectively. Minimum detection limits in a RIA ranged from 25–5000 pg PTH-rP 1-34 per tube. The three antibodies of highest avidity gave detection limits of approximately 30 pg PTH-rP 1-34 per tube in an RIA. Each of eight monoclonal antibodies examined showed no cross-reaction with 1 μg/tube PTH 1-34, suggesting that the antibody binding site may not be at the extreme amino-terminus. Monoclonal antibodies (coded 5A, 5C, 6C and 9D) were purified from ascitic fluid by chromatography on Protein A Sepharose CL-4B and then coupled to CNBr-activated Sepharose 4B for affinity purification of PTH-rP from conditioned medium from human keratinocytes. Two antibodies (coded 5C10 and 4E9) cross-reacted 77% and 75% (Fig. 1) respectively with affinity purified PTH-rP

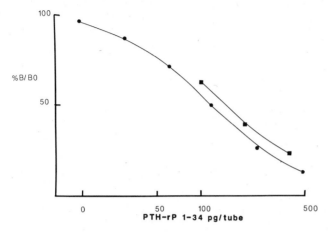

Fig. 1. RIA standard curve for PTH-rP 1-34 using monoclonal antibody 4E9. Affinity purified PTH-rP (■) was previously assayed by RIA with rabbit antiserum R4/2 and assigned a concentration in terms of PTH-rP 1-34. PTH 1-34 (3.9–1000 ng/tube) gave no inhibition of binding in this assay

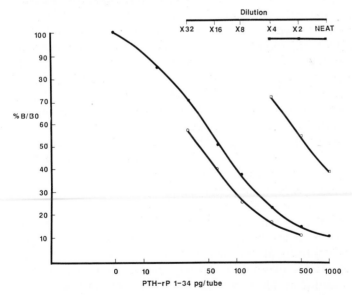

Fig. 2. RIA of PTH-rP 1-34 from keratinocyte culture fluid. Conditioned medium from human keratinocytes (□), immunoextracted culture fluid (■) and extracted PTH-rP (○) were assayed at a range of dilutions and compared with synthetic PTH-rP 1-34 as standard (●)

from keratinocytes which had previously been assayed in terms of PTH-rP 1-34 in a RIA with rabbit antiserum R4/2 (Fig. 2). These combined data provide evidence of cross-reaction with both authentic PTH-rP from keratinocytes and synthetic PTH-rP 1-34.

Studies are in progress to characterise these monoclonal antibodies in terms of their cross-reactivity with a range of sub-fragments of PTH-rP 1-34 to identify further their binding sites. Antibodies with non-overlapping epitopes will then be examined for their compatibility in a two-site assay. Studies are also continuing to produce antibodies to mid- and carboxy-terminal regions of PRP 1-141 for use in two-site assays for defined molecular species and to identify and quantitate secreted forms of PTH-rP.

Immunoextraction from Biological Fluids

Immunoextraction procedures have been developed to purify PTH-rP from biological fluids and tissue extracts and to concentrate PTH-rP before RIA. The immunoextraction procedure is technically simple and exploits the specificity of the monoclonal antibodies to selectively purify PTH-rP. It also avoids potential non-specific interferences in the RIA arising from unidentified components of serum or tissues.

The monoclonal antibody (9D) used was raised to PTH-rP 1-34 and has a titre in ascitic fluid of 1:70 000, an avidity constant of 1.4×10^9 l/M, and cross-reacts less than 0.05% by weight with PTH 1-34. Protein A purified antibody 9D was coupled to CNBr-activated Sepharose 4B (4–6 mg/g gel) by procedures recommended by Pharmacia.

In a typical column procedure for extraction of PTH-rP from biological fluids, 130 ml of pooled conditioned medium from cultures of human keratinocytes was passed slowly through a column containing 2 ml of affinity gel. After washing the column with saline, PTH-rP was eluted with 25 mM HCl. Parallelism of untreated keratinocyte culture fluid and affinity purified PTH-rP from culture fluid with standard PTH-rP 1-34 is shown in Fig. 2. PTH-rP 1-34 concentrations in untreated culture fluid and culture fluid after immunoextraction were 1.13 ng/ml (i.e. 147 ng/130 ml medium) and < 0.1 ng/ml, respectively, whereas 150 ng of immunoactive protein was recovered in the acid extract confirming that the immunoextraction was quantitative.

Fluids (e.g. 2–15 ml) such as serum, milk or culture fluid were affinity purified by a batch procedure using 100 μl of a 6.6% gel suspension with a 1–2 h period of mixing. Extraction efficiency was monitored by spiking a similar volume of an appropriate fluid with affinity purified keratinocyte PTH-rP. The extraction gel was poured into a disposable polystyrene mini-column and the gel retained by the filter was washed twice with assay diluent (4 ml). PTH-rP was eluted by addition of 25 mM HCl (150 μl), the gel washed with assay diluent (150 μl) and the combined acid and diluent eluates were recovered by centrifuging the column at 2000 g for 2 min and then assayed by RIA. The efficiency of immunoextraction of affinity purified PTH-rP added to serum was between 60%–80% for 8 and 4 ml serum, respectively (Table 2). The measured immunoreactivity in the extract was linearly related to the initial concentration of affinity purified keratinocyte PTH-rP added to serum after correction for extraction losses. Extraction of 10 ml serum and elution of PTH-rP in 0.3 ml produced a concentration factor of 33-fold. Thus the detection limit of the extraction RIA was between 1 and 3 ng PTH-rP 1-34 per litre serum, depending on the efficiency of the extraction and the sensitivity of the RIA.

Table 2. Immunoextraction of PTH-related protein from serum

| Serum Volume | PTH-rP[a] | | | |
| | Added | | Recovery | |
ml	pg/ml	pg total	pg	%
4	164	655	514	78
	246	984	788	80
8	246	1970	1388	70
	345	2758	1760	64

[a] PTH-rP was affinity purified from human keratinocyte conditioned medium and assayed by RIA with PTH-rP 1-34 as standard. Serum was from a blood donor

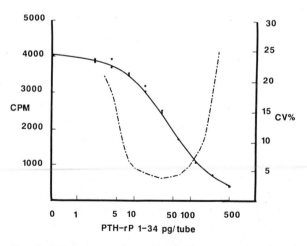

Fig. 3. RIA standard curve for PTH-rP 1–34. The standard curve is shown as a *solid line*, and the *broken line* represents the within-batch imprecision profile based on analysis by RIACalc software (Pharmacia) of the error distribution of at least 80 determinations in duplicate (includes standards and unknowns). The working range of this RIA was 12–430 pg/tube, corresponding to a within-batch CV of less than 10%

Radioimmunoassay

Standard PTH-rP 1-34 (100 μl) between 1.95 and 500 pg/tube was incubated with rabbit antiserum to PTH-rP 1-34 (code R4/2, 100 μl) at a final dilution of 1:500 000 and 15 000 cpm tracer (^{125}I-[Tyr^0]-PTH-rP 1-34, 100 μl). The diluent for all reagents consisted of 0.25% Polypep, 0.1% Triton X-100 and 0.01% sodium azide in 0.05 M phosphate buffered saline, pH 7.4. After incubating for 16 h at 4 °C, antibody-bound tracer was separated by adding a donkey anti-rabbit coated cellulose suspension (Sac-Cel, 100 μl). After incubation for 30 min at room temperature, 1 ml water was added and the tubes centrifuged at 3000 g for 15 min at 4 °C. The supernatant was aspirated and the precipitate counted. Specific binding of tracer was typically 40% with 1% non-specific binding.

The detection limit was 5 pg/tube when tracer and antiserum were added together initially. Improved sensitivity (1–3 pg/tube) was achieved by extending the incubation period to 3 days at 4 °C or by delaying addition of tracer for 1 day. A typical standard curve and within-batch imprecision profile is shown in Fig. 3. The cross-reactions of hPTH 1-34 and hPTH 1-84 were less than 0.025% and 0.01% by weight respectively.

PTH-rP Concentrations in Biological Fluids and Tissue Extracts

Keratinocyte Culture Fluid

PTH-rP immunoreactivity in conditioned medium from human keratinocytes diluted parallel to synthetic PTH-rP 1-34 standards in the RIA (Fig. 2). Fourteen specimens of medium harvested an average of 1.7 (range 0–8) days before confluence of the cells had a mean concentration of 1.8 (range 0.23–4.4) ng/ml. Seven specimens of medium harvested an average of 6.7 (range 2–11) days after confluence had a mean concentration of 0.69 (range < 0.1–1.4) ng/ml, indicating that more PTH-rP is secreted before the cells become confluent.

Human and Bovine Milk

PTH-rP immunoreactivity in human and pasteurised bovine milk was measured directly by RIA (Fig. 4) after centrifugation to remove lipid. The mean PTH-rP concentration in 21 specimens of human milk was 14 (range 0.8–96) ng/ml. The presence of PTH-rP in human milk was confirmed by immunoextraction of nine specimens of milk; on average 64% (range 19–105) of initial immunoreactivity was recovered in the extract after correction for the efficiency of extraction. Two samples of bovine milk assayed directly had PTH-rP concentrations of 40 and 42 ng/ml. PTH-rP immunoreactivity in

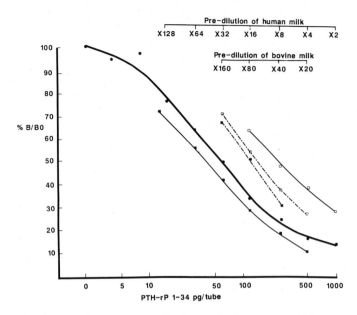

Fig. 4. RIA of PTH-rP 1-34 in bovine and human milk. Two specimens of human milk (■, □) and pasteurised cow's milk (■ --- ■, □ --- □) were centrifuged twice at 3000 g for 15 min to remove lipid, assayed by RIA at a range of dilutions and compared with synthetic PTH-rP 1-34 as standard (●)

bovine milk diluted parallel with the PTH-rP 1-34 standard, suggesting that like PTH the structure of bovine and human PTH-rP may be similar. The stability of bovine PTH-rP to pasteurisation, which involves heating at 73 °C for 15 s, is not unexpected since bioactive PTH-rP extracted from tumour tissue has been shown to be stable at 100 °C for at least 15 min (Stewart et al. 1983).

Serum

When serum (100 µl) from normal subjects was assayed directly by RIA, significant inhibition of binding was found. Similar apparent PTH-rP 1-34 concentrations were obtained for normal sera and sera from patients with primary hyperparathyroidism, hypoparathyroidism and hypercalcaemia of malignancy. On serum dilution, the immunoreactivity paralleled the synthetic PTH-rP 1-34 standard; however, the immunoactivity was not removed by the immunoextraction procedure described previously whereas authentic affinity-purified PTH-rP added to serum was quantitatively retained by the affinity gel. These findings suggest that serum components which differ from authentic PTH-rP cross-react in the direct assay, and confirm the need to extract PTH-rP from serum before assay to enhance specificity and sensitivity.

Immunoextraction reduced the minimum detection limit of the RIA to between 1 and 3 ng/l depending on the volume of serum extracted, the efficiency of extraction and the sensitivity of the RIA. Following extraction of 10 ml serum aliquots from several normal subjects PTH-rP levels were undetectable in an assay with a detection limit of 1.4 ng/l serum. This confirms that blood levels of PTH-rP are very low in normal subjects, and suggests that more sensitive immunometric assays, such as two-site immunometric assays, will be required to measure normal circulating concentrations. Studies are continuing with existing assays to examine PTH-rP concentrations in various pathological conditions, including humoral hypercalcaemia of malignancy.

Tissues

PTH-rP 1-34 immunoreactivity was demonstrated in an extract of a bronchial carcinoid associated with humoral hypercalcaemia (Fig. 5). This carcinoid tumour has previously been shown to contain multiple molecular forms of PTH-rP bioactivity (Docherty and Heath 1989). On dilution the immunoreactivity was non-parallel to standard PTH-rP, which may be explained in part by non-specific interference arising from the high protein content of the crude acetic acid extract and the presence of different molecular forms of PTH-rP. PTH-rP 1-34 immunoreactivity was also found in 0.1 M acetic acid extracts of a 19 week and a term human placenta, corresponding to 3.6 and 1.0 ng/g wet weight respectively. Previous studies in sheep have also reported higher placental PTH-rP bioactivity at mid-trimester than at term (Rodda et al. 1988).

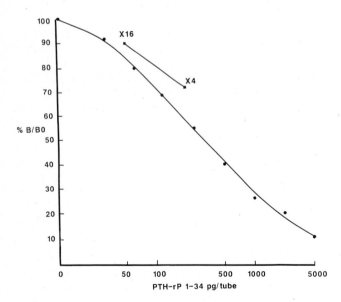

Fig. 5. RIA of acetic acid extract of a bronchial carcinoid tumour associated with humoral hypercalcaemia. A 33.7 g tumour was extracted in 155 ml 0.07 M acetic acid as described by Docherty and Heath (1989), and the extract was assayed at two dilutions (■) and compared synthetic PTH-rP 1-34 as standard (●)

Summary

The synthetic fragment PTH-rP 1-34 coupled to thyroglobulin was used to raise rabbit antisera and a panel of monoclonal antibodies. The selected rabbit antiserum and all monoclonal antibodies examined so far recognise authentic PTH-rP as well as PTH-rP 1-34, but do not cross-react significantly with PTH 1-34. A radioimmunoassay was developed using a rabbit antiserum to PTH-rP 1-34. This assay appears to be suitable for the direct assay of PTH-rP in medium from keratinocytes and also human and bovine milk. However, the direct assay of serum yielded high levels of immunoreactivity which were not extracted by an affinity gel. This suggests that unidentified components of serum cross-react in the direct assay. To avoid this cross-reactivity, and because the RIA lacks the sensitivity and specificity required for the direct measurement of PTH-rP in serum, an immunoextraction method was developed using a mono-clonal antibody linked to Sepharose. By extracting 10 ml serum and measuring PTH-rP in the extract, a detection limit of 1-3 ng PTH-rP per litre serum was achieved. Preliminary data suggest that serum PTH-rP concentrations in normal subjects are less than this detection limit and therefore lower than serum PTH levels. This may be consistent with PTH-rP having a minor physiological role in normal calcium homeostasis. The future development of two-site im-munometric assays using monoclonal antibodies together with the immunoex-traction method may provide the enhanced sensitivity required to measure physiological levels of the protein. Furthermore, the selection and application of monoclonal antibodies in region-specific two-site immunometric assays may provide valuable information on the molecular forms of PTH-rP in the circula-tion, tissues and tumours.

Initial interest in PTH-rP has focussed on its potential role as a mediator of HHM. So far however, the role of PTH-rP in HHM and the diagnostic value of serum assays in patients with hypercalcaemia remains to be established. Im-munohistochemical evidence suggests that antibodies to PTH-rP may be useful markers of tumour histogenesis.

The production of antisera to PTH-rP has allowed other potential roles to be investigated which may be equally important. High concentrations of PTH-rP have been measured in milk, suggesting its possible involvement in the mobilisation and/or transport of calcium into milk during lactation. The presence of the protein in placenta indicates that it may also be concerned in calcium homeostasis in the foetus since foetal calcium levels are higher than the maternal ones. Finally the demonstration of high PTH-rP concentrations in keratinocyte culture fluids raises the intriguing possibility that it has a role in normal dermal development.

Acknowledgements. We wish to thank Ms. A Blight, Birmingham Accident Hospital, for the generous provision of conditioned medium from keratinocytes, and Dr. H. Docherty for an extract of a tumour associated with hypercalcaemia. The collaboration of Dr. D.A. Heath and Dr. R.A.W. Stott, and the financial support of the Department of Health and the Endowment Fund, United Birmingham Hospitals is acknowledged.

References

Burtis WJ, Wu T, Bunch C, Wysolmerski JJ, Insogna KL, Weir EC, Broadus AE, Stewart AF (1987) Identification of a novel 17,000-dalton parathyroid hormone-like adenylate cyclase-stimulating protein from tumour associated with humoral hypercalcemia of malignancy. J Biol Chem 262:7151–7156

Burtis WJ, Wu T, Insogna KL, Stewart AF (1988) Humoral hypercalcemia of malignancy. Ann Intern Med 108:454–457

Danks JA, Ebeling PR, Hayman J, Chou ST, Moseley JM, Dunlop J, Kemp BE, Martin TJ (1989) Parathyroid hormone-related protein: immunohistochemical localisation in cancers and in normal skin. J Bone Min Res 4:273–278

Docherty HM, Heath DA (1989) Multiple forms of parathyroid hormone-like proteins in a human tumour. J Molec Endocrinol 2:11–20

Juppner H, Abou-Samra A-B, Uneno S, Gu W-X, Potts JT, Segre GV (1988) The parathyroid hormone-like peptide associated with humoral hypercalcaemia of malignancy and parathyroid hormone bind to the same receptor on the plasma membrane of ROS 17/2.8 cells. J Biol Chem 263:8557–8560

Mangin M, Ikeda K, Dreyer BE, Milstone L, Broadus AE (1988a) Two distinct tumor-derived parathyroid hormone-like peptides result from alternative ribonucleic acid splicing. Molec Endocrinol 2:1049–1055

Mangin M, Webb AC, Dreyer BE, Posillico JT, Ikeda K, Weir EC, Stewart AF, Bander NH, Milstone L, Barton DE, Francke U, Broadus AE (1988b) Identification of a cDNA encoding a parathyroid hormone-like peptide from a human tumor associated with humoral hypercalcemia of malignancy. Proc Natl Acad Sci USA 85:597–601

Martin TJ, Ebeling PR, Rodda CP, Kemp BE (1988) Humoral hypercalcemia of malignancy: involvement of a novel hormone. Aust NZ J Med 18:287–295

Merendino JJ, Insogna KL, Milstone LM, Broadus AE, Stewart AF (1986) A parathyroid hormone-like protein from cultured human keratinocytes. Science 231:388–390

Moseley JM, Kubota M, Diefenbach-Jagger HD, Wettenhall REH, Kemp BE, Suva LJ, Rodda CP, Ebeling PR, Hudson PJ, Zajac JD, Martin TJ (1987) Parathyroid hormone-related protein purified from a human lung cancer line. Proc Natl Acad Sci USA 84:5048–5052

Motokura T, Fukumoto S, Takahashi S, Watanabe T, Matsumoto T, Igarashi T, Ogata E (1988) Expression of parathyroid hormone-related protein in human T cell lymphotrophic virus type 1-infected T cell line. Biochem Biophys Res Commun 154:1182–1188

Mundy GR, Ibbotson KJ, D'Souza SM, Simpson EL, Jacobs J W, Martin TJ (1984) The hypercalcemia of cancer. N Engl J Med 310:1718–1727

Pizurki L, Rizzoli R, Moseley J, Martin TJ, Caverzasio J, Bonjour J-P (1988) Effect of synthetic tumoral PTH-related peptide on cAMP production and Na-dependent Pi transport. Am Physiol Soc 255:F957–F961

Rabbani SA, Mitchell J, Roy DR, Hendy GN, Goltzman D (1988) Influence of the amino-terminus on *in vitro* and *in vivo* biological activity of synthetic parathyroid hormone-like peptides of malignancy. Endocrinology 123:2709–2716

Ratcliffe WA, Ratcliffe JG, Heath DA (1988) Development of a radioimmunoassay for parathyroid hormone related protein (PRP). Ann Clin Biochem 25 Supplement: 171s–172s

Rodda CP, Kubota M, Heath JA, Ebeling PR, Moseley JM, Care AD, Caple IW, Martin TJ (1988) Evidence for a novel parathyroid hormone related protein in fetal lamb parathyroid glands and sheep placenta: comparisons with a similar protein implicated in humoral hypercalcaemia of malignancy. J Endocrinol 117:261–271

Stewart AF, Insogna KL, Goltzman D, Broadus AE (1983) Identification of adenylate cyclase stimulating activity and cytochemical glucose-6-phosphate dehydrogenase stimulating activity in extracts of tumours from patients with humoral hypercalcemia of malignancy. Proc Natl Acad Sci USA 80:1454–1458

Stewart AF, Wu T, Goumas D, Burtis WJ, Broadus AE (1987) N-terminal amino acid sequence of two novel tumor-derived adenylate cyclase-stimulating proteins: identification of parathyroid hormone like and parathyroid hormone-unlike domains. Biochem Biophys Res Commun 146:672–678

Strewler GJ, Stern PH, Jacobs JW, Eveloff J, Klein RF, Leung SC, Rosenblatt M, Nissenson RA (1987) Parathyroid hormone like protein from human renal carcinoma cells. J Clin Invest 80:1803–1807

Suva LJ, Winslow GA, Wettenhall REH, Hammonds RG, Moseley JM, Diefenbach-Jagger H, Rodda CP, Kemp BE, Rodriguez H, Chen EY, Hudson PJ, Martin TJ, Wood WI (1987) A parathyroid hormone-related protein implicated in malignant hypercalcaemia: cloning and expression. Science 237:893–896

Thiede MA, Strewler GJ, Nissenson RA, Rosenblatt M, Rodan GA (1988) Human renal carcinoma expresses two messages encoding a parathyroid hormone-like peptide: evidence for the alternative splicing of a single copy gene. Proc Natl Acad Sci USA 85:4605–4609

Thiede MA, Rodan GA (1988) Expression of a calcium mobilizing parathyroid hormone-like peptide in lactating mammary tissue. Science 242:278–280

Thompson DD, Seedor JG, Fisher JE, Rosenblatt M, Rodan GA (1988) Direct action of the parathyroid hormone-like human hypercalcemic factor on bone. Proc Natl Acad Sci USA 85:5673–5677

Wu TL, Insogna KL, Hough LM, Milstone L, Stewart AF (1987) Skin derived fibroblasts respond to human parathyroid hormone-like adenylate cyclase-stimulating proteins. J Clin Endocrinol Metab 65:105–109.

4 Cyclic AMP

Chapter 4.1

Plasma and Urinary Cyclic AMP, Assay and Clinical Application

F.P. ARMBRUSTER

Introduction

The nucleotide cyclic adenosine-3′,5′-monophosphate (cAMP) serves as a second messenger for the intracellular metabolic regulation of many hormones which cannot pass through the cell membrane or can do so only with difficulty. cAMP is formed from ATP through hormonal stimulation of the enzyme adenylate cyclase, which is located on the cell membrane. In the renal cortex the production of cAMP is stimulated mainly by parathyroid hormone (PTH). The amount of cAMP excreted into the urine by tubular cells depends not only on renal function but also on the PTH level in serum. The quantitative determination of cAMP in urine can thus be used for the clinical diagnosis and differentiation of primary and secondary hyperparathyroidism as well as of pseudohypoparathyroidism [14, 16–18]. Due to an increased metabolic turnover in tumor cells, which results in increased cAMP production and release into blood, the determination of cAMP in plasma can be used to localize a tumor. Ykio Miura et al. [10] demonstrated this in the case of a pheochromocytoma.

Handa and Bressan [8] proposed to measure cAMP by stimulation of protein kinase, a method that does not involve radioactivity. Goldberg [7] has described a radioimmunoassay (RIA) with ^{125}I-labeled cAMP as a tracer and an incubation period of 20–24 h; prior to the assay cAMP is acetylated. The cAMP RIA presented by Steiner et al. [20] requires trichloroacetic acid extraction for the determination of cAMP in plasma.

Methods which measure cAMP by competitive protein-binding analysis [13, 22] offer the following advantages: (a) ^{3}H-labeled cAMP with a long half-life period and low radiolysis (b) use of a binding protein which can be obtained more easily and cheaper than antibodies, and (c) a shorter incubation period [5, 6, 9, 21].

We present a cAMP protein-binding assay similar to that of Tovey et al. [21]. In our assay, however, binding protein from bovine myocardium is used instead of binding protein from bovine skeletal muscles.

This study shows that the optimal binding of cAMP to the binding protein depends on the protein content in the reaction mixture and that cAMP can be measured in urine, plasma, and buffer media without preceding extraction or derivatization on optimum assay conditions.

The use of immunoassay vials (see Chap. 1.4) with a total volume of 600 μl [19] for the reaction mixtures and for scintillation counting reduces the amount of reagents required, streamlines the assay, and lowers the amount of radioactive waste.

Materials and Methods

Material

The following materials were used: immunoassay vials (Walter Sarstedt Co., Rommelsdorf-Nümbrecht, FRG, cat. No. 73.1055); aluminum racks for 96 immunoassay vials (Sarstedt Co., cat. No. 95.1012); stoppers for immunoassay vials (Sarstedt Co., cat. No. 65.1375); a cooling centrifuge Roto-Silenta/K prepared for microtiter plates (Andreas Hettich Co., Tuttlingen, FRG, type 5500); and a liquid scintillation system LS 7000 (Beckman Instruments, Munich, FRG, cat. No. 960701).

Reagents

The following reagents were used: cAMP, crystallized free acid (Boehringer Mannheim GmbH, Mannheim, FRG, cat. No. 102300); ATP, crystallized disodium salt (Boehringer Co., cat. No. 126888); cGMP [guanosine-3:5'-cyclic monophosphate (G-3:5-MP)], monosodium salt (Boehringer Co., cat. No. 106305); GTP (guanosine-5'-triphosphate), disodium salt (Boehringer Co., cat. No. 106372); GppNHp [guanylyl-imidodiphosphate (GMP-PNP)], tetra-lithium salt (Boehringer Co., cat. No. 106402); [^{3}H]cAMP [(5',8'-^{3}H) adenosine 3',5'-cyclic phosphate ammonium salt], (Amersham Buchler GmbH & Co KG, Braunschweig, FRG, cat. No. TRK 559); histone (Sigma Chemie GmbH, Deisenhofen, FRG, cat. No. 38205); binding protein isolated from bovine myocardium according to the method described by Tovey et al. (1974) for the extraction of cAMP-binding protein from bovine skeletal muscles; HSA (human serum albumin), purest crystallized (Serva Feinbiochemica GmbH & Co, Heidelberg, FRG, cat. No. 11860); Norit A charcoal, practical (Serva Co., cat. No. 30890); and Pico-Fluor™15, high-efficiency scintillation solution for aqueous samples (Packard Instruments GmbH, Frankfurt, FRG, cat. No. 6013059).

All other reagents were purchased from E. Merck Company, Darmstadt, FRG, in a *pro analysi* grade.

Preparation of the Reagents

The buffers used were Tris HCl buffer, pH 7.4, 50 mmol/liter + 4 mmol/liter ethylenediaminetetraacetic acid (EDTA); assay buffer, 100 ml Tris HCl buffer pH 7.4 + 2 g HSA.

In order to test the protein dependence of cAMP protein binding, the standards, tracer, and binding protein were diluted in Tris HCl buffer with 0, 5, 10, 20, and 50 g/liter HSA; for other tests the dilution was as follows:

For the preparation of standards the nucleotides were diluted in assay buffer to obtain the desired concentration. The tracer was standardized to about 50 000 cpm/20 µl by diluting 250 µCi in 80 ml assay buffer. The binding protein was diluted 200 times in assay buffer. To prepare the charcoal suspension, 1 g Norit A was suspended in 100 ml assay buffer.

Standards, tracer, and binding protein can be stored frozen at $-20\,°C$ for several months without loss of quality. Urinary creatinine concentration was measured photometrically according to the Bartels and Böhmer [3] modification of the Jaffe method.

Sample Material and Preparation

For the determination of cAMP in plasma, blood was collected in EDTA tubes (0.2 g EDTA/ml blood), centrifuged at 4°C, and the plasma stored at $-20\,°C$ until assaying. For the assay the plasma was diluted in protein-free Tris HCl buffer $1 + 1$. During the collection period, the 24-h urine was stored in the refrigerator at a temperature of $4\,°C$, one aliquot being stored at $-20\,°C$ until assaying. For the assay the urine was diluted $1:40$ in assay buffer. Cell extracts must be diluted to a measurable concentration after their preparation in assay buffer. All standards and samples were measured in duplicate.

Pipetting Scheme

```
   50 µl   standard or sample
 + 20 µl   tracer
 + 20 µl   binding protein
           Incubate at 4 °C for 3 h
 + 100 µl  charcoal
           Incubate at 4 °C for 5 min
           Centrifuge at 1800 g for 10 min
```

100 µl supernatant is added to 300 µl scintillation fluid in immunoassay vials. The vials are firmly closed by stoppers, mixed well and counted in a liquid scintillation counter for 2 min.

Results

Isolation of the Binding Protein

The heart of a bullock is removed as soon as possible after slaughtering and brought to the laboratory in a bucket filled with ice water. The heart is cleaned of fatty tissue and the muscles are cut into small pieces; this should be done in an ice-water bath. 300 grams of muscle are added to 900 ml 4 mmol/liter EDTA (1.49 g/liter), homogenized in a mixer (e.g. a Sorvall Omnimix) for 10 min and then treated with an Ultraturrax homogenizer for 5 min. The entire homogenate is centrifuged at 12 000 g for 45 min (Sorvall RC 2-B, rotor GS-33, 45 min × 8500 rpm) and the supernatant, about 900 ml, is used for further processing.

The subsequent acetic acid precipitation as described by Miyamoto et al. [11] may be omitted according to Tovey et al. [21].

The next step is an ammonium sulfate precipitation of the cyclic AMP-binding proteins: pinches of finely ground ammonium sulfate are evenly and slowly added to the supernatant over a period of 45 min, being constantly stirred on a magnetic mixer (surrounded by a bowl with ice water) in order to avoid an uneven concentration. After 45 min the ammonium sulfate concentration should be 32.6 g/100 ml. The mixture is stirred for another 30 min in an ice

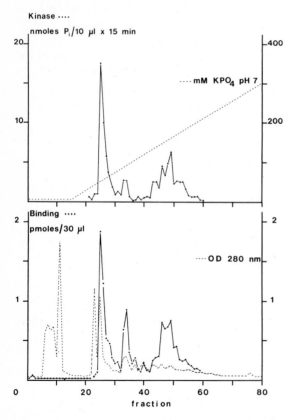

Fig. 1. Diethylaminoethanol-cellulose chromatography of the binding proteins for cyclic AMP from bovine myocardium. The elution was effected with potassium phosphate buffer, pH 7.0, from 5 to 400 mmol/liter (the figure only shows up to 300 mmol/liter). 20-milliliter fractions were collected

bath, then centrifuged at 12 000 g for 30 min and finally the supernatant is decanted carefully and discarded. The sediment contains the binding proteins for cyclic AMP. To the sediment is added 10 ml of 5 mmol/liter potassium phosphate buffer (3.48 g $K_2HPO_4/4$ liter) with   2 mmol/liter   EDTA (2.98 g/4 liters), pH 7.0, and dialysed against this buffer over night. The dialysate is loaded onto an ion-exchange column (DEAE-cellulose, Whatman DE 11, 1 mEq/g, column, Pharmacia Company, Uppsala, Sweden), which has been equilibrated with the potassium phosphate buffer (without EDTA). Elution occurs with a linear gradient of potassium phosphate, pH 7.0, of 5–400 mmol/liter (see Fig. 1).

Protein kinase activity was determined according to Miyamoto et al. [11], using histone as a substrate. The binding of [³H]cyclic AMP was tested with 4 pmol/reaction mixture. The binding protein (fraction 46-51) is frozen at − 20 °C in 1-ml portions. The number of binding sites for cyclic AMP can be increased by adding a so-called "inhibitor protein"—a protein which inhibits the transfer of $\gamma[^{32}P]ATP$ on histone by means of a cyclic-AMP-dependent protein kinase [1, 6]—or by adding serum albumin. Figure 2 illustrates the effects of inhibitor protein and serum albumin.

Figure 3 demonstrates the protein dependence of the cAMP protein binding. Up to 20 g/liter protein in the reaction mixture stimulates the binding activity,

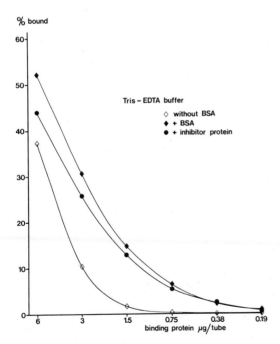

Fig. 2. Binding of [³H]cAMP to fraction 46-51 (peak II) of the binding protein in assay buffer (50 mmol/liter Tris, 4 mmol/EDTA, pH 7.4) without and with inhibitor protein or serum albumin

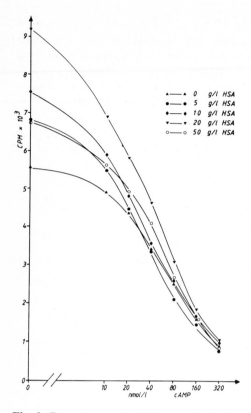

Fig. 3. Dependence of cAMP protein binding on the protein content in the reaction mixture: with 0, 5, 10, 20, and 50 g/liter human serum albumin added as a protein

whereas 50 g/liter partially inhibits the binding activity. All further assays were thus carried out in a 20 g/liter protein environment.

Protein-Binding Assay

Figure 4 shows a typical calibration curve of a reaction mixture with 20 g/liter human serum albumin. The detection limit, B_0-3S, is at 3.8 nmol/liter cAMP. The 80%, 50%, and 20% marks (related to the maximum binding) are found at 10, 38, and 150 nmol/liter cAMP. The linearity of the assay curve was examined in a dilution series of urine diluted 1:10 in assay buffer. As shown in Fig. 5, linearity is guaranteed over the total measuring range of the calibration curve, from approximately 5 to 300 nmol/liter cAMP. Cross-reactions with other nucleotides that are present in serum, urine, and cell extracts such as cGMP, ATP, GTP and the synthetic substance GppNHp are negligible up to 10^{-4} mol/liter nucleotide or do not occur at all (Fig. 6). The cAMP values of the control samples, which are measured in each assay, one plasma and one urine diluted

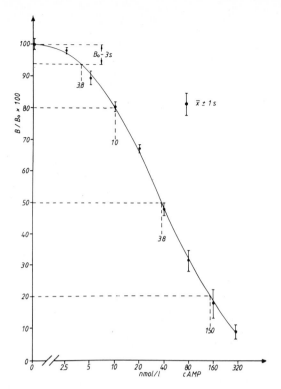

Fig. 4. Typical cAMP calibration curve of a reaction mixture with 20 g/liter protein. *B*, bound [³H]cAMP; $\bar{x}$, mean value; *s*, standard deviation

1:40 in assay buffer, were verified by adding known amounts of cAMP in equal volume parts to plasma and urine. The result was a calculated cAMP concentration value of 17 nmol/liter for the control plasma and 88 nmol/liter for the control urine (Fig. 7).

Intraassay reproducibility was verified by measuring 3 different samples 40 times each. The mean values of the determined cAMP concentrations were 18, 59, and 212 nmol/liter with *CV* values of 10.9%, 5.3%, and 6.8% (see Table 1). Table 2 shows that the mean values of the cAMP concentrations determined in the control samples, which were measured in each assay over a longer period, correspond to the results shown in Fig. 7. The control samples were measured in 32 consecutive assays and yielded a mean value of 17.5 nmol/liter cAMP with a *CV* value of 11.7% for the control plasma and a mean value of 90.1 nmol/liter with a *CV* value of 10.3% for the control urine. A collection of 24-h urines (*n* = 33) and EDTA plasma from healthy control persons (*n* = 35) aged between 18 and 45 years showed the following normal ranges: a normal range of 1.9–4.6 µmol cAMP/g creatinine for urinary excretion (see Table 3).

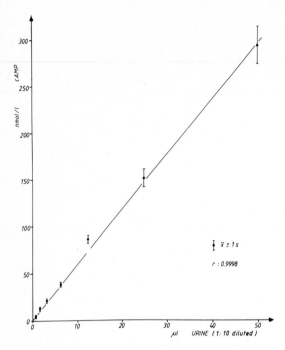

Fig. 5. Linearity testing of the cAMP-measuring system: $\bar{x}$, mean value; r, coefficient of correlation

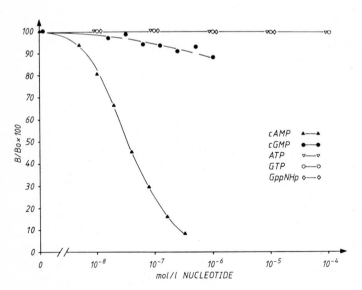

Fig. 6. Displacement curves of various nucleotides: cAMP, cGMP, ATP, GTP, and GppNHp

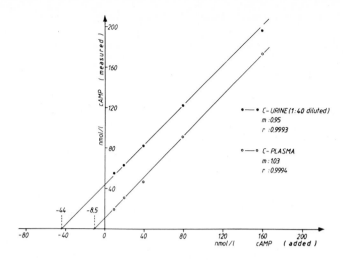

Fig. 7. Addition of known amounts of cAMP to the control urine and control plasma. *m*, slope; *r*, coefficient of correlation

Table 1. Intraassay variation of two different urine dilutions and one plasma, determined from $n = 40$ duplicates each

Sample	n	$\bar{x}$ (nmol/liter)	s (nmol/liter)	CV (%)
Plasma	40	18.1	2.0	10.9
Urine 1 (diluted 1:40)	40	58.8	3.1	5.3
Urine 2 (diluted 1:40)	40	211.8	14.5	6.8

$\bar{x}$, mean value; s, standard deviation; CV, coefficient of variation

Table 2. Interassay variation of the two control samples measured in each assay

Sample	n	$\bar{x}$ (nmol/liter)	s (nmol/liter)	CV (%)
Control plasma	32	17.5	2.0	11.7
Control urine (diluted 1:40)	32	90.1	9.3	10.3

n, number; $\bar{x}$, mean value; s, standard deviation; CV, coefficient of variation

The cAMP determination in plasma, using 50 µl plasma samples (excessive protein concentration), yielded a normal range of 9.9–33.5 nmol/liter with a mean value of 21.7 nmol/liter. We diluted the plasma samples with protein-free Tris HCl buffer at a 1:2 ratio (a protein concentration close to that of the

Table 3. Normal range of cAMP in urine, related to creatinine excretion, determined in the 24-h urines of 33 healthy persons

Sample	n	$\bar{x}$ (μmol/g)	2s (μmol/g)	$\bar{x} \pm 2s$ (μmol/g)	Range (μmol/g)
50 μl urine (diluted 1:40)	33	3.1	1.3	1.8–4.4	1.9–4.6

$\bar{x}$, mean value; s, standard deviation

Table 4. Comparison of the normal ranges of cAMP in plasma between 50 μl plasma samples and 50 μl plasma samples diluted 1:2 of 35 healthy control persons

Method	n	$\bar{x}$ (nmol/liter)	2s (nmol/liter)	$\bar{x} \pm 2s$ (nmol/liter)	Range (nmol/liter)
50 μl plasma	35	21.7	11.8	9.9–33.5	15–36
50 μl plasma (diluted 1:2)	35	16.7	8.9	7.8–25.6	8–28

$\bar{x}$, mean value; s, standard deviation

standards) and found a normal range for cAMP in plasma of 7.8–25.6 nmol/liter with a mean value of 16.7 nmol/liter (see Table 4).

As the recovery shown in Fig. 7 is excellent for plasma diluted 1:2, the higher concentrations found with undiluted plasma seem to be inappropriate (Table 4).

Discussion

When determining cAMP in samples having very different protein concentration such as plasma, urine, and cell extracts, the binding assay yields incorrect values unless the protein concentration in the samples is adjusted. The different protein contents of plasma, urine, and cell extracts have a different influence on the cAMP protein binding, depending on the protein concentration of the respective sample. By diluting the plasma samples with a protein-free buffer and the urine or cell extract samples with a protein-containing buffer, the protein concentrations of the samples to be analyzed can be adjusted. We selected 20 g/liter protein because this concentration leads to a maximum binding, as this chapter has shown. This is contradictory to the maximum binding with 0.5 g/liter protein in the reaction mixture and a declining binding capacity with a higher protein concentration, as described by Tovey et al. [21].

Adjusting the protein concentrations makes a direct measuring system possible. Preparation of an extract or of a derivative prior to the assay is unnecessary.

The cAMP method presented by us, with a detection limit of less than 4 nmol/liter, is still able to measure the cAMP level in plasma if the plasma has been diluted 1 + 1 with a buffer. The determined normal range for cAMP in plasma of 8–28 nmol/liter corresponds well to the normal ranges found by other research groups [2, 4]. The cAMP values measured in plasma without preceding dilution in a protein-free buffer are, however, approximately 5 nmol/liter higher, falsified by a reduced binding capacity of the [^{3}H]cAMP due to the excessive protein content of the reaction mixture. It is unlikely that an increase in the protein concentration results in a continuously reduced adsorption of free [^{3}H]cAMP to charcoal, since this would mean that the highest protein concentration would yield the highest counting rates. The protein concentration had no influence on the quench rate, as the constant quench numbers and channel ratios proved. The strongly differing cAMP values in urine can be adapted to the measuring range covered by the assay through previous dilution of the urine at a ratio of 1:40. The linearity of 5 to approximately 300 nmol/liter guarantees reliable results for strongly diluted as well as for concentrated urines, without the necessity to repeat the measurement in other dilutions. This assay yields a normal range of cAMP in urine, related to the creatinine excretion, of 1.9–4.6 µmol cAMP/g creatinine, and thus corresponds with the normal ranges described by Murad and Pak [12] and Sato et al. [15]. The intraassay and interassay CV values of approximately 10% and less are satisfactory. Apart from using this measuring system with binding protein extracted from bovine myocardium for the routine determination of cAMP in plasma and urine, it can also be employed for determining cAMP in cell extracts for research purposes. The nucleotides ATP and GTP, which are present in the cells besides cAMP, and the synthetically produced GppNHp show no cross-reaction up to 10^{-4} mol/liter; cGMP shows only a negligible cross-reaction. Therefore the cell extract samples do not yield falsely high cAMP concentration values either.

The use of immunoassay vials in 96-tube racks makes it possible to handle larger routine and research series economically and reduces the amount of reagents and material required. At the same time there is considerably less radioactive waste if immunoassay vials are employed for liquid scintillation counting instead of the formerly used 7-ml scintillation tubes.

References

1. Appleman MM, Birnbaumer L, Torres HN (1966) Factors affecting the activity of muscle glyogen synthetase. Arch Biochem Biophys 116:39–43
2. Barling PM, Albano JDM, Tomlinson S, Brown BL, O'Riordan JLH (1974) A saturation assay method for adenosine 3′:5′-cyclic monophosphate in plasma and its

use in studies of the action of bovine parathyroid hormone. Biochem Soc Trans 2:453–455

3. Bartels H, Böhmer M (1971) Eine Mikromethode zur Kreatininbestimmung. Clin Chim Acta 32:81–85

4. Broadus AE, Kaminsky NI, Hardman JG, Sutherland EW, Liddle GW (1970) Kinetic parameters and renal clearances of plasma adenosine 3′,5′-monophosphate and guanosine 3′,5′-monophosphate in man. J Clin Invest 49:2222–2236

5. Brown BL, Albano JDM, Ekins RP, Sgherzi AM, Tampion W (1971) A simple and sensitive saturation assay method for the measurement of adenosine 3′:5′-cyclic monophosphate. Biochem J 121:561–562

6. Gilman AG (1972) Protein binding assays for cyclic nucleotides. In: Advances in cyclic nucleotide research, vol 2. Eds Greengard P, Robison GA, Paoletti R. Raven, New York, pp 9–24

7. Goldberg ML (1977) Radioimmunoassay for adenosine 3′,5′-cyclic monophosphate and guanosine 3′,5′-cyclic monophosphate in human blood, urine and cerebrospinal fluid. Clin Chem 23:576–580

8. Handa AK, Bressan RA (1980) Assay of adenosine 3′,5′ cyclic monophosphate by stimulation of protein kinase: a method not involving radioactivity. Anal Biochem 102:332–339

9. Madsen SN, Badawi I, Skovsted L (1975) A simple competitive protein-binding assay for adenosine-3′,5′-monophosphate in plasma and urine. Acta Endocrinol (Copenh) 81:208–214

10. Miura Y, Nezu M, Kimura S, Yoshinaga K, Endoh M (1984) Localisation of pheochromocytoma by measurement of plasma cyclic AMP. N Engl J Med 311:676

11. Miyamoto E, Kuo JF, Greengard P (1969) Cyclic nucleotide-dependent protein Kinases. J Biol Chem 244:6395–6402

12. Murad F, Pak CYC (1972) Urinary excretion of adenosine-3′,5′-monophosphate and guanosine-3′,5′-monophosphate. N Engl J Med 286:1382–1387

13. Nagel W, Schmidt-Gayk H, Förster P, Wahl HD, Voll R (1978) Grundlagen des Radioimmunoassay (RIA) und der competitiven Protein-Bindungs-Analyse (CPBA). Medizintechnik 98:36–44

14. Potts JT Jr (1987) Diseases of the parathyroid gland and other hyper- and hypocalcemic disorders. In: Harrison's principles of internal medicine. McGraw-Hill, New York, pp 1870–1889

15. Sato T, Saito K, Takezawa J, Fujishima T, Iijima T, Kuninaka A, Yoshina H (1981) Urinary excretion of cyclic nucleotides and principal electrolytes in healthy humans of different ages. Clin Chim Acta 110:215–225

16. Schmidt-Gayk H, Röher HD (1973) Urinary excretion of cyclic adenosine monophosphate in the detection and diagnosis of primary hyperparathyroidism. Surg Gynecol Obstet 137:439–444

17. Schmidt-Gayk H, Seitz H, Stengel R, Ritz E (1975) Secondary hyperparathyroidism of gastrointestinal and renal origin: influence of renal function on urinary cyclic AMP. In: 12th International Congress of Internal Medicine, Tel Aviv. Karger, Basel, pp 130–134

18. Schmidt-Gayk H, Stengel R, Haueisen H, Hüfner M, Ritz E, Jakobs KH (1977). Hyperparathyoidism: influence of glomerular filtration rate on urinary excretion of cyclic AMP. Klin Wochenschr 55:275–281

19. Schmidt-Gayk H, Wahl M, Limbach HJ, Walch S (1979) Ein spezielles Gefäß zur Durchführung des Radioimmunoassays (RIA). Medizintechnik 99:103–104

20. Steiner AL, Wehmann RE, Parker CW, Kipnis DM (1972) Radioimmunoassay for the measurement of cyclic nucleotides. In: Advances in cyclic nucleotide research, vol 2, Eds Greengard P, Robison GA, Paoletti R. Raven, New York, pp 51–61
21. Tovey KC, Oldham KG, Whelan JAM (1974) A simple direct assay for cyclic AMP in plasma and other biological samples using an improved competitive protein binding technique. Clin Chim Acta 56:221–234
22. Zettner A (1973) Principles of competitive binding assays (saturation analyses). I Equilibrium techniques. Clin Chem 19:669–705

5 Vitamin D: Assays of 25-Hydroxyvitamin D (Calcidiol) and 1,25-Dihydroxyvitamin D (Calcitriol)

Chapter 5.1

Simultaneous Determination of 25-Hydroxyvitamin D_2 and 25-Hydroxyvitamin D_3 by High-Performance Liquid Chromatography

E. Mayer and H. Schmidt-Gayk

Introduction

Vitamin D_3, biosynthesized in the skin or ingested in the diet along with vitamin D_2, is bound to vitamin D-binding protein (DBP) and transported to the liver to be 25-hydroxylated [21]. The resulting metabolites, namely 25-OH-D_2 and 25-OH-D_3, represent major circulating forms of the vitamin and therefore their serum concentrations are a good measure for the vitamin D status of the individual. Under normal circumstances, the serum concentration of 25-OH-D_2 is low in comparison to 25-OH-D_3 even in countries where food products are fortified with vitamin D_2. In fact, Hughes et al. [12] reported that the vitamin D_2 metabolite contributed less than 5% to the 25-OH-D serum concentration in healthy American blood donors. On the other hand, as expected, patients on high-dose vitamin D_2 treatment had very high levels of 25-OH-D_2.

As well as in individuals with low vitamin D intake or insufficient exposure to sunlight, low levels of 25-OH-D were found in patients with severe parenchymal or cholestatic liver disease [16], in patients with malabsorption syndrome, and in patients with nephrotic syndrome. The latter have marked proteinuria and thus lose DBP along with its ligand 25-OH-D into the urine [24]. Also, low levels of 25-OH-D were reported in patients on long-term antiepileptic therapy with phenytoin and phenobarbital [10]. These drugs appear to inactivate vitamin D and its metabolites through enzyme activation in the liver.

The first assays for 25-OH-D_3 included a chromatographic step and quantitation of the metabolite by competitive protein-binding analysis [1, 9]. Several modifications of these methods, some omitting the chromatographic step, have been reported since [2, 3, 5, 6, 20, 22, 25]. Also, the determination of 25-OH-D_3 by applying isotope dilution-mass fragmentography has been described [4]. A third type of assay for 25-OH-D uses high-performance liquid chromatography [7, 8, 11, 13-15, 18, 19, 23, 26, 27]. Because 25-OH-D_2 is slightly less polar than 25-OH-D_3 (for chemical structures of vitamin D metabolites, see Fig. 1), application of HPLC allows the simultaneous quantitation of 25-OH-D_2 and 25-OH-D_3.

All HPLC methods reported involve extraction of the vitamin D metabolite into organic solvents, followed by one or more chromatographic steps using Sephadex LH 20, silic acid, or celite prior to HPLC. Then, final purification and

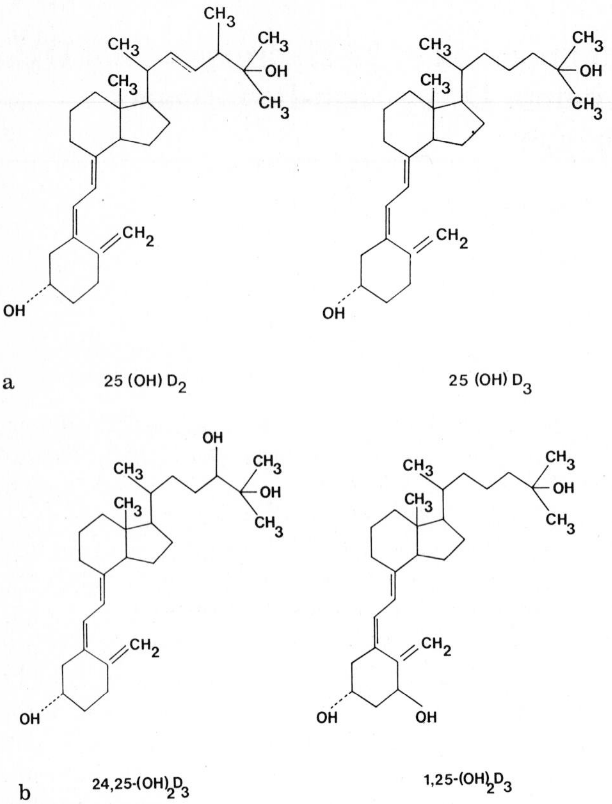

Fig. 1a,b. Chemical structures of 25-OH-D$_2$ and 25-OH-D$_3$, 24,25-(OH)$_2$D$_3$ and 1,25-(OH)$_2$D$_3$

quantitation of the metabolites is achieved by measurement of their UV absorption following HPLC chromatography.

In this chapter we describe an assay for the simultaneous determination of 25-OH-D$_2$ and 25-OH-D$_3$, applying HPLC with UV detection of the compounds, which enables the metabolites to be quantified in 0.5-ml serum samples when a detection limit of 20 nmol/liter is applied.

Experimental Procedures

Instruments and Chemicals

High-performance liquid chromatography was carried out with a Waters Model 6000 A equipped with a detector, Model 440 nm (Waters Associates, Milford, MA, United States). A µPorasil column (0.39 × 30 cm, Waters) was used for metabolite separation. Sephadex LH 20 was purchased from Pharmacia Fine Chemicals, Uppsala, Sweden. All solvents were obtained *pro analysi* grade from E. Merck Co., Darmstadt, Federal Republic of Germany; 25-OH-D_2 was kindly provided by Dr. J. Babcock, Upjohn Co., Kalamazoo, MI, United States and 25-OH-D_3 by Dr. H. Rust, Albert-Roussel Co., Wiesbaden, Federal Republic of Germany; 25-OH-[26,27-H^3]-D_3 (specific radioactivity 110 Ci/mmol) was purchased from Amersham-Buchler GmbH, Frankfurt, Federal Republic of Germany.

Methods

Samples

Plasma or serum samples from healthy blood donors collected in June were pooled. To parts of this pool either 25-OH-D_2 (8, 20, 40, or 80 ng/0.5 ml) or 25-OH-D_3 (20, 50, 100, or 200 ng/0.5 ml) were added. In addition, sera from healthy blood donors ($n = 15$), from hypoparathyroid patients on high-dose vitamin D_2 or D_3 therapy, and from a patient with nutritional osteomalacia were assayed for their 25-OH-D_2 and 25-OH-D_3 content. Finally, a sample of a healthy individual on vitamin D intake (15000 units/day) for a period of 2 weeks was analyzed.

Extraction

Sera (0.5 ml) were pipetted into conical glass tubes and [^{3}H]25-OH-D_3 (5000 cpm in 10 µl ethanol) was added. Following an equilibration period of 30 min at room temperature, 3 ml cold methyl alcohol/dichloromethane (2:1, v/v) was added (10). After mixing, the samples were allowed to stand for 15 min at 4 °C. Then, 1 ml dichloromethane was added followed by centrifugation of the samples for 10 min at 500 g. Using Pasteur pipettes, the lower layers were removed and the upper layers were reextracted with 1 ml dichloromethane. The organic layers were pooled and subsequently evaporated to dryness under nitrogen in a water bath at 37 °C.

Sephadex LH 20 Chromatography

The residues were redissolved in 500 µl LH solvent (*n*-hexane/chloroform/ methyl alcohol, 9:1:1, v/v) and applied to Sephadex LH 20 columns (0.6 × 16 cm). Columns were equilibrated and eluted with the solvent systems described above. The fraction eluted from 5 to 10 ml was collected and evaporated to dryness under nitrogen. The column had been calibrated previously with [^{3}H]-D_3, [^{3}H]25-OH-D_3, and [^{3}H]24-25(OH)$_2$–D_3.

High-Performance Liquid Chromatography

The fraction containing 25-OH-D was redissolved in 50 µl HPLC solvent and applied to a µPorasil column, which was eluted with 4% isopropyl alcohol in *n*-hexane. The flow rate used was 1.5 ml/min, the sensitivity of the UV detector 0.01 Absorbance Units Full Scale (AUFS). At min 6 of each run, the speed of the recorder was increased from 0.5 cm/min to 3 cm/min in order to improve the precision of the determination of the area under the peaks. The retention times of 25-OH-D$_2$ and 25-OH-D$_3$ were determined using authentic standards.

Recovery

The fraction containing 25-OH-D$_3$ was collected, evaporated to dryness under nitrogen, and redissolved in 200 µl ethanol. Samples were transferred into a Pico-Plastik vial (Packard Instruments, Frankfurt, FRG) and counted in a liquid scintillation counter (model LS 7000, Beckman Instruments Inc., Fullerton, CA, United States) using a scintillation cocktail of 4 ml Pico-Fluor™15 (Packard Instruments). To calculate recovery the amount of radioactivity recovered was related to that originally added.

Quantitation of 25-OH-D$_2$ and 25-OH-D$_3$

Ultraviolet absorbance after separation of the metabolites by HPLC was quantitated in the samples. The quantity of metabolite was determined by comparison with standard curves derived from chromatography of various amounts of 25-OH-D$_2$ and 25-OH-D$_3$, respectively. The plasma concentration of the metabolites was then calculated by the following equation:

$$\text{nmol/liter} = \frac{\text{nmol in sample tube}}{(0.5 \text{ ml plasma sample}) \times (\text{recovery of } [^3\text{H}]25\text{-OH-D}_3)}$$

Table 1. Flow chart of procedures used for the simultaneous quantitation of 25-OH-D$_2$ and 25-OH-D$_3$ by HPLC with UV detection

---

Serum (0.5 ml) + [^{3}H]25-OH–D$_3$ (5000 cpm)

Extraction using dichloromethane/methyl alcohol (1:2, v/v)

Sephadex LH 20 chromatography (column size 0.6 × 16 cm, solvent system: *n*-hexane/chloroform/methyl alcohol (9:1:1, v/v)

High-performance liquid chromatography (HPLC) (10 µm µPorasil column (0.39 × 30 cm), solvent system: *n*-hexane/isopropyl alcohol (96:4, v/v)

Integration of the area under the 25-OH-D$_2$ and 25-OH-D$_3$ peaks

---

Results

Extraction

Ninety-eight percent of the $[^3H]$25-OH-D_3 initially added was recovered after extraction with dichloromethane/methyl alcohol.

Sephadex LH 20 Chromatography

The initial chromatographic step, elution of 25-OH-D in hexane/chloroform/ methyl alcohol (9:1:1, v/v) from Sephadex LH 20 columns, removed the bulk of interfering lipids from 25-OH-D. Applying 0.6×16-cm columns, $[^3H]$25-OH-D_3 was eluted from 5 to 10 ml (see Fig. 2). This fraction was evaporated to dryness under nitrogen at 37 °C in a water bath and subsequently subjected to HPLC. After extraction and Sephadex LH 20 chromatography, recovery averaged 77%.

High-Performance Liquid Chromatography

Final purification and quantitation of the metabolites was achieved by HPLC with UV detection. The elution profile of synthetic 25-OH-D is shown in Fig. 3. In all samples processed, at 8 min a UV-absorbing peak not related to vitamin D appeared which slightly contaminated the 25-OH-D_3 region. Since this area can easily be subtracted from that under the 25-OH-D_3-peak, we did not change our

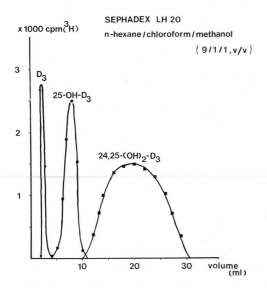

Fig. 2. Elution profile of tritiated vitamin D_3, 25-OH-D_3, and 24,25(OH)$_2$D$_3$ from Sephadex columns

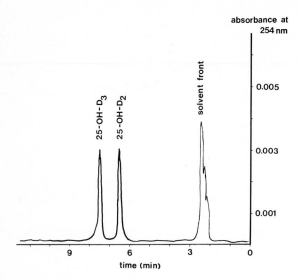

Fig. 3. High-performance liquid chromatography with UV detection of 25-OH-D$_2$ and 25-OH-D$_3$ standards (for conditions see text)

procedure. Complete separation from this contaminant can be achieved by using a somewhat less polar solvent system, e.g., 3% isopropyl alcohol in *n*-hexane. Of course this procedure is more time consuming.

Accuracy

Various amounts of 25-OH-D$_2$ [8–80 ng (19–194 pmol)/0.5 ml] or 25-OH-D$_3$ [20–200 ng (50-500 pmol)/0.5 ml] were added to pool sera from healthy volunteers. The amount recovered, corrected for losses using [^{3}H]25-OH-D$_3$ as internal standard, followed a linear pattern (see Fig. 4). These samples were assayed in triplicate. As can be seen from Fig. 4, the results obtained for both compounds were well reproducible at any concentration.

Clinical Samples

The range of 25-OH-D$_3$ levels in plasma samples from a group of 15 healthy individuals was 28–160 nmol/liter with an average of 68 $\pm$ 22 (SD) nmol/liter. No. 25-OH-D$_2$ was detectable in any of these samples. The elution profile of a sample derived from a healthy person on oral intake of vitamin D$_2$ is shown in Fig. 5. In fact, this individual, a 19-year-old member of an Army Medical Corps, had served as one of the volunteers. To our surprise 25-OH-D$_2$ was easily detectable in his plasma, he agreed that he had taken in 2 weeks 15 000 units vitamin D$_2$/day plus vitamin C (Calcium Frubiase forte) because of its good taste. Furthermore, a sample of a patient with nutritional osteomalacia was

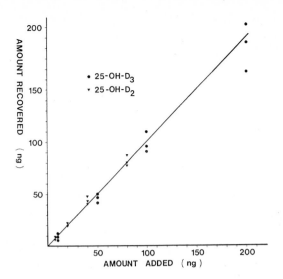

Fig. 4. Recovery of 25-OH-D_2 or 25-OH-D_3 added to parts of a plasma pool (healthy blood donors) before extraction

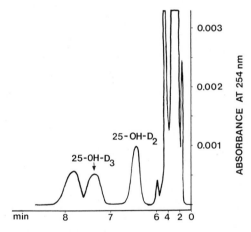

Fig. 5. High-performance liquid chromatography with UV detection of 25-OH-D_2 and 25-OH-D_3 isolated from serum of a normal individual on oral intake of 15000 units vitamin D_2 for 2 weeks

assessed. 25-OH-D in either form of the vitamin was not detectable (see Fig. 6). The detection limit of the method is 20 nmol/liter when 0.5 ml serum is extracted. Also, 25-OH-D_2 and 25-OH-D_3 were measured in sera from two hypoparathyroid patients treated with high-dose vitamin D_2 or D_3 to maintain normocalcemia. 25-OH-D_2 was not detectable in the serum from the patient on vitamin D_3 therapy and was measured at 1850 nmol/liter in the patient treated

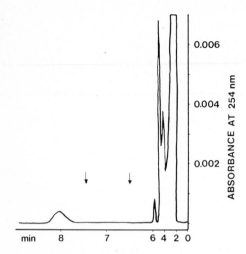

Fig. 6. High-performance liquid chromatography of a plasma sample from a patient with nutritional osteomalacia

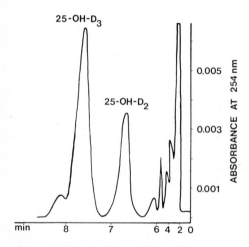

Fig. 7. High-performance liquid chromatography and UV detection of 25-OH-D$_2$ and 25-OH-D$_3$ isolated from a normal serum where 40 ng (97 pmol) 25-OH-D$_2$ and 100 ng (250 pmol) 25-OH-D$_3$ had been added before extraction

with vitamin D$_2$. In the patient on high-dose vitamin D$_3$ treatment, a 25-OH-D$_3$ concentration of 418 nmol/liter was detected and a level of 32 nmol/liter in the D$_2$-treated patient. Finally, in Fig. 7 the HPLC elution profile of a sample from a healthy volunteer is shown, where 40 ng (97 pmol) 25-OH-D$_2$ and 100 ng (250 pmol) 25-OH-D$_3$ had been added before the assay.

Discussion

Based on the report by Horst et al. [11], we have developed an assay for the simultaneous determination of 25-OH-D_2 and 25-OH-D_3 by quantitation of their UV absorbance following HPLC chromatography. Using Sephadex LH 20 chromatography as did Horst et al. [11], but omitting the additional purification steps on Lipidex 5000 and yet another Sephadex LH 20 column, we found that this single chromatographic step is sufficient as prepurification prior to HPLC. Also, for reasons of practicability, we used a higher polarity of the HPLC solvent system eluting 25-OH-D_3 at 10 ml (versus 25 ml in Horst's assay), with 25-OH-D_2 and 25-OH-D_3 still being well separated. The 25-OH-D_3 region was constantly slightly contaminated by a more polar compound not related to vitamin D. Since this did not complicate the determination of the area under the 25-OH-D_3 peak, we decided not to change our solvents used for HPLC. If complete separation of this compound is desired, it can easily be done by applying a somewhat less polar system (e.g., 3% isopropyl alcohol in *n*-hexane). Of course this procedure is more time consuming.

The mean 25-OH-D_3 concentration measured in 15 healthy subjects was 68 nmol/liter. This agrees with reports applying isotope dilution-mass fragmentography [4], competitive protein-binding assay [1, 9], or similar methods to ours using HPLC with UV detection [7, 15]. No. 25-OH-D_2 was detected in the samples from volunteers. Since in Germany food products are not fortified with vitamin D, this result was expected. In the United States, where this has been done for decades, 25-OH-D_2 contributes about 5% to the plasma 25-OH-D as reported by Hughes et al. [12].

In summary, the assay method for the simultaneous determination of 25-OH-D_2 and 25-OH-D_3 is accurate, reproducible, and highly specific. Also, in contrast to other methods applying HPLC which have been reported, small sample volumes (0.5 ml) are sufficient and a detection limit of 20 nmol/liter is adequate. However, even in this simplified version, the method is quite laborious in comparison to competitive protein-binding assays for 25-OH-D and is therefore not suitable as a routine method for clinical purposes. On the other hand, it may well serve as a reference method. In fact, we have applied this assay for samples used for an interlaboratory comparison of 25-OH-D determination within Europe [17].

References

1. Belsey RE, DeLuca HF, Potts JT jr (1971) Competitive binding assay for vitamin D and 25-OH-vitamin D. J Clin Endocrinol Metab 33:554–557
2. Belsey RE, DeLuca HF, Potts JT jr (1974) A rapid assay for 25-OH-vitamin D_3 without preparative chromatography. J Clin Endocrinol Metab 38:1046–1051

3. Bishop JE, Norman AW, Coburn JW et al. (1980) Determination of the concentration of 25-hydroxyvitamin D, 24,25-dihydroxyvitamin D and 1,25-dihydroxyvitamin D in a single 2 ml plasma sample. Miner Electrolyte Metab 3:181–189
4. Björkhem J, Holmberg I (1976) A novel specific assay for 25-hydroxyvitamin D_3. Clin Chim Acta 68:215–219
5. Bouillon R, van Kerkhove P, DeMoor P (1976) Measurement of 25-hydroxyvitamin D_3 in serum. Clin Chem 22:364–368
6. Edelsteins S, Charman M, Lawson DEM, Kodicek E (1974) Competitive protein-binding assay for 25-hydroxycholecalciferol. Clin Sci Mol Med 46:231–240
7. Eisman JA, Shepard RM, DeLuca HF (1977) Determination of 25-hydroxyvitamin D_2 and 25-hydroxyvitamin D_3 in human plasma using high-pressure liquid chromatography. Anal Biochem 80:298–305
8. Gilbertson TJ, Stryd RP (1977) High-performance liquid chromatographic assay for 25-hydroxyvitamin D_3 in serum. Clin Chem 23:1700–1704
9. Haddad J, Chyu KJ (1971) Competitive protein-binding radioassay for 25-hydroxycholecalciferol. J Clin Endocrinol Metab 33:992–995
10. Hahn JJ, Birge SJ, Sharp CR (1972) Phenobarbital-induced alterations in vitamin D metabolism. J Clin Invest 51:741–748
11. Horst HL, Shepard RM, Jorgensen NA, DeLuca HF (1979) Assay for vitamin D and its metabolites. In: Norman AW et al. (eds) Vitamin D; basic research and its clinical application. de Gruyter, Berlin, pp 213–220
12. Hughes MR, Baylink DJ, Jones PG, Haussler MR (1976) Radioligand receptor assay for 25-hydroxyvitamin D_2/D_3 and $1\alpha,25$-dihydroxy-vitamin D_2/D_3. J Clin Invest 58:61–70
13. Jones G (1978) Assay of vitamins D_2 and D_3, and 25-hydroxyvitamins D_2 and D_3 in human plasma by high-performance liquid chromatography. Clin Chem 24:287–298
14. Koshy KT, Van der Slik AL (1977) High-performance liquid chromatographic method for the determination of 25-hydroxycholecalciferol in human serum. Anal Lett 10:523–537
15. Lambert PW, Syverson BJ, Arnaud CD, Spelsberg TC (1977) Isolation and quantitation of endogenous vitamin D and its physiologically important metabolites in human plasma by high-pressure liquid chromatography. J Steroid Biochem 8:929–937
16. Long RG, Skinner RK, Meinhard E, Wills MR, Sherlock S (1976) Serum 25-OH-D values in liver disease and hepatic osteomalacia. Gut 17:824–827
17. Mayer E, Schmidt–Gayk H (1984) Interlaboratory comparison of 25-hydroxyvitamin D determination. Clin Chem 30:1199–1204
18. Mayer E, Schmidt–Gayk H, Gartner R, Knuppen R (1981) Simultaneous assay of 25-OH-vitamin D_2 and 25-OH-vitamin D_3 by HPLC. Acta Endocrinol [Suppl] (Copenh) 240, (96): A44
19. Mayer E, Schmidt–Gayk H, Lichtwald K et al. (1981) Simultane Bestimmung von 25-Hydroxy-Vitamin-D_2 und 25-Hydroxy-Vitamin-D_3 durch Hochdruckflüssigkeitschromatographie. Ärztl Lab 27:89–94
20. Morris JF, Peacock M (1976) Assay of plasma 25 hydroxyvitamin D. Clin Chim Acta 72:383–391
21. Norman AW, Roth J, Orci L (1982) The vitamin D endocrine system: steroid metabolism, hormone receptors, and biological response (calcium binding proteins). Endocr Rev 3:331–366

22. Preece MA, O'Riordan JLH, Lawson DEM, Kodicek E (1974) A competitive protein-binding assay for 25-hydroxycholecalciferol and 25-hydroxyergocalciferol in serum. Clin Chim Acta 54:235–242
23. Schaefer PC, Goldsmith RS (1978) Quantitation of 25-hydroxycholecalciferol in human serum by high-pressure liquid chromatography. J Lab Clin Med 91:104–108
24. Schmidt–Gayk H, Grawunder C, Tschöpe W et al. (1977) 25-Hydroxyvitamin D in nephrotic syndrome. Lancet II:105–108
25. Schmidt–Gayk H, Nagel W, Martiskainen I et al. (1977) Sättigungsanalyse für 25-Hydroxy-Vitamin-D. Ärztl Lab 23:111–123
26. Shepard RM, Horst RL, Hamstra AJ, DeLuca HF (1979) Determination of vitamin D and its metabolites in plasma from normal and anephric man. Biochem J 182:55–69
27. Stryd RP, Gilbertson TJ (1978) Some problems in development of a high-performance liquid chromatographic assay to measure 25-hydroxyvitamin D_2 and 25-hydroxyvitamin D_3 simultaneously in human serum. Clin Chem 24:927–930

Chapter 5.2

Competitive Protein-Binding Assay for the Diagnosis of Hyper- and Hypovitaminosis D

V. Bothe and H. Schmidt-Gayk

Introduction

Vitamin D is absorbed from the diet and produced in the skin by UV light radiation. It is then metabolized by the liver to a more potent compound, 25-hydroxyvitamin D (25-OH-D), which is the major metabolite in plasma. A large number of binding assays for 25-OH-D have been published, as shown in Table 1. Using the competitive binding assay described by Belsey et al. (1974), a shortcoming in the assay was observed to be insufficient binding of [^{3}H]25-OH-D to the binding protein, with fairly high coefficients of variation. Therefore, the conditions of the assay were reevaluated. As will be shown, the result was an assay entirely different from the published ones. The extraction, binding protein, gelatin concentration, and tracer solvent differ from those in the published methods. In addition, this assay circumvents the need for evaporation of the extract.

Materials and Methods

25-Hydroxy [23,24 (n)^{3}H] cholecalciferol (code TRK.558) was obtained from Amersham Buchler (3300 Braunschweig, FRG). Specific activity was about 85 Ci/mmol. The unlabeled 25-OH-D$_3$ was obtained from Albert-Roussel (6200 Wiesbaden, FRG). 24,25-Dihydroxyvitamin D$_3$ and 1,25-dihydroxyvitamin D$_3$ were obtained from Duphar B.V., (P.O. Box 900, 1380 Da Weesp, Holland). Gelatin was obtained from E. Merck (6100 Darmstadt, FRG). All other reagents were obtained pro analysi from E. Merck. Charcoal was obtained from Serva-Technik (6900 Heidelberg, FRG).

The assay was performed in immunoassay vials (Chap. 1.4), obtained from Sarstedt (5223 Nümbrecht, FRG). Picofluor™15 scintillation fluid was obtained from Packard Instruments (6000 Frankfurt/M., FRG).

Binding Protein. Serum from a vitamin D deficient patient and serum with low 25-OH-D content obtained from a rabbit was stored frozen at −30°C. Before use in an assay, an aliquot was diluted with 0.06 mol/liter phosphate buffer,

Table 1. Details on extraction, chromatography, incubation conditions and separation of bound and free from published 25-hydroxyvitamin D assays

Author/ reference	Year of publication	Extraction	Chromatography	Binding protein	Incubation Time	Incubation Volume	Recovery	Solubilizing/ stabilizing agents	Separation technique
Belsey et al [2]	1971	CHCl₃/MeOH	Activated SA	Rat serum D(−)	Days	0.8 ml	75–85%	Lipoprotein (human)	Centrifugation after precipitation of lipoprotein
Haddad and Chyu [14]	1971	Ether	SA	Kidney cytosol D(−)rat	60 min 25°C	1.1 ml	64.1%	7% EtOH	DCC
Bayard et al. [1]	1972	CHCl₃/MeOH	TLC	Human serum D(−)	BP + Std 14 h, 4°C + tracer 4–6 h	1 ml	20–25%	2% EtOH	Florisil
Edelstein et al. [10]	1974	CHCl₃/MeOH	LH20	Purified D(−) rat serum	30 min RT	1.1 ml	80%	7% EtOH	DCC
Preece et al. [38]	1974	CHCl₃/MeOH	SA	D(−)rat serum	Over night 4°C	0.5 ml	90%	2%EtOH in BSA-buffer	DCC
Belsey et al. [3]	1974	EtOH	–	D(−)rat serum	2 h	1 ml	95–100%	1% EtOH	DCC
Offermann et al. [33]	1974	EtOH	–	Kidney cytosol D(−)rat	1 h 4°C	1 ml	97–100%	1% EtOH	DCC
Bouillon et al. [6]	1976	CH₂Cl₂/MeOH	LH20	D(−)rat serum	1 h 0°C	1 ml	82%	8% EtOH lipoprotein	DCC
Shimotsuji [46]	1976	CHCl₃/MeOH	LH20	D(−)rat serum	30 min	1 ml	91.6%	6.5% EtOH	DCC

Table 1. Continued

Author/reference	Year of publication	Extraction	Chromatography	Binding protein	Incubation Time	Incubation Volume	Recovery	Solubilizing/stabilizing agents	Separation technique
Justova et al. [20]	1976	(NH$_4$)$_2$SO$_4$/MeOH/Toluene	—	D(−)human serum	2 h 4°C	1.5 ml	95–110%	1.3% EtOH	DCC
Pettifor et al. [37]	1976	EtOH	—	D(−)rat serum	3 h 4°C	1 ml	96–102%	1% EtOH	DCC
Garcia-Pascual et al. [12]	1976	EtOH	—	D(−)rat serum	2 h 4°C	1 ml	91%	9% EtOH	DCC
Morris and Peacock [31]	1976	EtOH	—	D(−) human serum	2 h 4°C	1 ml	83%	10% EtOH	DCC
Ellis and Dixon [11]	1977	EtOH	SA	Human serum	90 min + tracer 60 min	1 ml	—	10% EtOH Tris—buffer containing Triton X-405	DCC
Mason and Posen [29]	1977	EtOH	SA	Rat kidney cytosol	2 h 4°C	2.46 ml	95.3%	6.1% EtOH	DCC
Schmidt-Gayk et al. [43]	1977	EtOH	—	D(−)rat serum	1 h 0°C	1.07 ml	90%	6.5% EtOH	DCC
Keck and Krüskemper [21]	1981	CH$_2$Cl$_2$/MeOH	LH20 HPLC	Kidney homogenate D(−)rat	2 h 25°C	1.1 ml	50%	4.5% EtOH	DCC
Toss [48]	1981	CH$_2$Cl$_2$/MeOH	LH20	D(−)rat serum	60 min 4°C	1.28 ml	—	6.2% EtOH 1.7% Gelatin	DCC
Wood [51]	1983	EtOH	—	rabbit serum	2 h, 4°C	570 µl	—	12.3% EtOH	DCC

	Year		Sep-Pak						
Hummer et al. [16]	1984	Aceto-nitrile	Sep-Pak	rabbit anti-serum	20 h, 4°C	550 µl	93.7% – 115.1%	4.5% EtOH	DCC
Bothe et al. [5]	1984	Aceto-nitrile	—	D(–)rabbit serum	1 h, 4°C	435 µl	92%	0.2% Gelatin 8% Acetonitrile	DCC
Bouillon et al. [7]	1984	a) EtOH b) n-Hexane c) Cyclohex./ ethyl-acet.	—	a) D(–) rat serum b) rabbit antibody	1 h, 4°C 1 h, 4°C	550 µl 550 µl	101% – 103%	0.01% Ovalb. 9.1% EtOH 0.01% Ovalb. 9.1%EtOH	DCC DCC
Prószynska et al. [39]	1985	Extrelut	—	D(–)rat serum	2–20 h, 4°C	570 µl	99% – 108%	12.3% EtOH	DCC
Hollis and Napoli [15]	1985	Aceto-nitrile	—	rabbit anti-serum	2 h, 4°C	550 µl	108%	9.1% EtOH 0.04% Gelatin	DAB

Abbreviations: EtOH, ethanol
MeOH, methanol
LH20, Sephadex LH20 column chromatography
SA, silicic acid column chromatography
TLC, thin layer chromatography
HPLC, high performance liquid chromatography
D(–), vitamin D deficient serum

RT, room temperature
BSA, bovine serum albumin
DCC, dextran coated charcoal
BP, binding protein
Std, standard
DAB, double antibody separation

pH 8.4, containing 1 g sodium azide/liter. The concentration of the binding protein was 400 µl/liter phosphate buffer (working solution).

Standards. Crystalline 25-OH-D$_3$ was dissolved in ethanol to a concentration of 25 µmol/liter. The concentration of this solution was checked by measurement of the absorbance at 254 and 265 nm (absorbance should be 0.402 at 254 and 0.450 at 265 nm). Furthermore, an aliquot of the solution was injected into a Waters (6236 Eschborn, FRG) HPLC and a peak eluted at the usual time after 7 min. The HPLC method was performed according to chap. 5.1 (30). The stock solution of 25 µmol/liter was added to vitamin D-deficient human serum which had been prepared by charcoal incubation and oscillation (60 cycles/min) for 48 h, as described by Kruse (1979). This highest standard concentration in human serum (800 nmol/liter) was diluted with the vitamin D-deficient serum to yield the concentrations of 400, 200, 100, 50, 25, and 12.5 nmol/liter.

Incubation Buffer. A buffer of 0.06 mol/liter sodium phosphate was prepared from E. Merck solution No. 6587 (disodium hydrogen phosphate) and E. Merck solution No. 4875 (potassium dihydrogen phosphate). This solution was heated to 80 °C. Two grams of gelatin was added per liter, and the solution was mixed until all particles were dissolved.

After cooling to room temperature, 1 g sodium azide and 200 µl Brij-35 (No. 10522, E. Merck) were added to 1 liter buffer to prevent bacterial growth and to increase the solubility of 25-OH-D.

Binding Protein Buffer. Four hundred microliters normal rabbit serum with a low 25-OH-D concentration was diluted with 1 liter phosphate buffer, pH 8.4, containing 1 g sodium azide/liter.

Dextran-coated Charcoal Suspension. The charcoal-dextran suspension was prepared by mixing 12.5 g Norit A and 1.25 g dextran T70 with 1 liter phosphate buffer, pH 8.4. This suspension was stored at 4 °C.

Scintillation Fluid. Two milliliters of the scintillation fluid was required for a 400-µl aliquot from the incubation mixture to achieve a counting efficiency of 30% for tritium.

Assay Procedure. The assay was carried out at 4 °C in RIA vials

Extraction. Plasma (50 µl) was mixed with acetronitrile (200 µl) and left at 4 °C for 30 min. Upon centrifugation (3000 rpm for 10 min, 2000 g) at 4 °C, 25 µl aliquots of the extract were transferred to another rack with immunoassay vials. Then [^{3}H]25-OH-D (about 18 000 cpm in 10 µl acetonitrile) was added to the acetonitrile extract. Thereafter, 300 µl incubation buffer (containing gelatin, sodium azide, and Brij-35) was added. Binding protein (100 µl phosphate buffer pH 8.4 containing sodium azide) was added to this mixture. The tubes were covered with adhesive tape, and the rack was mixed, centrifuged for 30 s to clear the adhesive tape, and incubated for 60 min at 4 °C. Then the charcoal/dextran suspension (100 µl) was added by a rapid dispensor. This charcoal/dextran suspension was placed in an ice-water bath. During the time of charcoal addition, the aluminum rack with the immunoassay vials was also placed in an ice-water bath. The tubes were again closed by adhesive tape, mixed, and placed into the ice-water bath for another 5 min. Thereafter, the tubes were mixed again and centrifuged for 10 min 2000 g at 4 °C. Then the rack was placed in an ice-water bath, and 400 µl supernatant was transferred to scintillation vials. These were counted for 2 min or until 10 000 counts were accumulated.

Nonspecific Binding. Nonspecific binding of labeled 25-OH-D_3 in the absence of binding protein was determined in the same way by replacing the binding protein solution by phosphate buffer, pH 8.4, containing 1 g sodium azide/liter. Total counts of [^{3}H]25-OH-D were determined by adding 10 µl tracer solution to scintillation vials. The acetonitrile was evaporated to dryness. Thereafter, 2 ml scintillation fluid was added and the total counts determined. Usually, total counts yielded 18 000 cpm/10 µl tracer solution.

Calculations. The standard curves were constructed by plotting the counts per minute of [^{3}H]25-OH-D bound (minus nonspecific bound) on the y-axis and the concentration of 25-OH-D on a logarithmic scale on the x-axis.

Normal subjects and Patients. The serum samples of 37 normal subjects were assayed. Sera were collected in September. The age of the normal subjects ranged from 20 to 70 years. Throughout the year, serum was collected in healthy men ($n = 728$) and women ($n = 690$) aged 20–40 years, participants of the "Heidelberg Study." In addition, serum samples of 6 healthy volunteers aged 20–40 years were taken monthly for 12 months to establish a seasonal profile. Furthermore, in the age groups below 10, 11–20, 21–40, 41–60, and 61–80 years, serum was collected during wintertime (December to January) in 8–10 apparently healthy persons from each group.

1. Serum was also collected from the following patient groups: 100 geriatric patients and 22 patients with femoral neck fractures. The age of the latter group ranged from 61–79 years. (We are indebted to Dr. Oster, Bethanien-Krankenhaus, Heidelberg, for collecting the samples.)
2. In 28 children at the hemodialysis unit of the University of Heidelberg, Department of Pediatrics. (We are indebted to Prof. Mehls, Department of Pediatrics, for collecting the samples.)
3. In 33 adult patients with nephrotic syndrome (urinary protein above 3.5 g/24 h) and in 4 patients with proteinuria (urinary protein below 3.5 g/24 h). (We are indebted to Prof. Ritz, Department of Nephrology, for collecting the samples.)
4. Furthermore, in 146 patients on chronic anticonvulsant therapy. (We are indebted to Prof. Krause, Department of Neurology, for collecting the samples.)

Results

Influence of pH on Buffer Solution. The influence of pH on the standard curves is shown in Fig. 1, the standard curve being most sensitive at pH 8.4. Therefore, all further experiments were performed at pH 8.4.

Binding Proteins. Human and rabbit serum were used as binding protein in several different dilutions for the assay of 25-OH-D. The results are shown in Fig. 2, which shows that rabbit serum (NRS) diluted to 400 μl/liter phosphate buffer, pH 8.4, yielded the steepest standard curve. Rat serum was similar to human serum (data not shown).

Buffer Solutions. To investigate the effect of gelatin on the assay performance, an assay with ethanol extraction (50 μl serum was mixed with 200 μl ethanol; procedure as for acetonitrile) was performed. Gelatin was added in different concentrations to the incubation buffer. The results with 2, 10, and 17 g/liter and the control experiment without gelatin are shown in Fig. 3, which shows that the highest binding was observed at the gelatin concentration of 2 g/liter at pH 8.4. The same experiment was repeated with the acetonitrile extraction method. The

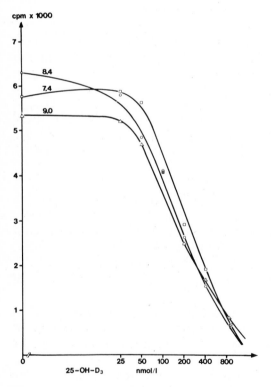

Fig. 1. Influence of pH 7.4, 8.4 and 9.0 on binding and displacement of [^{3}H]25-OH-D. The extraction was performed with ethanol

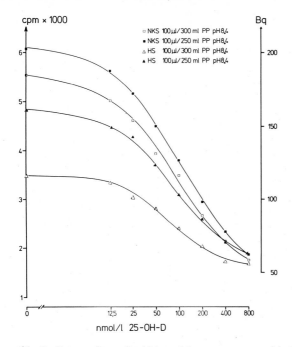

Fig. 2. Comparison of rabbit and human serum as binding protein in different dilutions at pH 8.4 with ethanol extraction, NKS, normal rabbit serum; HS, human serum

result is shown in Fig. 4, which shows that again a gelatin concentration of 2 g/liter yielded the most sensitive standard curve and the highest binding at zero concentration. In addition, acetonitrile extraction without evaporation of the transferred extract resulted in higher binding of [^{3}H]25-OH-D than the ethanol extraction. This was confirmed in a separate experiment. The results are shown in Fig. 5, where it can be seen that the acetonitrile extraction—without evaporation of transferred extract—using buffer containing gelatin (2 g/liter, pH 8.4) yielded a more sensitive standard curve than ethanol extraction and evaporation of the ethanolic extract. In an additional experiment, the ethanol extraction was repeated without evaporation of the transferred extract. No difference between the standard curves with or without evaporation was observed. The detection limit of the acetonitrile extraction method combined with the assay containing gelatin buffer is 8 nmol/liter (Bo-2SD).

Recovery Experiments. A total of 250 nmol/liter 25-OH-D was added to vitamin D-deficient serum. The recovery of the metabolite was determined in 26 different assays. Using ethanol extraction without gelatin, a mean recovery of 90% was observed. The interassay coefficient of variation was 10.3%. In the assay employing acetonitrile extraction and incubation with a gelatin-containing buffer (2 g/liter, pH 8.4), a recovery of 92% and a coefficient of variation of 4.2% were observed.

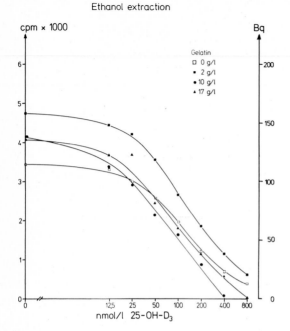

Fig. 3. Influence of gelatin (0, 2, 10, and 17 g/liter) on binding and displacement of ^{3}H-25-OH-D. The extraction was performed with ethanol

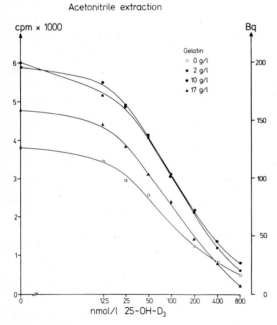

Fig. 4. Influence of gelatin (0, 2, 10, and 17 g/liter) on binding and displacement of [^{3}H]-25-OH-D. The extraction was performed with acetonitrile

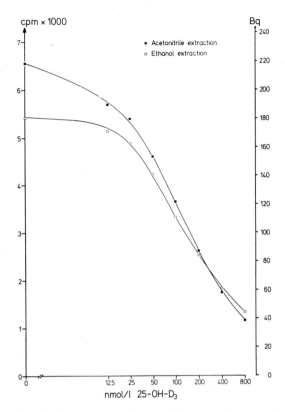

Fig. 5. Comparison of acetonitrile and ethanol extraction at optimum pH (8.4) and gelatin concentration (2 g/l)

Specificity. To charcoal-treated serum, 25-OH-D$_2$ (125 nmol/liter), 24,25-(OH)$_2$D$_3$ (250 nmol/liter) and 1,25(OH)$_2$D$_3$ (250 nmol/liter) were added; 25-OH-D$_2$ and 24,25-(OH)$_2$D$_3$ interfered 60% and 100%, respectively, while 1,25-(OH)$_2$D$_3$ did not interfere.

Clinical Results

Results in Normal Subjects and Patients. The mean 25-OH-D concentration in 37 normal subjects in September was 109 nmol/liter with a median of 89 nmol/liter. The range was 14–383 nmol/liter. Thirty-five of the normal subjects had levels ranging from 15 to 270 nmol/liter. In December to January, 46 normal subjects of different age groups, as shown in Fig. 7, displayed a normal range from < 8–120 nmol/liter.

Seasonal Profile. The seasonal profile of 25-OH-D in six healthy volunteers aged 20–40 years is shown in Fig. 6, which shows markedly elevated levels from July to September and relatively low levels from January to March. The daily intake of 1000 IU vitamin D$_3$ in one person (starting in November) increased the

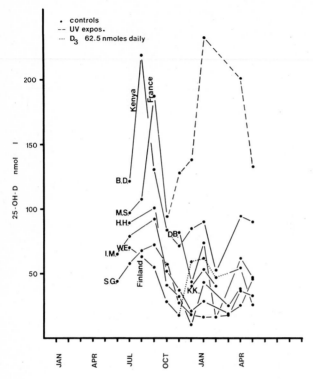

Fig. 6. Seasonal profile of 25-OH-D in six healthy volunteers. Person W.E. started in November with a daily intake of 1000 IU vitamin D_3, and person M. S. was exposed to artificial UV light from November to March

25-OH-D by about 40–50 nmol/liter. UV exposure by artificial UV radiation in another person from November to March increased the level of 25-OH-D by more than 100 nmol/liter.

Age Dependency. In different age groups of apparently healthy people, serum was collected during the winter (December to January). The serum concentration of 25-OH-D in these persons is shown in Fig. 7. In the age group 60–80 years a low mean 25-OH-D level was found. One of these ten persons had a high concentration of 25-OH-D as a consequence of vitamin D intake prescribed by his family physician.

Patient Groups. Calcium, phosphate, alkaline phosphatase, and 25-OH-D were measured for the following groups:

1. Geriatric Patients. In 100 consecutive patients admitted to a geriatric hospital (mean age 77 years; 67 women, 33 men) during the winter months, blood was taken for measurement. Of the patients, 8% showed a low level of serum calcium (below 2.2 mmol/liter), and 28% of serum phosphate (below 0.8 mmol/liter); 37% had a substantially increased alkaline phosphatase

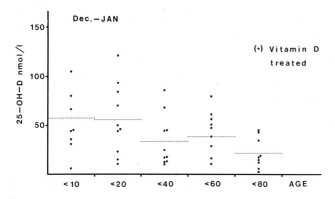

Fig. 7. Age dependency of 25-OH-D. One person in the group aged 60–80 years was on a vitamin D prescription

(above 200 IU/liter; normal range 60–170 IU/liter); 78% had a 25-OH-D concentration below 50 nmol/liter, which is a low normal amount according to Fig. 6, and in 41% of the patients 25-OH-D was below 15 nmol/1, which means true vitamin D deficiency. This was substantiated by serum calcium, phosphate, and alkaline phosphatase results (Oster et al. 1983).

2. Patients with Femoral Neck Fracture. In 10 patients with femoral neck fracture and 10 patients with fracture from severe trauma (traffic accidents) in January and in 12 patients with femoral neck fracture and 12 patients with fracture from severe trauma (traffic accidents) in July measurements were performed. The results are shown in Table 2. Very low levels of 25-OH-D are found in the femoral neck fracture group in January and also in July. These are significantly different from the traffic accident group ($p < 0.05$). Phosphorus in serum was significantly lower in the femoral neck fracture group only in January. Calcium and alkaline phosphatase were not significantly different.

3. Children on Hemodialysis. In 28 children at the hemodialysis unit, serum calcium and 25-OH-D were determined. The result is shown in Fig. 8, which shows a positive relationship of 25-OH-D to serum calcium.

4. Patients with Nephrotic Syndrome and Proteinuria. In 33 adult patients with nephrotic syndrome (urinary protein > 3.5 g/24 h) and in 4 patients with proteinuria (urinary protein < 3.5 g/24 h) the levels of 25-OH-D in serum were determined. The results are shown in Fig. 9, which also contains the upper and lower limits of normal, derived from the seasonal profile in healthy persons.

All patients with nephrotic syndrome exhibit low levels of 25-OH-D (mean 19, range < 8–41 nmol/liter), whereas the patients with proteinuria fit into the normal range. The dependence of 25-OH-D on urinary protein is shown in Fig. 10, which indicates that an increase in urinary protein decreases the serum level of 25-OH-D. Serum concentrations of Gc globulin—

Table 2. 25-OH-D in patients with femoral neck fracture and controls. Data from 10 and 12 patients in each group in January and July, respectively

| | January | | | July | | |
	FNF	TRA	p	FNF	TRA	p
age (years)						
Mean	84	49		78	45	
range	73–94	16–90		54–92	22–68	
25-OH-D (nmol/1)						
mean	9	26	< 0.05	19	45	< 0.05
range	5–14	12–52		4–17	18–79	
Ca (mmol/1)						
mean	2.25	2.33		2.24	2.26	
range	2.1–2.4	2.2–2.6		1.5–2.6	2.0–2.5	
P (mmol/1)						
mean	0.71	1.06	< 0.05	0.86	1.03	
range	0.4–1.0	0.8–1.3		0.5–1.3	0.7–1.9	
AP (IU/1)						
mean	136	145		167	150	
range	26–280	65–330		81–459	60–305	

FNF, femoral neck fracture; TRA, fracture by traffic accident; P, phosphorus, inorganic (phosphate); AP, alkaline phosphatase

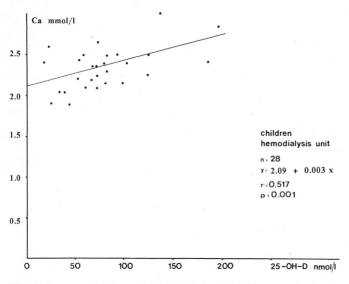

Fig. 8. Serum calcium and 25-OH-D in 28 children at the hemodialysis unit. Linear regression analysis and the coefficient of correlation are shown

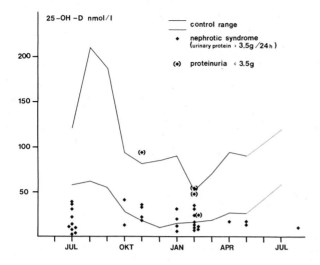

Fig. 9. 25-OH-D in 33 patients with nephrotic syndrome and in 4 patients with proteinuria < 3.5 g/24 h. The upper and lower limits of the seasonal profile are marked

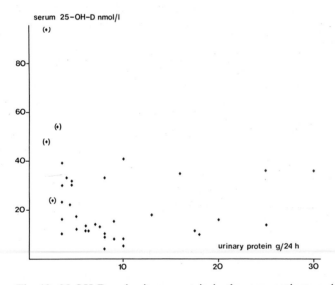

Fig. 10. 25-OH-D and urinary protein in the same patients as in Fig. 9

the binding protein for vitamin D (DBP) and its metabolites—were significantly lower in patients with the nephrotic syndrome ($p < 0.001$, mean 340 mg/liter, range 190–480 mg/liter) than in nonproteinuric controls (mean 440 mg/liter, range 376–510 mg/1, measured by radial immunodiffusion).

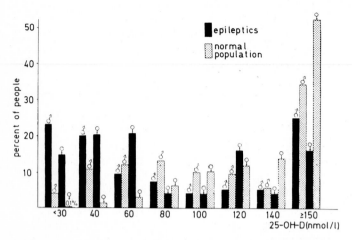

Fig. 11. 25-OH-D in 146 epileptics and in 1418 healthy controls grouped according to the level of 25-OH-D

In contrast to nonproteinuric urine, the urine of all nephrotic syndrome patients contained a large amount of 25-OH-D binding capacity; DBP was detected in each urine after concentration. Scatchard analysis of the urine demonstrated the presence of a low-affinity and a high-affinity binding protein (tentatively identified as albumin and DBP) (Schmidt-Gayk et al. 1977).

5. Patients on Chronic Anticonvulsant Therapy. Serum 25-OH-D was determined in 146 epileptics, 95 men and 49 women, aged 20–40 years. In addition, the results were compared with healthy controls from the "Heidelberg Study," who were of the same age (728 men and 690 women). Most patients were treated with a combination of the following anticonvulsants for at least 1 year: phenytoin ($n = 60$), primidone ($n = 55$), carbamazepine ($n = 42$), sodium valproate ($n = 33$), phenobarbital ($n = 14$), ethosuximide ($n = 13$), CHP-phenobarbital ($n = 12$), clonazepam, mesuximide, mephenytoin, sulthiam, and trimethadione. The results are shown in Fig. 11 (Krause et al. 1982), which shows that the epileptic patients on chronic anticonvulsant therapy tend to low levels of 25-OH-D.

Discussion

Protein Precipitation and Extraction. The results of this study indicate that acetonitrile is superior to ethanol for extraction of 25-OH-D from serum. Most assays published to date rely on ethanol, chloroform/methanol, dichloromethane/methanol, ether, or a combination of ammonium sulfate and methanol/toluene for extraction [1–3, 6, 10–12, 14, 20, 21, 29, 31, 33, 37, 38, 43, 46, 48]. There has been a recent increase in interest in acetonitrile, which has been used by few authors [15, 17, 28, 41].

The recovery of $[^3H]$25-OH-D after acetonitrile extraction is similar to that after ethanol extraction. Data on its accuracy are reported in Chap. 5.4 (interlaboratory comparison of 25-hydroxyvitamin D determination).

Risco and coworkers compared the standard method for the extraction of lipid-soluble metabolites, the Bligh and Dyer method [4], with the acetonitrile method. The Bligh and Dyer method yielded recoveries of 82.5%, and the acetonitrile method 84%. Furthermore, the latter method was more reproducible and is also much easier and faster to use. Column chromatography increases the specificity of the assay [1, 2, 6, 10, 11, 14, 21, 29, 38, 46, 48], circumventing interference of 24,25-$(OH)_2$D or other polar metabolites. However, column chromatography has not been used by all authors and is not indispensible for assay procedures applied for the diagnosis of hypo- or hypervitaminosis D. Of course, assays without chromatography overestimate the concentration of 25-OH-D due to specific interference of other vitamin D metabolites, especially in patients under treatment with vitamin D. In normal persons the levels of 24,25-$(OH)_2$D are about 2–10 nmol/liter and about 9% of the concentration of 25-OH-D [22].

Binding protein. Whereas serum from vitamin D-deficient rats is used as binding protein in most of the assays published [2, 3, 6, 10, 12, 37, 38, 42, 46, 48], rabbit serum yielded more sensitive standard curves than rat or human serum. As a stabilizing agent, Toss [48] introduced a 17 g/liter gelatin-containing buffer. We tested different gelatin concentrations and found 2 g/liter to give the highest increase in binding of 25-OH-D without increasing nonspecific binding. In addition, 2 g/liter is more convenient to use than 17 g/liter, because of the tendency of the latter to form a gel at low temperature.

Specificity. From data on the samples with added 24,25-$(OH)_2D_3$ and 25-OH-D_2, it can be concluded that this assay, as other nonchromatographic assays, overestimates the true 25-OH-D_3 serum concentration. This, however, is not important for the diagnosis of hypo- or hypervitaminosis D, which can be assessed by this assay. Therefore, we prefer to declare this assay suitable for the diagnosis of hypo- and hypervitaminosis D, and not for measurement of true 25-OH-D_3. The 1,25-$(OH)_2D_3$ level is fairly constant and therefore less representative for the nutritional state unless severe 25-OH-D deficiency occurs.

Normal Range. As can be seen in Table 3, there is a marked seasonal variation, a geographical influence, and a correlation to the specific method employed. For the nonchromatographic competitive protein-binding assays, we adopted 50–250 nmol/liter as a normal range for the summer months (similar to [3]), as shown in Fig. 6, and 25–125 nmol/liter for the winter months (similar to [9]).

What should be considered as the safe lower limit of 25-OH-D in serum? For this purpose, we looked at calcium, phosphorus, alkaline phosphatase, 25-OH-D, and parathyroid hormone levels in 100 patients on long-term antiepileptic treatment [23]. We found in these patients that a level of 25-OH-D below 25 nmol/liter was associated with a lowered level of serum calcium and an increase in parathyroid hormone (C-terminal fragment). For nonchromatographic assays, we regard 25 nmol/liter as the safe lower limit of normal.

Table 3. Normal range of 25–OH–D in serum, as described in the literature

Author	Year	n Persons	Country	range nmol/1	Mean ± SD	Remarks
Bayard	1972	18	France	25–60	38	
Belsey	1974	15	USA	50–250	88	
Bouillon	1976	51	Belgium		33 ± 10	May
Dabek	1981	10	Finland	20–120	30	Nov. -May,
Dabek	1981	16	Finland	33–120	64	May-Oct., HPLC
Edelstein	1974	18	England		38 ± 14	Chromatogr.
Garcia-P.	1976	18	Suisse	62–153	100 ± 24	
Gilbertson	1977	24	USA	14–60	38 ± 13	HPLC, February
Haddad	1971	40	USA	28–138	68 ± 27	May and June
Hollis	1985	50	USA		65 ± 28	HPLC
Jones	1978	25	Canada	23–60	40 ± 10	December, HPLC
Justova	1976	30	CSSR	50–105	72 ± 13	May to September
Keck	1981	17	BRD		30 ± 15	Oct., HPLC + CPBA
Keck	1981	17	BRD		8,2 ± 2,3	April, HPLC + CPBA
Lambert	1977	10	USA, MN		63 ± 5	September, HPLC
Mason	1977	?	Australia	33–110	72 ± 20	fall season
Morris	1976	35	England	13–181	67	Nov.-Dec., 20–40 y
Morris	1976	15	England	0–104	27	May-June, 65–75 y
Nayer	1977	11	Belgium	40–93	58 ± 17	
Offermann	1974	50	Berlin/West		90 ± 42	
Parviainen	1981	16	Finland		55 ± 12	Oct.-Nov., HPLC
Pettifor	1976	286	South Africa		77 ± 25	children 1–18 y
Preece	1974	38	England	10–55	30 ± 14	adults, early winter
Preece	1974	14	England	10–50	28 ± 12	children, early winter
Stryd	1979	10	USA, MI	20–60	33 ± 15	January, HPLC
Stryd	1979	10	USA, MI	52–117	78 ± 25	June, HPLC
Trafford	1981	11	England		60 ± 28	August, HPLC
Turnbull	1982	24	England		50 ± 19	April-July, HPLC

Bouillon and coworkers [7] compared values of the nonchromatographic competitive protein-binding assay with those obtained by two different chromatographic methods. The direct competitive protein-binding assay over-estimated the true 25-OH-D concentration by about 20 %, but this percentage was constant from 5 to 600 µg/liter (= 12.5–1500 nmol/liter). Overestimation by a direct radioimmunoassay employing an antiserum against 25-OH-D was less than 10%. As is shown in Fig. 7, there is an age correlation of serum 25-OH-D, with a fairly large proportion of low 25-OH-D concentrations in elderly people. This is also confirmed by Morris and Peacock [31], as shown in Table 3.

25-OH-D in Geriatric Patients. In 41 of 100 consecutive patients admitted to a geriatric hospital, 25-OH–D in serum was below 15 nmol/liter. In addition, our results from the femoral neck fracture group demonstrated that vitamin D deficiency is fairly common in elderly people during the winter months in the Federal Republic of Germany. This was also demonstrated by Offermann [34]. These results suggest that the policy of the USA and Canada, who fortify milk with vitamin D_3 (400 IU/liter), should be adopted in the Federal Republic of Germany and, as may be deduced from Table 13, in England too. As an alternative, other methods of preventing a vitamin D deficiency in the aged may also be adopted.

Hemodialysis and 25-OH-D. In Fig. 8, a significant relationship between 25-OH-D and serum calcium is described in children on hemodialysis. This seems remarkable, as these children may not synthesize adequate amounts of $1,25(OH)_2D_3$. However, there may be some production of $1,25(OH)_2D_3$ by bone cells and keratinocytes [40]. Recent studies have reported low circulating concentrations of $1,25(OH)_2D_3$ (4–16 ng/liter = 10–40 pmol/liter) in the majority of anephric patients who either were untreated or were treated with vitamin D.

Recently, Coratelli and coworkers [8] reported that the serum level of 25-OH-D exerted a marked influence on parathyroid hormone concentration in serum. Low levels of 25-OH-D were associated with high levels of parathyroid hormone and vice versa. From our data in these children and from Coratelli's results, levels of 25-OH-D below 50 nmol/liter should be avoided in hemodialysis patients.

25-OH-D in Nephrotic Syndrome. Low levels of 25-OH-D were found in patients with the nephrotic syndrome [43]. This fall in serum 25-OH-D level is accompanied by urinary loss of the vitamin D-binding globulin (DBP, or Gc globulin) and usually, but not consistently, by low serum levels of DBP. A similar mechanism may be operating in patients on continuous ambulatory peritoneal dialysis [45]. Practically, both groups of patients should be administered vitamin D until normal levels of 25-OH-D are obtained.

25-OH-D in Patients on Chronic Anticonvulsant Therapy. It can be seen in Fig. 11 that epileptic patients on chronic anticonvulsant therapy tend to have low levels of 25-OH-D and that a substantial proportion of these values is below 30 nmol/liter, which means that these patients are prone to antiepileptic osteopathy. It is recommended that at least during the winter the serum level of 25-OH-D be determined for patients on long-term antiepileptic treatment, to avoid levels of 25-OH-D below 25 nmol/liter, as these low levels of 25-OH-D have been associated with low levels of serum calcium and increases in parathyroid hormone.

In a study on the prophylactic treatment of epileptic patients with vitamin D_2 or vitamin D_3 we observed that a prophylactic administration of 1300 IU of vitamin D_2 or D_3 was not sufficient in all patients to raise the level of 25-OH-D into the normal range (above 25 nmol/liter, [24]).

Conclusion

The extraction of 25-hydroxyvitamin D and incubation conditions in a competitive protein-binding assay for this vitamin D metabolite were evaluated. Comparison of ethanol and acetonitrile as solvents for the extraction of the vitamin D metabolite from serum showed that acetonitrile was superior and made it possible to perform a direct assay. No evaporation of the extract was necessary. By comparing pH values of the incubation buffer, pH 8.4 was found superior to pH 7.4 or 9.0. Of the different gelatin concentrations tested (0, 2, 10, and 17 g/liter), 2 g/liter yielded the highest binding of $[^3H]$25-hydroxyvitamin D_3 without increasing nonspecific binding. Tracer dissolved in acetonitrile was slightly superior to tracer dissolved in ethanol. Comparison of human and rabbit serum binding proteins revealed that steeper standard curves were obtained by use of the latter.

Data on normal subjects (a seasonal profile and the age correlation) are presented. We demonstrate the clinical utility by reporting the application of this assay on serum samples from 100 geriatric patients, 22 patients with femoral neck fractures, 33 patients with nephrotic syndrome, and 146 patients with antiepileptic treatment. Vitamin D deficiency is common in these patient groups, at least in the winter.

References

1. Bayard F, Bec P, Louvet JP (1972) Measurement of plasma 25-hydroxycholecalciferol in man. Eur J Clin Invest 2:195–198
2. Belsey R, DeLuca HF, Potts JT jr (1971) Competitive binding assay for vitamin D and 25-OH vitamin D. J Clin Endocrinol Metab 33:554–557
3. Belsey RE, DeLuca HF, Potts JT jr (1974) A rapid assay for 25-OH-vitamin D_3 without preparative chromatography. J Clin Endocrinol Metab 38:1046–1051
4. Bligh EG, Dyer WJ (1959) A rapid method of total lipid extraction and purification. Can J Biochem Physiol 37:911–917
5. Bothe V, Schmidt-Gayk H, Armbruster FP, Mayer E (1984) Assay for the diagnosis of hyper- and hypovitaminosis D. Ärztl Lab 30:151–156
6. Bouillon R, Van Kerkhove P, De Moor P (1976) Measurement of 25-hydroxyvitamin D_3 in serum. Clin Chem 22:364–368
7. Bouillon R, Van Herck E, Jans I, Keng Tan B, Van Baelen H, De Moor P (1984) Two direct (nonchromatographic) assays for 25-hydroxyvitamin D. Clin Chem 30:1731–1736
8. Coratelli P, Buongiorno E, Petrarulo F, Corciulo R, Giannattasio M, Passavanti G, Antonelli G (1989) Pathogenetic aspects of uremic cardiomyopathy. Miner Electrolyte Metab 15:246–253
9. Dabek JT, Härkönen M, Wahlroos Ö, Adlercreutz H (1981) Assay for plasma 25-hydroxyvitamin D_2 and 25-hydroxyvitamin D_3 by "high-perfomance" liquid chromatography. Clin Chem 27:1346–1351

10. Edelstein S, Charman M, Lawson DEM, Kodicek E (1974) A competitive protein-binding assay for 25-hydroxycholecalciferol. Clin Sci Mol Med 46:231–240

11. Ellis G, Dixon K (1977) Sequential-saturation-type assay for serum 25-hydroxyvitamin D. Clin Chem 23:855–862

12. Garcia-Pasqual B, Peytremann A, Courvoisier B, Lawson DEM (1976) A simplified protein-binding assay for 25-hydroxycholecalciferol. Clin Chim Acta 68:99–105

13. Gilbertson TJ, Stryd RP (1977) High-performance liquid chromatographic assay for 25-hydroxyvitamin D_3 in serum. Clin Chem 23:1700–1704

14. Haddad JG, Chyu KJ (1971) Competitive protein-binding radioassay for 25-hydroxycholecalciferol. J Clin Endocrinol Metab 33:992–995

15. Hollis BW, Napoli JL (1985) Improved radioimmunoassay for vitamin D and its use in assessing vitamin D status. Clin Chem 31:1815–1819

16. Hummer L, Nilas L, Tjellesen L, Christiansen C (1984) A selective and simplified radioimmunoassay of 25-Hydroxyvitamin D_3. Scand J Clin Lab Invest 44:163–167

17. Hummer L, Tjellesen L, Christiansen C (1983) Simplified assay of 25(OH)D_3 and 25(OH)D_2 using a combination of specific radioimmunoassay and a competitive protein binding assay. Calcified Tissue Suppl., Abstract 201, p. A52

18. Hummer L, Tjellesen L, Rickers H, Christiansen C (1984) Measurement of 25-hydroxyvitamin D_3 and 25-hydroxyvitamin D_2 in clinical settings. Scand J Clin Lab Invest 44:595–601

19. Jones G (1978) Assay of vitamins D_2 and D_3, and 25 hydroxyvitamins D_2 and D_3 in human plasma by high-performance liquid chromatography. Clin Chem 24:287–298

20. Justova V, Starka L, Wilczek H, Pacovsky V (1976) A simple radioassay for 25-hydroxycholecalciferol without chromatography. Clin Chim. Acta 70:97–102

21. Keck E, Krüskemper HL (1981) Protein binding assays for 25-hydroxy, 24,25-dihydroxy and 1,25-dihydroxy metabolites of vitamin D in human plasma. J Clin Chem Clin Biochem 19:1043–1050

22. Korhonen RT, Savolainen KE, Mäenpää PH (1983) High performance liquid chromatographic determination of 24,25-dihydroxyvitamin D_3 in serum. J Chromatogr 275:418–422

23. Krause KH, Prager P, Schmidt-Gayk H, Ritz E (1977) Diagnostik der Osteopathia antiepileptica im Erwachsenenalter. Dtsch Med Wochenschr 102:1872–1877

24. Krause KH, Bohn T, Schmidt-Gayk H, Prager R, Ritz E (1978) Zur prophylaktischen Gabe von Vitamin D_2 und D_3 bei Anfallskranken. Nervenarzt 49:174–180

25. Krause KH, Berlit P, Bonjour JP, Schmidt-Gayk H, Schellenberg B, Gillen J (1982) Vitamin status in patients on chronic anticonvulsant therapy. Internat J Vit Nutr Res 52:375–385

26. Kruse V (1979) Removal of endogenous ligands from a high affinity antiserum for a radioimmunoassay. Scand J Clin Lab Invest 39:533–541

27. Lambert PW, Syverson BJ, Arnaud CD and Spelsberg TC (1977) Isolation and quantitation of endogenous vitamin D and its physiologically important metabolites in human plasma by high pressure liquid chromatography. J Steroid Biochem 8:929–937

28. Lindbäck B, Berlin T, Björkhem (1987) Three commercial kits and one liquid-chromatographic method evaluated for determining 25-hydroxy vitamin D_3 in Serum. Clin Chem 33: 1226–1227

29. Mason RS, Posen S (1977) Some problems associated with assay of 25-hydroxycalciferol in human serum. Clin Chem 23:806–810

30. Mayer E, Schmidt-Gayk H, Lichtwald K, Kraas E, Knuppen R (1981) Simultane Bestimmung von 25-Hydroxy-Vitamin-D$_2$ und 25-Hydroxy-Vitamin-D$_3$ durch Hochdruckflüssigkeitschromatographie. Ärztl. Lab 27:89–94
31. Morris JF, Peacock M (1976) Assay of plasma 25-hydroxyvitamin D. Clin Chim Acta 72:383–391
32. Nayer Ph De, Thalasso M, Beckers C (1977) Radioimmunoassay and related procedures in medicine. International Atomic Energy Agency, Proceedings Series: Radioimmunoassay and Related Procedures in Medicine, Vol. II:199–209
33. Offermann G, Dittmar F (1974) A direct protein-binding assay for 25-hydroxy-cholecalciferol. Horm Metab Res 6:534
34. Offermann G, Biehle G (1978) Vitamin-D-Mangel und Osteomalazie beim alten Menschen. Ptsch. Med. Wochenschr. 103:415–419
35. Oster P, Tabouillot WV, Nold F, Schmidt-Gayk H, Schlierf G (1983) Prävalenz pathologischer Vitamin-D- und Parathormonspiegel bei geriatrischen Patienten. Akt. Gerontol 13:221–222
36. Parviainen MT, Savolainen KE, Korhonen PH, Alhava EM, Visakorpi JK (1981) An improved method for routine determination of vitamin D and its hydroxylated metabolites in serum from children and adults. Clin Chim Acta 114:233–247
37. Pettifor JM, Ross FP, Wang J (1976) A competitive protein-binding assay for 25-hydroxyvitamin D. Clin Sci Mol Med 51:605–607
38. Preece MA, O'Riordan JLH, Lawson DEM, Kodicek E (1974) A competitive protein-binding assay for 25-hydroxyergocalciferol in serum. Clin Chim Acta 54:235–242
39. Proszynska K, Lukaszkiewicz J, Jarocewicz N and Lorenc RS (1985) Rapid method for measuring physiological concentrations of 25-hydroxyvitamin D levels in blood serum. Clin Chim Acta 153:85–92
40. Reichel H, Koeffler HP, Norman AW (1989) The role of the vitamin D endocrine system in health and disease. N Eng J Med 320:980–991
41. Risco F, Babé M and Traba ML (1987) Simple method for extracting vitamin D metabolites from biological samples. Clin Chem 33:720
42. Schmidt-Gayk H, Nagel W (1977) Sättigungsanalyse für 25-Hydroxy-Vitamin-D. Ärztl Lab 23:111–123
43. Schmidt-Gayk H, Schmitt W, Grawunder C, Ritz E, Tschöpe W, Pietsch V, Andrassy K and Bouillon R (1977) 25-Hydroxy-vitamin D in nephrotic syndrome. The Lancet II:105–108
44. Schmidt-Gayk H, Wahl R, Jung JJ, Goossen J, Röher HD (1978) Vitamin-D-Mangel bei Schenkelhalsfrakturen. Münch Med Wochenschr 100:1167–1171
45. Shany S, Rapoport J, Goligorsky M, Yankowitz N, Zuili I, Chaimovitz C (1984) Losses of 1,25- and 24,25-Dihydroxycholecalciferol in the peritoneal fluid of patients treated with continuous ambulatory peritoneal dialysis. Nephron 36:111–113
46. Shimotsuji T, Seino Y, Yabuuchi H (1976) A competitive protein-binding assay for plasma 25-hydroxyvitamin D$_3$ in normal children. Tohuku J Exp Med 118:233–240
47. Stryd RP, Gilbertson TJ and Brunden MN (1979) A seasonal variation study of 25-hydroxyvitamin D$_3$ serum levels in normal humans. J Clin Endocrinol Metab 48:771–775
48. Toss G (1981) An evaluation of stabilizing agents in competitive protein-binding assay for 25-hydroxyvitamin D. Clin Chim Acta 117:361–364
49. Trafford DJH, Seamark DA, Turnbull H, Makin HLJ (1981) High-performance

liquid chromatography of 25-hydroxyvitamin D_2 and 25-hydroxyvitamin D_3 in human plasma. J Chromatogr 226:351–360

50. Turnbull H, Trafford DJH and Makin HLJ (1982) A rapid and simple method for the measurement of plasma 25-hydroxyvitamin D_2 and 25-hydroxyvitamin D_3 using Sep-Pak C_{18} cartridges and a single high-performance liquid chromatographic step. Clin Chim Acta 120:65–76

51. Wood WG (1983) A simple competitive binding assay for serum 25-hydroxyvitamin D_3 metabolites. Ärztl Lab 29:352–356

Chapter 5.3

A Competitive Protein-Binding Assay with Second Antibody Separation for the Diagnosis of Hyper- and Hypovitaminosis D

H. Birringer and H. Schmidt-Gayk

Introduction

As is shown in Chap. 5.2, Table 1, numerous assays for the measurement of 25-hydroxy vitamin D have been published in the last two decades. In all of the competitive protein-binding assays and in nearly all the radioimmunoassays mentioned above, charcoal or hydroxylapatite separation are used to separate the bound from free ligand. Only Hollis and Napoli (1985) introduced a radioimmunoassay for 25-hydroxy vitamin D with second antibody separation. However, second antibody separation for assays of vitamin D metabolites may be a very sophisticated procedure, as shown in Chap. 5.6. In the case of vitamin D metabolites only vitamin D binding protein (DBP) free solutions of first and second antibody may be employed, otherwise the metabolite will bind to DBP as well and will only partially be precipitated by the second antibody.

We solved this problem as outlined below.

By using human DBP (hDBP) as a binding protein and an IgG-fraction of rabbit anti-DBP, a complex was formed that will be precipitated by an IgG fraction of swine anti-rabbit IgG. This principle is outlined in Fig. 1, which shows 25-hydroxy vitamin D bound to hDBP, the latter bound by anti-DBP from a rabbit (r-a-hDBP), and this complex is precipitated by a second antibody (anti-rabbit IgG from swine, s-a-r-IgG).

Materials and Methods

All substances are used as outlined in Chap. 5.2. For the buffer for diluting DBP, anti-DBP, and anti-rabbit IgG: 0.06 mol/liter phosphate buffer, pH 8.4, is prepared first. Then 900 ml of this buffer are warmed to 80 °C on a heated magnetic stirrer, adding 2 g of gelatin and stirring the solution until the gelatin is dissolved. Then the solution is stirred without heating, until room temperature is reached. Finally 1 g of sodium azide is added and phosphate buffer is added up to 1000 ml. The pH is tested, and if necessary, readjusted to pH 8.4. This buffer is designated "PPGN."

25-OH-D   CPBA-DAB

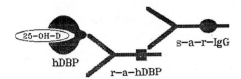

Fig. 1. 25-hydroxy vitamin D competitive protein-binding assay with double antibody separation (25-OH-D CPBA-DAB). 25-OH-D is bound to human vitamin D binding protein (hDBP), and the latter is bound to rabbit anti-hDBP (r-a-hDBP), which is then precipitated by an IgG fraction of swine anti-rabbit IgG (s-a-r-IgG)

Assay Buffer. A total of 50 g polyethylenlyglycol (PEG 6000, obtained from Serva, Heidelberg, FRG) is dissolved in about 900 ml of buffer PPGN by mixing with a magnetic stirrer. Then 200 µl of a solution of Brij-35 (obtained from E. Merck, Darmstadt, FRG) are added and PPGN buffer is added up to 1000 ml. The pH is again checked and adjusted to 8.4, if necessary. This buffer is designated "PPGNPB."

DBP. A pool of vitamin D-deficient human serum is made from several patient sera that are below the detection limit of the 25-hydroxy vitamin D assay (below 8 nmol/liter or 3.2 ng/ml). This pool is divided into 0.2 ml amounts and stored frozen at $-30\,°C$. For the assay, this pool is diluted 1:500 with PPGN buffer.

Anti-human-DBP. The anti-hDBP (anti-Gc-globulin) from rabbits is obtained from Dakopatts (Glostrup, Denmark) as an IgG fraction. For use in the assay, it is diluted 1:125 in PPGN buffer.

Second Antibody. Anti-rabbit IgG, produced in swine, is also obtained from Dakopatts as an IgG fraction. For use in the assay, it is diluted 1:12.5 in PPGN buffer.

Standards. These are prepared as outlined in Chap. 5.2.

Wash Solution. In second antibody procedures, the precipitate is washed normally once. For this purpose, physiological saline (9 g/liter), with Brij-35, 1 ml/liter, is used.

Assay Procedure. The assay is carried out at $4\,°C$ in immunoassay vials (Chap. 1.4).

Extraction. Plasma (50 µl) was mixed with acetonitrile (200 µl) and left at $4\,°C$ for 30 min. Upon centrifugation (3000 rpm for 10 min, 2000 g at $4\,°C$) 25 µl aliquots of the extract were transferred to another rack with immunoassay vials. Then [³H]25-OH-D (about 18 000 cpm in 10 µl acetonitrile) was added to the acetonitrile extract. Thereafter, 300 µl incubation buffer PPGNPB was added. Binding protein (50 µl DBP, serum pool, diluted 1:500 in PPGN) was added to this mixture, followed by anti-human-DBP (50 µl, diluted 1:125 in PPGN) and second antibody (50 µl, diluted 1:12.5 in PPGN). The tubes were covered with adhesive tape, and the rack was mixed, centrifuged for 30 s to clear the adhesive tape and incubated overnight at 4°C. Thereafter, the tubes were centrifuged for 10 min 2000 g at 4°C. The supernatants were aspirated by a device (Sarstedt, Nümbrect, FRG) to remove the fluid from 12 tubes simultaneously. Then 400 µl washing fluid with Brij-35 was added, the tubes centrifuged again, and the supernatants aspirated; 10 µl of sodium hydroxide, 1 mol/liter, were added to the sediment; and the rack was mixed and incubated for 10 min at room temperature to liquify the protein precipitates. Then 250 µl of scintillation fluid were added, the tubes closed with a firmly impressed stopper, the racks containing the tubes mixed carefully, and the tubes counted for 1 min.

Calculations. These are performed as in Chap. 5.2.

Results

DBP. In initial experiments, the amount of DBP was optimized. The concentrations used in Chap. 5.2 served as a guideline. A total of 50 µl DBP diluted 1:500 with PPGN buffer yielded a steep standard curve with sufficient binding.

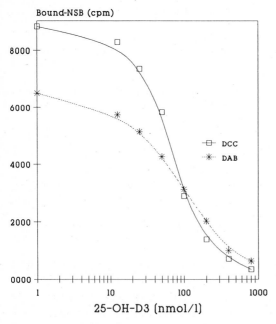

Fig. 2. Standard curves of the assay with dextran-coated charcoal (DCC) and double antibody (DAB) separation. The *y-axis* depicts the cpm bound minus nonspecific bound, the *x-axis* the concentration of unlabeled 25-hydroxy vitamin D_3

pH. The pH 8.4 was again compared with pH 7.4 and, as in Chap. 5.2, pH 8.4 proved to be superior (better binding, steeper standard curve). Then, pH 8.4 was compared with pH 8.6, and in the second antibody assay, pH 8.4 was slightly superior (data not shown).

PEG. The concentration of PEG was tested in steps of 1 g/liter from zero up to 10 g/liter in PPGNPB buffer; 5% proved to be the optimum concentration. A standard curve with the optimized reagents is shown in Figs. 2 and 3, which show both the competition curve of the assay with charcoal separation, as outlined in Chap. 5.2, and the second antibody separation. The curves are similar if B/B_0 is plotted on the y-axis and the concentration of the competitor on the x-axis, as shown in Fig. 3.

Comparison of Second Antibody with Charcoal Separation. In 39 patients the results from a routine assay, which at that time was performed with charcoal separation, were compared with the assay described here with second antibody separation. The result is shown in Fig. 4, which shows that both assays yield about the same results.

The coefficient of variation, determined for the 39 duplicates shown in Fig. 4, was 8.0%. The interassay coefficient of variation, determined in 32 routine assays with second antibody separation, was 10.5% at a concentration of 250 nmol/liter.

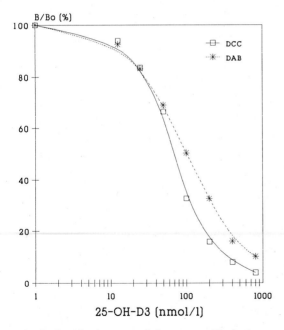

Fig. 3. Standard curves of the assay with dextran-coated charcoal (DCC) and double antibody (DAB) separation. The *y-axis* depicts the ratio of bound/bound at zero concentration (B/Bo), the *x-axis* the concentration of unlabeled 25-hydroxy vitamin D_3

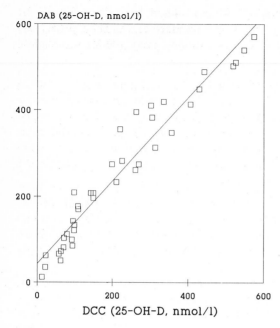

Fig. 4. Comparison of the double antibody (DAB, *y-axis*) with the charcoal separation method (DCC, *x-axis*). A linear regression analysis is performed

Discussion

Second antibody separation of bound and free ligand seems to be very advantageous, as this method is nondisruptive. In contrast, charcoal may disturb the equilibrium obtained. In addition, charcoal may not be added simultaneously to all tubes to achieve phase separation, thereby "stripping" counts from the binding protein. This will lower the count rate in the tubes incubating for longer time with charcoal. This critical timing in charcoal addition prohibits the measurement of long series of samples or introduces a systematic error (drift). In contrast, second antibody separation is nondisruptive and very large numbers of samples may be processed.

Hollis and Napoli (1985), who published a radioimmunoassay for 25-hydroxy vitamin D with second antibody separation, also noted that it is important to remove α-globulins (DBP) from the immune serum, thus eliminating the possibility of its interference in competing with the antibody for binding of the 25-hydroxy vitamin D in the assay solution.

The main advantages of the assay we present here are in our opinion:

1. Large series may be handled, because there is no critical timing.
2. Only very small amounts of radioactive waste are produced (1000 tubes yield about 1 liter).

3. Only very small amounts of scintillation fluid (250 µl) are needed.
4. The technique is less cumbersome than the charcoal handling and one manual step, the transfer of the supernatant, is omitted.

In the future, this system may be combined with the "scintillation proximity reagent" (Amersham, Frankfurt, FRG). This technique is very convenient as a separation step, centrifugation and washing no longer being necessary. Using this technique, the number of pipetting steps is also reduced (no transfer of a supernatant, as with charcoal), thereby making it possible to increase the precision.

In conclusion, a second antibody separation was introduced into the competitive protein-binding assay for 25-hydroxy vitamin D. This is more convenient than charcoal separation and large series of samples may be handled because there is no critical timing. The radioactive waste and the consumption of scintillation fluid are greatly reduced. In the future, introduction of the "scintillation proximity reagent" would make a separation step unnecessary.

Reference

1. Hollis BW, Napoli JL (1985) Improved radioimmunoassay for vitamin D and its use in assessing vitamin D status. Clin Chem 31:1815–1819

Chapter 5.4

Interlaboratory Comparison of Calcidiol Determination*

E. MAYER

Introduction

Vitamin D must be metabolized before it exerts biological effects. The first step, 25-hydroxylation, is believed to occur mainly in the liver [21]. Subsequently, 25-hydroxyvitamin D (25-OH-D) is further processed in the kidney to $1,25(OH)_2D$, the biologically most active vitamin D metabolite, or to $24,25(OH)_2D$ [18, 22]. Because the concentration of 25-OH-D in serum is believed to reflect the vitamin D nutritional state of the individual, its quantification has become important in diagnosing and managing patients with disorders of calcium and phosphorus homeostasis, including rickets, osteomalacia, renal osteodystrophy, and vitamin D intoxication. Two forms of the vitamin, vitamin D_2 and vitamin D_3, occur naturally, and despite the small difference in the side chain of these molecules they are metabolized in an identical fashion and have equivalent biological effects in humans [11]. The first assays for 25-OH-D_3 [1, 9] included a chromatographic step and quantification of the metabolite by competitive protein-binding assay. Belsey et al. [2] later reported an assay for 25-OH-D_3 without chromatography. Several modifications of these methods have since appeared [4, 7, 8, 20, 23, 25], all of which include use of the natural serum transport protein for vitamin D (DBP) as a binding protein in the assay. This protein from various species shows similar characteristics, so that the choice of source is wide [6]. The relative displacement potency of 25-OH-D_2 and 25-OH-D_3 is identical for DBP derived from mammals [10, 13], while that for avian DBP is 15-fold less for 25-OH-D_2 [2]. Because routine competitive protein-binding assays of 25-OH-D tend not to discriminate between 25-OH-D_2 and 25-OH-D_3, but instead measure total 25-OH-D, use of avian DBP in the assay will result in underestimation of the 25-OH-D content of the sample if 25-OH-D_2 is present.

Alternatively, 25-OH-D in serum can be quantified by its absorbance of ultraviolet light after separation by high-performance liquid chromatography (HPLC) [5, 12, 15–17]. Because 25-OH-D_2 is somewhat less polar than 25-OH-D_3 in the solvent systems usually applied, 25-OH-D_2 and 25-OH-D_3 can be determined simultaneously. A third type of assay for 25-OH-D involves isotope dilution-mass fragmentography [5], a laborious and expensive method

---

*This chapter has partly been published in Clinical Chemistry (1984) 30: 1199–1204.

that clearly is suitable only as a reference method.

To evaluate the performance of 25-OH-D measurement in various laboratories interested in calcium-regulating hormones, the European Parathyroid Hormone Study Group (EPSG) performed an interlaboratory comparison of 25-OH-D determination in 1980. Concomitantly, an interlaboratory comparison of parathyroid hormone (parathyrin) [19] and calcitonin [24] determination was carried out. The 15 participating laboratories were asked to measure 25-OH-D in 23 serum samples in one series, using their routine assays. In addition, for comparison, we measured 25-OH-D$_2$ and 25-OH-D$_3$ simultaneously by HPLC [16, 17].

Here we report the results of this study and propose reasonable steps to improve the validity of the various assay systems applied.

Materials and Methods

Chemicals. 25-Hydroxyvitamin D$_2$ was kindly provided by Dr. J. Babcock, Upjohn Co., Kalamazoo, MI, United States. All other vitamin D compounds were donated by Dr. M. Uskokovic, Hoffmann-La Roche, Nutley, NJ, United States. All compounds were in ethanolic solution and exhibited the characteristic ultraviolet absorption, with a maximum at 265 nm and a minimum at 228 nm, indicative of the vitamin D 5,6-*cis*-triene chromophore and of the purity of the compounds. Their concentration was calculated from their absorption at 265 nm, assuming a molar absorptivity [21] of 18 300.

Removal of Endogenous Vitamin D from Bovine Serum. We shook 1 liter bovine serum horizontally, at room temperature, with 120 g activated charcoal (Norit A; Serva Chemicals, Heidelberg, FRG) for 48 h. The charcoal was then allowed to sediment and the supernatant was centrifuged (5000 g, 30 min). After filtration, we again centrifuged and filtered the serum. The clear filtrate was divided into 11 equal parts, to which we added defined amounts of 25-OH-D$_3$, 25-OH-D$_2$, vitamin D$_3$, 24, 25(OH)$_2$D$_3$, or 1,25(OH)$_2$D$_3$. The sera were carefully mixed and allowed to equilibrate for 1 h. Then, 2-ml aliquots were stored at $-20\,°C$.

Test Sera (Table 1). We distributed 23 numbered sera, frozen in Styrofoam boxes containing solid CO_2. Besides the samples mentioned above, we included sera collected in March from healthy volunteers (members of the medical staff of the hospital) and two serum samples from patients being treated with high doses of vitamin D$_2$ or D$_3$.

Study Arrangement. Fifteen independent laboratories in eight European countries were asked to evaluate a test set of 23 samples in their routine assays for 25-OH-D. The collaborating laboratories are listed by number here and so remain anonymous. Table 2 lists the technical details of the methods for quantifying serum 25-OH-D as described by the collaborating laboratories.

Table 1. Description of the serum samples distributed to the laboratories participating in this study

Sample No.	Source
1, 4	Healthy volunteer (G.L.)
2, 5	Healthy volunteer (F.K.)
3, 6	Healthy volunteer (A.W.)
7, 20	Hypoparathyroid patient (E.K.) receiving high-dose vitamin D_3
8	Bovine serum, charcoal treated
9	Plus 25[a]
10	Plus 50
11	Plus 100
12	Plus 200
13	Plus 400
14	Plus 800
15	Plus vitamin D_3, 250 nmol/liter
16	No. 8 plus 1,25 $(OH)_2D_3$, 250 nmol/liter
17	No. 8 plus 24,25 $(OH)_2D_3$, 250 nmol/liter
18	No. 8 plus 25–OH–D_2, 125 nmol/liter
19	Healthy volunteer (J.B.) plus 25–OH–D_3, 200 nmol/liter
21	Equal volumes of 7 and 22
22	Healthy volunteer (C.H.)
23	Hypoparathyroid patient (E.B.) receiving high-dose vitamin D_2

[a] In 9–14, quantity of 25-OH-D_3 added to sample No. 8 is indicated

Seven of the laboratories included a chromatographic purification step (Sephadex LH 20, silicic acid), seven omitted chromatography, and in one Sep-Pak SIL was used for prepurification. The vitamin D-binding proteins used are shown in Table 2.

In addition, we quantified all 23 samples by ultraviolet absorbance after prepurification on columns of Sephadex LH 20 and separation by HPLC according to Horst et al. [12], and modified by Mayer et al. (Chap. 5.1) [16, 17]. The procedure, in short, was as follows. Sera were extracted with six volumes of dichlormethane/methanol (1/2, by vol) and chromatographed on a 0.6 × 16-cm column of Sephadex LH 20 (solvent system: n-hexane/chloroform/methanol, 9/1/1, by vol). The material eluting from 5 to 8 ml was evaporated under nitrogen, and the redissolved residue was chromatographed on a 0.4 × 30-cm column of μPorasil (Waters Associates, Milford, MA, United States), with n-hexane/isopropanol (96/4 by vol) as eluent. By monitoring the absorbance at 265 nm we found that 25-OH-D_2 and 25-OH-D_3 were eluted at 6.5 and 7.8 min, respectively. We quantified the vitamin D compounds by peak integration, correcting for sample losses by measuring the recovery of [³H]25-OH-D_3 initially added to the samples. We evaluated all test samples in duplicate. In addition, the 25-OH-D_2 and 25-OH-D_3 content of serum samples from 15 healthy volunteers was determined with this method.

Table 2. Technical characteristics of the assay methods applied, as communicated by the collaborating laboratories

Lab. No.	Extraction	Prepurification	Specific activity of tracer[a] (kCi/mol)	Source of DBP	Reference
1	Cyclohexane/ethylacetate	Sephadex LH 20	10	Rat	Bouillon et al. [7]
2	Ethanol	–	102	Rabbit	
3	Methanol/diethyl ether	Silicic acid	9	Human	Morris and Peacock [20]
4	Methanol	–	22	Human	
5	Ethanol	–	22	Human	
6	Ethanol	–	8	Human	
7	Ethanol	–	22	Rat	Belsey et al. [3]
8	Chloroform/methanol/H_2O	Silicic acid	10	Rat	
9	Ethanol	–	12	Rat	
10	Methanol/chloroform	Silicic acid	90	Rat	Preece et al. [23]
11	Methanol/dichlormethane	Silicic acid	22	Human	Preece et al. [23]
12	Ethanol	Sep-Pak Sil	102	Rabbit	Schmidt-Gayk et al. [25]
13	Ethanol	Sephadex LH 20	102	Human	
14	Methanol/dichlormethane	Sephadex LH 20	102	Chick	
15	Chloroform/methanol/H_2O	Silicic acid	9	Rat	Preece et al. [23]
RM[b]	Dichlormethane/methanol	Sephadex LH 20	102	–	Mayer et al. [16, 17]

[a] Tracer = [^{3}H] 25-OH-D_3

[b] RM, reference method: ultraviolet quantification after HPLC separation

Results

Reproducibility. To investigate the reproducibility of the assays used, we included samples 1–3 (sera from healthy volunteers) and sample No. 7 (sample from a patient with hypoparathyroidism on treatment with vitamin D_3) twice in the set of sera (labeled 4, 5, 6, and 20, respectively). Figure 1 depicts the 25-OH-D_3 assay results for samples 4 and 1. This serum test was assayed only twice, so an intraassay CV cannot be given. Nevertheless, it is apparent that the intraassay variation was quite low in most laboratories; almost identical results were obtained. In this respect, the results for the other set-duplicated samples were comparable (see Table 3)

Accuracy. Because we had no sera devoid of any vitamin D and its metabolites, we treated bovine serum with charcoal to remove endogenous vitamin D. After a procedure that included shaking the serum at room temperature for 48 h, filtering, and centrifugation, a small amount of 25-OH-D_3 was still present. We measured in this sample (sample No. 8) a concentration of 21 nmol 25-OH-D_3/liter with the reference method.

This serum was divided into 11 equal parts, either increasing amounts of 25-OH-D_3 or a single concentration of vitamin D_3, 25-OH-D_2, 24,25(OH)$_2$D$_3$, or 1,25(OH)$_2$D$_3$ was added. The presence of the 25-OH-D_3 serum standard curve was well recognized by the assays of most laboratories (see Fig. 2, Table 4).

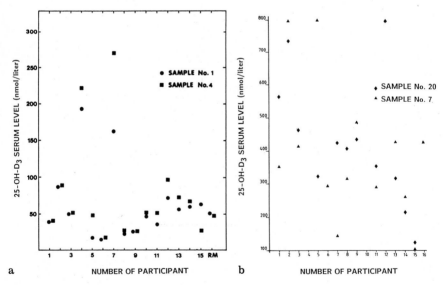

Fig. 1a,b. Reproducibility of the various assay systems used for the measurement of 25-OH-D. **a** samples 1 (●) and 4 (■), **b** samples 7 (▲) and 20 (◆) were identical (see Table 1). Participant (lab.) number corresponds to that in Tables 2–4

Table 3. Reproducibility and accuracy of the assays for 25-OH-D

Lab. No.	Sample No.											
	1	2	4	5	3	6	22	7	20	21	[c]	23
1	40[a]	21	42	22	24	27	60	353	563	206	259	1054
2	88	30	89	47	25	46	89	798	735	285	428	2000
3	50	32	52	34	37	38	141	415	469	250	291	790
4	194	130	224	112	160	160	200	2320	2000	927	1180	NA[d]
5	19	18	49	14	25	21	25	800	322	235	293	256
6	18	1	15	1	10	5	85	294	383	160	212	550
7	162	95	270	125	142	160	175	145	425	437	230	437
8	24	23	29	13	28	NA	NA	316	408	312	–	545
9	27	17	27	14	16	17	11	488	437	437	237	725
10	47	28	51	28	38	34	223	380	512	452	334	1150
11	36	26	52	20	28	19	124	290	355	224	223	950
12	73	25	98	29	42	83	113	800	800	800	456	800
13	57	55	74	55	61	59	119	430	317	195	246	940
14	60	35	69	35	65	27	80	262	216	131	159	575
15	64	18	28	18	21	7	4	103	125	4	59	125
RM[b]	52	42	49	37	44	50	160	418	NA	269	289	1850/32[e]
Mean	47[f] / 83[g]	30 / 45	50 / 110	28 / 49	38 / 60	30 / 70	107 / 100	318 / 806	370 / 728	222 / 468	224 / 433	766 / 794
SD	13 / 70	12 / 48	17 / 99	13 / 50	17 / 63	16 / 66	69 / 70	104 / 717	149 / 589	130 / 290	91 / 343	336 / 622
CV (%)	28 / 84	40 / 99	34 / 90	46 / 99	45 / 105	53 / 94	64 / 70	33 / 88	40 / 81	59 / 62	40 / 79	44 / 78

[a] 25-OH-D values (nmol/liter)
[b] RM, reference method (HPLC method)
[c] Mean of results of samples No. 7 and 20 were averaged with result of sample no. 22
[d] NA, not analyzed
[e] Simultaneous quantification of 25-OH-D$_2$/25-OH-D$_3$ content
[f] Assay with chromatography
[g] Assay without chromatography

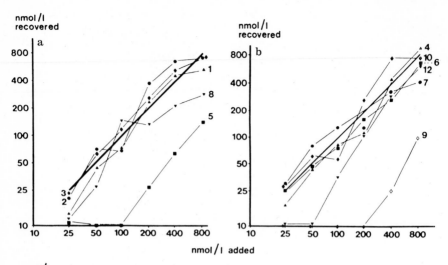

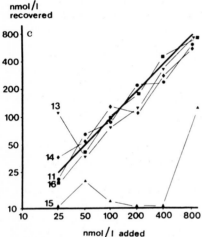

Fig. 2a–c. Analytical recovery of various amounts of 25-OH-D$_3$ added to charcoal-treated bovine serum (samples 8–14), as measured by laboratories 1–16

Indeed, the overall mean values obtained for samples 8–14 almost approach the true concentrations. However, the large average CV (55%) reflects the poor agreement among results obtained by the various laboratories. This is also illustrated by the results reported in Table 3 and Fig. 1, e.g., the 25-OH-D concentrations for sample 1 range from 18 to 194 nmol/liter, those of sample 7 from 193 to 2320 nmol/liter. Comparable results indicative of a low accuracy of the assay system being applied were obtained for the remaining samples from healthy volunteers and patients on treatment with pharmacological doses of vitamins D$_3$ or D$_2$.

Sample 21 was an equivolume mixture of samples 7 and 22. The latter was derived from a healthy volunteer with a high (for this country) 25-OH-D$_3$ concentration, 160 nmol/liter. The former was from a hypoparathyroid patient on high-dose vitamin D$_3$ treatment, and the concentration was 418 nmol/liter.

Table 4. Analytical recovery of added 25-OH-D₃, and specificity for 25-OH-D

Sample No.	8	9	10	11	12	13	14	15	16	17	18	19
Concentration added, (nmol/liter)	0	25	50	100	200	400	800	250	250	250	125	200
Compound added	25-OH-D₃							D₃	1,25	24,25	25-OH-D₂	25-OH-D₃
Lab. No.												
1	10ᵃ	23	53	82	235	459	634	18	7	6	20	240
2	23	43	90	90	392	673	728	21	30	396	90	291
3	37	59	98	152	283	540	757	38	38	39	165	315
4	24	41	68	116	146	448	962	26	19	192	NAᵇ	968
5	5	11	5	10	32	67	144	5	5	40	15	227
6	12	37	56	88	180	270	650	0	11	15	83	166
7	15	45	95	145	200	400	425	14	24	400	125	412
8	13	24	40	154	144	232	300	17	25	123	42	231
9	7	7	6	11	32	107	362	6	7	107	7	275
10	31	57	91	88	283	775	807	72	71	602	292	502
11	35	55	100	128	248	273	647	35	42	40	132	203
12	25	25	25	50	120	301	702	25	25	510	29	800
13	32	153	69	110	181	370	778	10	10	138	113	220
14	32	69	83	162	141	318	610	17	29	27	48	131
15	24	21	44	36	1	34	125	10	1	56	56	111
RMᶜ	21	40	61	122	206	506	731	26	34	20	141/32ᵈ	254
Mean	21ᵉ 15ᶠ	58 30	72 49	114 73	190 157	375 323	582 567	27 14	28 17	61 237	108 58	244 448
SD	10 8	43 16	24 37	51 44	95 122	221 208	273 243	21 10	23 10	50 197	89 48	122 310
CV (%)	37 50	74 53	33 75	70 39	50 78	59 64	48 42	78 71	82 59	82 83	82 83	50 69

ᵃ 25-OH-D values (nmol/liter)
ᵇ NA, not analyzed.
ᶜ RM, reference method (HPLC method)

ᵈ Quantification of 25-OH-D₂/25-OH-D₃ content
ᵉ Assay with chromatography
ᶠ Assay without chromatography

1,25 = 1,25(OH)₂D₃
24,25 = 24,25(OH)₂D₃

The results from 8 of 14 laboratories came close to the calculated values (range, 30%). In contrast, the CV (60%) calculated for the 25-OH-D values as assessed for sample 21 by the 15 laboratories (mean 332, SD 238 nmol/liter) was large. Altogether, these results point to wide interlaboratory variation in 25-OH-D measurement, while on the other hand the precision was good for most of these laboratories.

On analyzing the data obtained by assays including a chromatographic step versus methods with no chromatography, it becomes apparent that the latter measures about twice as much apparent 25-OH-D in all serum samples not pretreated with charcoal. This twofold difference appears to be independent of the actual 25-OH-D concentration, because it can be observed in samples both from normal subjects and from patients with very high 25-OH-D concentrations as a result of treatment with pharmacological doses of vitamin D_3 or vitamin D_2 (see Table 3). To prepare test sample No. 19, we had added synthetic 25-OH-D_3 to the serum of healthy subject (endogenous 25-OH-D_3 concentration: 37 nmol/liter) to increase the 25-OH-D_3 by 200 nmol/liter. The identical amount of 25-OH-D_3 had been added to charcoal-treated serum (sample No. 12). From the results obtained by the various laboratories for samples 12 and 19 it is evident that nonchromatographic methods overestimated the amount of 25-OH-D_3 added to the sample from the normal subject (448 vs. 244 nmol/liter) but not in the charcoal-treated test sample (190 vs. 157 nmol/liter). Also 25-OH-D assay in the remaining charcoal-treated and 25-OH-D_3-fortified samples revealed comparable results by chromatographic and nonchromatographic methods.

Specificity

To test the interference of vitamin D_3 or vitamin D metabolites in the assays for 25-OH-D, we fortified samples 15–18 with either D_3 (250 nmol/liter), $24,25(OH)_2D_3$ (250 nmol/liter), $1,25(OH)_2D_3$ (250 nmol/liter), or 25-OH-D_2 (125 nmol/liter).

Vitamin D_3 and $1,25(OH)_2D_3$, even at a concentration of 250 nmol/liter, showed no cross-reactions in the assays of any participant. Sample 17 contained 250 nmol/liter of $24,25(OH)_2D_3$/liter. This metabolite greatly interfered in the assays of those laboratories omitting a chromatographic step (mean, 237 nmol/liter), but only slightly in the assay systems including chromatography (mean, 56 nmol/liter). Of course, this high a concentration of $24,25\text{-}(OH)_2D_3$ will not be reached under physiological conditions [normal value in humans, 7.3 (SD 2.2)nmol/liter][14], but it documents the known interference of $24,25(OH)_2D_3$ in assays for 25-OH-D without chromatography. Also, it is worth mentioning that in vitamin D intoxication a concentration of $24,25(OH)_2D_3$ of 535 nmol/liter was reported in serum [26].

Addition of 125 nmol/liter 25-OH-D_2/liter to the charcoal-treated serum resulted in similar analytical recovery of the metabolite by chromatographic and nonchromatographic methods.

Validity of the Data. The 25-OH-D concentration in serum is representative of the vitamin D nutritional state of the individual. Consequently, high concentrations of this metabolite are detected in vitamin D intoxication, low ones in vitamin D deficiency. To test the validity of the 25-OH-D assays applied by the various collaborating laboratories, we included in the set of sera samples with high 25-OH-D_3 or 25-OH-D_2 content (derived from patients on vitamin D_3 or D_2 treatment) subnormal concentration (charcoal-treated bovine serum) and samples from healthy volunteers. The results (Fig. 3) show that all laboratories were able to distinguish between 25-OH-D concentrations in the high-dose samples and those from normal subjects, but only eight laboratories discriminated normal from subnormal values.

Reference Method. Simultaneous quantification of 25-OH-D_2 and 25-OH-D_3 by its ultraviolet absorbance after HPLC: We simultaneously determined 25-OH-D_2 and 25-OH-D_3 in the 23 test sera by quantification of their ultraviolet absorbance after separation by HPLC, for reference purposes (see Tables 3, 4). This method proved to be an appropriate reference method, because it is reproducible, accurate, precise, and highly specific. For 15 normal subjects, serum 25-OH-D_3 concentration ranged from 28 to 160 nmol/liter with a mean of 68 (SD 22) nmol/liter. No 25-OH-D_2 was detected in the samples from healthy volunteers, a patient on high-dose vitamin D_3 treatment, or the charcoal-treated bovine sera. As expected, a high concentration of 25-OH-D_2

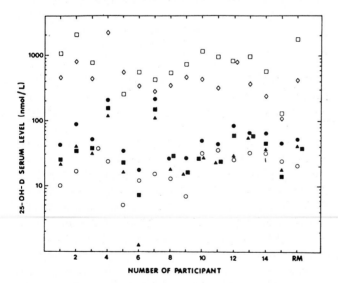

Fig. 3. 25-Hydroxyvitamin D concentrations measured in charcoal-treated bovine serum (○), sera from healthy volunteers (●,▲,■), and sera from hypoparathyroid patients on high-dose treatment with vitamin D_2 (□) or vitamin D_3 (◇). *RM*, reference method: ultraviolet quantification after HPLC. Participant number corresponds to that in Tables 2–4

(1850 nmol/liter) and a normal concentration of 25-OH-D$_3$ (32 nmol/liter) were present in the serum from a patient on high-dose vitamin D$_2$ therapy.

Discussion

Jongen et al. [14] reported results of a study on the interlaboratory variation of vitamin D metabolite measurements. They included two concentrations of 25-OH-D$_3$ in ethanol and three different sera in their set of samples. The results for the serum samples showed substantially higher interlaboratory variation of 25-OH-D measurement as compared with results for 25-OH-D$_3$ in ethanol [26]. These authors concluded that this discrepancy must originate from the different extraction and purification procedure used for the serum samples.

In our study, the 15 laboratories evaluated a test set of 23 sera, using their routine assays for 25-OH-D. The results show good reproducibility of 25-OH-D values in most laboratories, and all could distinguish between normal and grossly above-normal 25-OH-D concentrations. In contrast, a sample with a subnormal 25-OH-D$_3$ content was reported to be within the normal range by seven laboratories, a result we believe is ascribable to nonspecific interference. Certainly, the subnormal range should be clearly distinguishable from normal for diagnosis of vitamin D deficiency.

The presence of compounds nonspecifically interfering at the DBP-binding site is most clearly evident when methods were applied that omitted any chromatographic preassay purification. In this case, values were accurate for samples consisting of different amounts of 25-OH-D$_3$ added to charcoal-treated bovine serum, but the 25-OH-D content of sera from healthy subjects or patients on high-dose vitamin D treatment was overestimated about twofold. Charcoal treatment of serum not only removes most endogenous 25-OH-D$_3$, but also other substances such as Na$^+$, Cl$^-$, parathyroid hormone, insulin, folic acid, uric acid, creatinine, and triiodothyronine (unpublished observation)—a list that obviously includes material interfering in nonchromatographic assays for 25-OH-D. This is most clearly illustrated by the results obtained by the various laboratories for samples 12 and 19. When the 25-OH-D$_3$ was increased by 200 nmol/liter in charcoal-treated serum or in serum from a normal subject, direct assays measured 25-OH-D$_3$ equally as well as chromatographic methods in charcoal-treated samples, but overestimated by twofold the 25-OH-D$_3$ concentration in the samples from a normal subject. Thus a chromatographic step (e.g., with silicic acid, Sephadex LH 20) apparently is desirable before radioassay for 25-OH-D$_3$. A direct assay would be an important improvement for routine 25-OH-D measurement, because it would be far less laborious and expensive. This, however, would require elimination of the nonspecifically interfering material present in serum extracts. Bouillon [6] published a preliminary report that nonspecific interference could be eliminated by an extraction procedure including saponification followed by extraction with *n*-hexane and including a 25-OH-D$_3$ standard curve prepared by using serum freed from vitamin D by affinity chromatography. When this method was compared with a chromatographic procedure, the values correlated well ($r = 0.96$), but the absolute values were about 20% higher. Of course, in this assay system still other vitamin D metabolites such as $24,25\text{-}(OH)_2D$, $25,26(OH)_2D$ and 25-OH-D-26,23-lactone will interfere. However, their concentrations in plasma are 20–100 times lower than those of 25-OH-D, and so in routine screening for vitamin D deficiency and vitamin D intoxication this slight overestimate as a consequence of specific interferences in the assay is not of major concern.

25-Hydroxyvitamin D_2 was not detectable in 15 sera from healthy volunteers as evaluated by an HPLC procedure for the simultaneous quantification of $25\text{-}OH\text{-}D_2$ and $25\text{-}OH\text{-}D_3$. However, this compound reached a very high concentration in serum from a patient being treated with pharmacological doses of vitamin D_2 (sample 23, see Table 3).

All but one laboratory used in their assays DBP (from rat, rabbit, or human), which equally recognizes $25\text{-}OH\text{-}D_2$ and $25\text{-}OH\text{-}D_3$ [10, 13]. Thus, in fact, even when established for $25\text{-}OH\text{-}D_3$, their assays actually measure total 25-OH-D. One laboratory uses chick serum as the source of DBP. Chick DBP reportedly recognizes $25\text{-}OH\text{-}D_2$ 15 times less strongly than it does $25\text{-}OH\text{-}D_3$ [3]. Therefore, if differentiation between $25\text{-}OH\text{-}D_2$ and $25\text{-}OH\text{-}D_3$ is sought, chick DBP might be the protein of choice, but when measurement of total 25-OH-D is desired, DBP from human, rat, or rabbit is preferable.

As an alternative approach to measure 25-OH-D, we applied HPLC and subsequent quantification of $25\text{-}OH\text{-}D_2$ and $25\text{-}OH\text{-}D_3$ by their ultraviolet absorbance, finding the method to be accurate, precise, and specific. Results compared well with those using the best chromatographic-competitive protein-binding assays. Furthermore, simultaneous separate determination of 25-OH-D_2 and $25\text{-}OH\text{-}D_3$ was possible. This method is laborious and expensive, so it is not applicable for routine 25-OH-D measurement, but it served well as a reference method for this study.

From the results reported in this chapter it is evident that interlaboratory variation in the measurement of 25-OH-D is too wide for a comparison of assay results reported by different laboratories to be valid. To improve interlaboratory variation, we propose either standardization of the methods applied or the introduction of reference sera to control thereby each assay carried out. Because the latter procedure appears more promising to us, we prepared a set of reference sera, which will be sent on request to laboratories interested in 25-OH-D measurement.

In conclusion, this interlaboratory study on determination of 25-hydroxy vitamin D (25-OH-D) in serum involved 15 laboratories in eight European countries. All distinguished between normal (50 ± 31 nmol/liter, mean $\pm$ SD) and grossly increased concentrations, but for eight laboratories the results for serum samples with low and normal 25-OH-D content overlapped. In general, values were well reproducible, but interlaboratory variation in 25-OH-D measurement was large, $24,25(OH)_2D_3$ interfering in most of the assays. We present evidence in favor of chromatography before assay, as opposed to nonchromato-graphic methods. Liquid chromatography with ultraviolet detection for quantifying 25-OH-D$_2$ and 25-OH-D$_3$ appears to be an appropriate reference method, whereas competitive protein-binding assay is the method of choice for routine determinations. Control sera with subnormal, normal, and above-normal concentrations of 25-OH-D$_3$ are needed for use in standardization of 25-OH-D assays.

Participating Laboratories. R. Ardaillou, Paris, France; R. Bouillon, Leuven, Belgium; H. Brauman, Brussels, Belgium; V. lo Cascio, G. Galvanini, and D. Tartarotti, Verona, Italy; M. Cecchettin, Brescia, Italy; M. A. Dambacher, Zürich, Switzerland; S. A. Duursma and H. Bosch, Utrecht, The Netherlands; E. Leicht and C. Biro, Homburg/Saar, Federal Republic of Germany; H. v. Lilienfeld-Toal, Bonn, Federal Republic of Germany; E. Mayer and H. Schmidt-Gayk, Heidelberg, Federal Republic of Germany; G. Offermann, Berlin, Federal Republic of Germany; M. Paillard, Colombes, France; A. Rapado and M. L. Traba, Madrid, Spain; P. O. Schwille, Erlangen, Federal Republic of Germany; W. Woloszcuk and R. Willvonseder, Vienna, Austria.

Acknowledgments. We wish to thank Byk-Mallinckrodt Co., Dietzenbach, FRG, for sending the frozen serum samples to the laboratories participating in this study. This work was supported by the Deutsche Forschungsgemeinschaft (Schm 400/5).

References

1. Belsey RE, DeLuca HF, Potts JT Jr (1971) Competitive binding assay for vitamin D and 25-OH-vitamin D. J Clin Endocrinol Metab 33:554–557
2. Belsey RE, DeLuca HF, Potts JT Jr (1974) A rapid assay for 25-OH-vitamin D$_3$ without preparative chromatography. J Clin Endocrinol Metab 38:1046–1051
3. Belsey RE, DeLuca HF, Potts JT (1974) Selective binding properties of vitamin D transport in chick plasma in vitro. Nature 274:208–209
4. Bishop JE, Norman AW, Coburn JW et al. (1980) Determination of the concentration of 25-hydroxyvitamin D, 24,25-dihydroxyvitamin D and 1,25-dihydroxyvitamin D in a single 2 ml plasma sample. Miner Electrolyte Metab 3:181–189
5. Björkhem J, Holmberg I (1976) A novel specific assay of 25-hydroxyvitamin D$_3$. Clin Chim Acta 68:215–219
6. Bouillon R (1983) Radiochemical assays for vitamin D metabolites: technical possibilities and clinical application. J Steroid Biochem 19:921–927
7. Bouillon R, van Kerkhove P, DeMoor P (1976) Measurement of 25-hydroxyvitamin D$_3$ in serum. Clin Chem 22:364–368
8. Edelstein S, Charman M, Lawson DEM, Kodicek E (1974) Competitive protein-binding assay for 25-hydroxycholecalciferol. Clin Sci Mol Med 46:231–240
9. Haddad J, Chyu KJ (1971) Competitive protein-binding radioassay for 25-hydroxy-cholecalciferol. J Clin Endocrinol Metab 33:992–995

10. Haddad JG, Hillmann L, Rojanasathit S (1976) Human serum binding capacity for 25-hydroxyergocalciferol and 25-hydroxycholecalciferol. J Clin Endocrinol Metab 43:86–91

11. Holick MF, Potts JT (1980) Vitamin D. In: Isselbacher KJ et al. (eds) Harrison's principles of internal medicine. McGraw-Hill, New York, pp 1843–1849

12. Horst HL, Shepard RM, Jorgensen NA, DeLuca HF (1979) Assays for vitamin D and its metabolites. In: Norman AW et al. (eds) Vitamin D; basic research and its clinical application. de Gruyter, Berlin, pp 213–220

13. Jones G, Byrnes B, Palma F et al. (1980) Displacement potency of vitamin D_2 analogs in competitive protein-binding assays for 25-hydroxyvitamin D_3, 24,25-dihydroxyvitamin D_3 and 1,25-dihydroxy-vitamin D_3. J Clin Endocrinol Metab 50:773–775

14. Jongen MJM, van der Vigh WJF et al. (1982) Interlaboratory variation of vitamin D metabolite measurements. J Clin Chem Clin Biochem 20:753–756

15. Lambert PW, Syverson BJ, Arnaud CD, Spelsberg TC (1977) Isolation and quantitation of endogenous vitamin D and its physiologically important metabolites in human plasma by high-performance liquid chromatography. J Steroid Biochem 8:929–937

16. Mayer E, Schmidt-Gayk H, Gartner R, Knuppen R (1981) Simultaneous assay for 25-OH-vitamin D_2 and 25-OH-vitamin D_3 by HPLC. Acta Endocrinol [Suppl] (Copenh) 240:96 (abstr no 44)

17. Mayer E, Schmidt-Gayk H, Lichtwald K et al. (1981) Simultane Bestimmung von 25-Hydroxy-Vitamin D_2 und 25-Hydroxy-Vitamin D_3 durch Hochdruckflüssigkeitschromatographie. Ärztl Lab 27:89–94

18. Mayer E, Kadowaki S, Williams G, Norman AW (1984) The mode of action of 1,25-dihydroxyvitamin D. In: Kumar R (ed) Vitamin D. Nijhoff, Boston, pp 259–302

19. Minne HW (1984) Quality control in parathyroid hormone radioimmunoassays: a multicentre study performed by the European Parathyroid Hormone Study Group. Eur J Clin Invest 14:16–23

20. Morris JF, Peacock M (1976) Assay of plasma 25-hydroxyvitamin D. Clin Chim Acta 72:383–391

21. Norman AW (1979) Vitamin D, the calcium homeostatic steroid hormone. Academic Press, New York

22. Norman AW, Roth J, Orci L (1982) The vitamin D endocrine system; steroid metabolism, hormone receptors and biological response (calcium binding proteins). Endocr Rev 3:331–366

23. Preece MA, O'Riordan JLH, Lawson DEM, Kodicek E (1974) A competitive protein-binding assay for 25-hydroxycholecalciferol and 25-hydroxyergocalciferol in serum. Clin Chim Acta 54:235–242

24. Raue F (1982) Interlaboratory comparison of radioimmunological calcitonin determination. J Clin Chem Clin Biochem 20:157–161

25. Schmidt-Gayk H, Nagel W, Martiskainen I et al. (1977) Sättigungsanalyse für 25-Hydroxy-Vitamin D. Ärztl Lab 23:111–123

26. Shepard R, DeLuca HF (1980) Plasma concentrations of vitamin D_3 and its metabolites in the rat as influenced by vitamin D_3 or 25-hydroxyvitamin D_3 intakes. Arch Biochem Biophys 202:43–53

Chapter 5.5

A Sensitive Radioimmunoassay for 1,25-Dihydroxyvitamin D$_3$ (Calcitriol) after High-Performance Liquid Chromatography of Plasma or Serum Extracts

S. SCHARLA and H. REICHEL

Introduction

Vitamin D is produced either in the skin from the precursor 7-dehydrocholes-terol or ingested with food [46]. When entering the circulation it is bound to vitamin D-binding protein (DBP) and transported to the liver, where it is hydroxylated to 25-hydroxyvitamin D (25-OH-D), the major circulating form of the vitamin. Further hydroxylation takes place in the kidney to yield 1,25-dihydroxyvitamin D [1,25(OH)$_2$D] or 24,25-dihydroxyvitamin D [24,25(OH)$_2$D]. The biologically most active metabolite is 1,25(OH)$_2$D, which fulfills all the criteria of a classical hormone. It plays an important role in calcium homoeostasis and the maintenance of a healthy skeleton. 1,25(OH)$_2$D exerts its effects via binding to specific receptors in cells of intestine, bone, and kidney [36]. In recent years typical receptors for 1,25(OH)$_2$D have also been found in cells from other normal or neoplastic tissues, indicating that 1,25(OH)$_2$D may have functions beyond those of calcium metabolism, such as the modulation of the immune system [42] and cell differentiation [38]. Therefore, the measurement of 1,25(OH)$_2$D is of increasing importance in the evaluation and management of patients with a wide variety of clinical disorders.

Because the normal circulation levels of 1,25(OH)$_2$D are 100- to 1000-fold less than the levels of 25-OH-D, assays for 1,25(OH)$_2$D are technically difficult to perform and require extensive sample purification to remove lipids and cross-reacting metabolites of vitamin D. Several methods have been applied to the measurement of 1,25(OH)$_2$D$_2$ and 1,25(OH)$_2$D$_3$, the two naturally occurring forms of the hormone. In 1974, Brumbaugh et al. [6] reported a cytosol-chromatin radioreceptor assay for 1,25(OH)$_2$D$_3$, utilizing chick intestinal mucosa. This method included chromatography of serum extracts on Sephadex LH 20, silicic acid, and Celite. A second radioreceptor assay was developed by Eisman et al. [12], who introduced final purification of 1,25(OH)$_2$D$_3$ by high-performance liquid chromatography (HPLC) following prepurification on Sephadex LH 20 columns. Several modifications of these methods have been reported since [1, 8, 10, 11, 13, 22, 24, 26, 28, 30, 45, 48]. Blayau et al. [3] proposed the use of a cytosolic receptor from bovine-lactating mammary gland, a material easier to obtain than intestinal mucosa from rachitic chickens.

Apart from a sensitive bioassay [47], an assay based on isotope dilution-mass fragmentography [2], and a cytoreceptor assay [29], several reports on radioimmunoassays (RIAs) for 1,25(OH)$_2$D$_3$ [4, 5, 7, 9, 16, 17, 39, 43] and 1,25(OH)$_2$D$_2$ [14] have appeared. Most of them applied extraction steps with organic solvents, and further purification by HPLC was necessary because of the low specificity of the antisera for 1,25(OH)$_2$D$_3$ or 1,25(OH)$_2$D$_2$. Few authors developed monoclonal antibodies for 1,25(OH)$_2$D$_3$ [31, 40].

The improvement of the cytosol radioreceptor assay employing 1,25(OH)$_2$D receptor from calf thymus by Reinhardt et al. [41] was widely recognized. This receptor preparation provided both high specificity and sensitivity, making possible the use of a two-step solid-phase extraction of plasma samples without the necessity of further HPLC purification. Hollis [20] introduced a novel single-cartridge extraction and purification procedure applying phase-switching of organic solvents followed by the calf thymus receptor assay. Hartwell and Christiansen [18] showed that the calf thymus assay is more precise and sensitive than the intestinal receptor assay. Although the thymus receptor assay made the measurement of 1,25(OH)$_2$D possible for laboratories not equipped with an HPLC system, the solid-phase extraction is still time consuming and the thymus receptor is not as stable as an antibody used for RIA.

In addition, cross-reaction and interference of other vitamin D metabolites is not excluded when samples with high concentrations of 25-OH-D are measured. For this reason HPLC purification is still used [3, 18, 25] and it is recommendable especially for research purposes.

In the following we describe a rapid and simple solid-phase extraction of plasma or serum samples using "Extrelut-1" minicolumns, final purification with HPLC, and quantitation of 1,25(OH)$_2$D$_3$ by a sensitive RIA.

Materials and Methods

Chemicals

1,25(OH)$_2$[23,24(n)-^{3}H]D$_3$ (specific activity, 158 Ci/mmol), 25-OH[23,24(n)-^{3}H]D$_3$ (specific activity, 85 Ci/mmol), 24,25(OH)$_2$[23,24(n)-^{3}H]D$_3$ (specific activity, 90 Ci/mmol), and 25,26(OH)$_2$[23,24(n)-^{3}H]D$_3$ (specific activity, 90 Ci/mmol) were purchased from Amersham Co. (Amersham, UK). 1,25(OH)$_2$-24-oxo-D$_3$ and 1,23,25(OH)$_3$-24-oxo-D$_3$ were prepared as described previously [35] and kindly provided by Dr. Anthony W. Norman, Riverside, United States. 25-OH-26,23-Lactone D$_3$ was chemically synthesized in the laboratory of Dr. Dudley Williams, Cambridge, United Kingdom, and all remaining vitamin D compounds in the laboratory of Dr. Milan Uskokovic, Nutley, NJ, United States. Collectively, all unlabeled vitamin D metabolites were generously made available to us by Dr. Anthony W. Norman (Riverside, CA, United States). Charcoal (Norit A) and bovine serum albumin were obtained from Serva Co.

(Heidelberg, FRG); dextran T 70 was purchased from Roth KG (Karlsruhe, FRG). All solvents were purchased from Merck Co. (Darmstadt, FRG).

Serum Samples

Serum samples were obtained from 30 healthy members of the staff of our hospital (9 females and 21 males; mean age, 25 years; range, 18–40 years), who did not regularly use medicaments, and from 35 employees of a factory, who underwent a routine examination (12 females and 23 males; mean age, 44 years; range, 20–65 years). In the latter group no detailed information concerning diseases or medication was available. $1,25(OH)_2D_3$ was also determined in sera from 55 elderly patients (37 females and 18 males; mean age, 77 years; range, 60–92 years) and in 3 patients with chronic renal failure on $1,25(OH)_2D_3$ treatment. In addition, we assessed the serum $1,25(OH)_2D_3$ concentration in ten patients with chronic renal failure who were not receiving $1,25(OH)_2D_3$ drug therapy. Finally, both serum $1,25(OH)_2D_3$ and creatinine were determined in a patient with renal failure from days 4–12 after kidney transplantation. Plasma samples from 12 apparently healthy blood donors were pooled; part of this pool was fortified with 120 pmol/liter $1,25(OH)_2D_3$. Charcoal-treated sera were prepared as described by Mayer et al. [32]. These samples were used as control sera for each assay carried out.

Extraction Procedure

One milliliter of serum or plasma was transferred onto an Extrelut-1 minicolumn (Merck Co.). Following an equilibration period of 20 min at room temperature, $1,25(OH)_2D_3$ was eluted by the addition of two aliquots of 5 ml diisopropylether. The eluate was collected in conical glass tubes and evaporated to dryness under nitrogen in a water bath at 37 °C. To each batch of samples two 1-ml samples of plasma spiked with 10 000 decays per minute (dpm) $1,25(OH)_2[^3H]D_3$ were added. After vortex-mixing and equilibration for 30 min, the spiked samples were processed in a manner identical to the patient samples.

This method can be modified according to Schilling et al. [44] as follows: after equilibration of the column $1,25(OH)_2D_3$ was stepwise eluted with diisopropylether, adding 1 ml at a time up to a total of 5 ml.

Purification of Extracts by HPLC

The residues were redissolved in 200 µl HPLC solvent (n-hexane/isopropanol/methanol, 87/10/3, v/v), aspirated into gas-tight syringes (Hamilton Co., Reno, NE, United States), and subsequently subjected to HPLC [Model 6000A solvent delivery system, Model 440 detector monitoring ultraviolet absorbance at 254 nm, RCM-100 Radial Compression Separation System equipped with a µPorasil Radial-Pak cartridge (10 µm), all purchased from Waters Assoc.,

Milford, MA, United States]. Alternatively the redissolved extracts (200 µl) were transferred to autosampler vials and injected by an autosampler system (WISP 710A, Waters). The suitable and programmable fraction collector (Foxy™) was obtained from Isco Inc. (Lincoln, NE, United States). The HPLC apparatus was operated at a constant flow rate of 2 ml/min; solvents were filtered and then degassed in a sonicator in vacuo before use. Under these conditions operating pressure was about 100 psi at a flow rate of 2 ml/min. Before each assay run the retention time was determined with $1,25(OH)_2[^3H]D_3$. The fraction eluted between 6 and 7.5 min from the column contained $1,25(OH)_2D_3$ and was collected for RIA (see Fig. 1). For estimation of recovery of $1,25(OH)_2[^3H]D_3$,

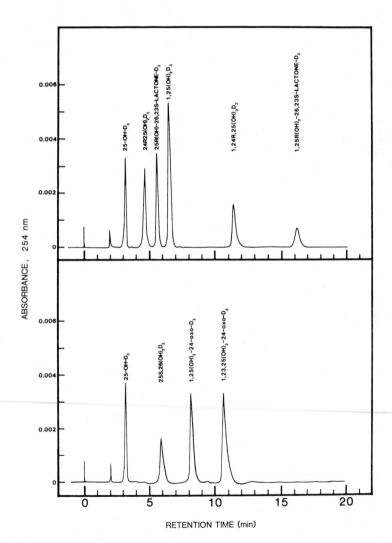

Fig. 1. Elution profile of several vitamin D₃ metabolites

the two spiked samples were collected in a liquid scintillation vial, whereas the patient samples were collected in conical glass tubes. For RIA, these fractions were evaporated to dryness under nitrogen and redissolved in 250 µl ethanol.

Radioimmunoassay for 1,25(OH)$_2$D$_3$

The antiserum used had been raised by immunization of rabbits with a 3-hemisuccinate derivative of 1,25(OH)$_2$D$_3$ linked to bovine serum albumin (BSA) (code: KH 090478, kindly supplied by Dr. Bouillon, Leuven, Belgium). Phosphate buffer (pH 7.5, 0.06 mol/liter) containing BSA (1 g/liter), sodium azide (1 g/liter), and ethylenediaminetetraacetic acid (EDTA) (0.4 g/liter) was used for dilution of the antiserum. This buffer was labeled "PPPNE." The antiserum was diluted 1:50 000 (working solution) and then 5 ml normal rabbit serum/liter antiserum working solution was added. The incubation was carried out under sequential saturation conditions.

Duplicate 100-µl portions of the redissolved fraction obtained from HPLC were transferred into assay tubes and evaporated to dryness under a stream of nitrogen. Twenty microliters each of ethanolic standard solutions were pipetted in the corresponding tubes and not evaporated. Then, 100 µl antiserum working solution was added along with 300 µl PPPNE buffer. The tubes were incubated for 16 h at 4 °C. Then, 1,25(OH)$_2$[^{3}H]D$_3$ (10 000 dpm in 20 µl ethanol) was added using a Hamilton Repeating Dispenser (Hamilton Co., Reno, NE, United States). The samples were incubated for a further 48 h at 4 °C. Thereafter, ice-cold dextran-coated charcoal (1.25 g charcoal/100 ml and 0.125 g dextran T 70/100 ml), 100 µl/tube, was added, the tubes closed, vortexed, and allowed to stand for another 10 min in a refrigerator at 4°C. Thereafter, the tubes were vortex-mixed again and centrifuged for 10 min at 1200 g in a refrigerated centrifuge. The supernatants were transferred into Pico-plastic vials (Packard Instruments, Frankfurt, FRG). All radioactivity measurements were carried out

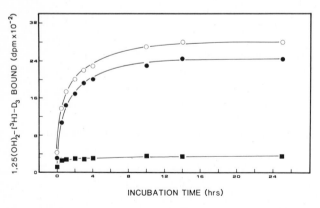

Fig. 2. Association of 1,25(OH)$_2$[^{3}H]D$_3$ to the antibody binding site: ○——○, total dpm bound; ●——●, dpm specifically bound; ■——■, dpm nonspecifically bound

in a liquid scintillation counter (Model LS 7000, Beckman Instruments Inc., Fullerton, CA, United States) using a scintillation cocktail of 4 ml Pico-Fluor™15 (Packard Instruments, Frankfurt, FRG).

Kinetic Experiment

To determine the time point when equilibrium binding is reached, steroid association experiments were carried out. Following a time course (see Fig. 2), dpm totally bound as well as nonspecifically bound were determined by incubating $1,25(OH)_2[^3H]D_3$ and antiserum in the absence or presence of a 300-fold molar excess of $1,25(OH)_2D_3$. Dpm specifically bound was calculated by subtracting dpm nonspecifically bound from totally bound dpm.

Results

Extraction

Sera were transferred onto Extrelut-1 minicolumns and $1,25(OH)_2D_3$ was extracted by eluting the columns with diisopropylether. Recovery for $1,25(OH)_2[^3H]D_3$ after this initial step was 86.6% $\pm$ 1.4% (mean $\pm$ SD, $n = 8$). The extraction of $1,25(OH)_2D_3$ using Extrelut-1 minicolumns proved to be a good prepurification step, since recovery of $25-OH[^3H]D_3$, $24,25(OH)_2[^3H]D_3$, and $25,26(OH)_2[^3H]D_3$ was 20.8% $\pm$ 0.2% (mean $\pm$ SD, $n = 8$), 24.3% $\pm$ 0.4% (mean $\pm$ SD, $n = 8$), and 28% $\pm$ 1.5% (mean $\pm$ SD, $n = 8$), respectively.

High-Performance Liquid Chromatography

Final purification before assay was achieved using a radial compression separation system equipped with a μPorasil cartridge. The column was eluted with a ternary solvent system of n-hexane/isopropanol/methanol (87/10/3, v/v) at a flow rate of 2 ml/min. The fraction eluted from 6–7.5 min was collected for $1,25(OH)_2D_3$ RIA; this system allowed 4 HPLC runs/h to be carried out. While $25-OH-D_3$, $24,25(OH)_2D_3$, $25-OH-26,23$-lactone D_3, and their corresponding 1α-hydroxylated analogs were completely separated by this procedure, 20% of the $25,26(OH)_2D_3$ subjected to HPLC was still contained in the $1,25(OH)_2D_3$ fraction (see Fig. 1).

Since extracts obtained after the Extrelut-1 prepurification step were fairly clean, a single μPorasil cartridge was useable for the purification of at least 500 samples with no shifting or broadening of the retention volumes occurring. Furthermore, no specific or nonspecific RIA-interfering material was accumulated during the purification of 35 identical samples chromatographed in sequence; no increase was observed in the $1,25(OH)_2D_3$ values obtained after RIA.

Using the manual injection technique, recovery for $1,25(OH)_2[^3H]D_3$ after Extrelut-1 and HPLC chromatography was $77\% \pm 2.6\%$ (mean $\pm$ SD, $n = 51$). With automated injection the recovery was lower, $60\% \pm 6\%$ (mean $\pm$ SD, $n = 26$). Since the recovery for $1,25(OH)_2D_3$ after HPLC was very reproducible, the addition of $1,25(OH)_2[^3H]D_3$ to each sample was omitted. Instead, to each batch two samples were added, which were fortified with $1,25(OH)_2[^3H]D_3$ (10 000 dpm) for monitoring recovery after HPLC.

Kinetic Studies

Figure 2 shows the results of steroid association experiments for evaluation of the steady state of equilibrium binding of $1,25(OH)_2[^3H]D_3$ to the antiserum at $2°C$. Dpm nonspecifically bound were subtracted from a total dpm bound to yield dpm specifically bound. Equilibrium was reached at 16 h incubation and consequently this period was used for the subsequent equilibrium-binding experiments.

Assay Curve

Two different techniques, equilibrium binding (16 h) versus sequential incubation [16 h preincubation with unlabeled and an additional 48 h after the addition of tritiated $1,25(OH)_2D_3$], were compared with respect to assay sensitivity. Evaluations of each point of the standard curve measured sevenfold in one assay showed that the sequential type of incubation had resulted in a four times greater sensitivity: addition of 0.8 pg/tube reduced binding of $1,25(OH)_2[^3H]D_3$ significantly ($P < 0.001$) when compared with tubes containing no $1,25(OH)_2D_3$. The standard curves are depicted in Fig. 3.

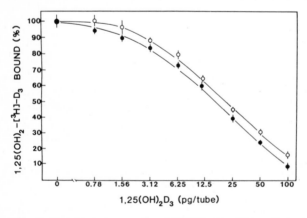

Fig. 3. Standard curves for $1,25(OH)_2D_3$ RIA using equilibrium-binding kinetics ($\bigcirc$——$\bigcirc$, incubation period: 16 h) or a sequential type of incubation ($\bullet$——$\bullet$, 16 h preincubation with unlabeled $1,25(OH)_2D_3$ and another 48 h following addition of $1,25(OH)_2[^3H]D_3$).

These evaluations were repeated twice on different days with virtually identical results.

Antiserum Specificity

The specificity for 1,25(OH)$_2$D$_3$ of the antiserum used was assessed by comparing the displacement of 1,25(OH)$_2$[^{3}H]D$_3$ by 1,25(OH)$_2$D$_3$ to the displacement by several other metabolites of vitamin D$_3$ (see Fig. 4).

The metabolite concentration at 50% displacement of 1,25(OH)$_2$[^{3}H]D$_3$ was used for this comparison. It is apparent that absence of the C-1 hydroxyl in the steroid molecule decreases the binding affinity to the antibody-binding site markedly, the relative order of displacement being 25-OH-D$_3$(2.5%) > 25,26(OH)$_2$D$_3$(1.1%) > 24,25(OH)$_2$D$_3$(0.5%) > 25-OH-26,23-lactone D$_3$(0.1%). Since the antiserum was raised against a 3-hemisuccinate derivative of 1,25(OH)$_2$D$_3$, thus maximally exposing the steroid side chain, its binding affinity was also diminished by modifications on the steroid side chain. Metabolites of 1,25(OH)$_2$D$_3$ with substitution of either a hydroxyl or a ketone group at C-24, namely 1,24,25(OH)$_3$D$_3$(20%) and 1,25(OH)$_2$-24-oxo-D$_3$(25%), displaced the radioligand somewhat less when compared with 1,25(OH)$_2$D$_3$. Further, when two side chain carbons were involved in the structural modification of the steroid side chain as in 1,25(OH)$_2$-26,23-lactone D$_3$ (0.1%) and 1,23,25(OH)$_3$-24-oxo-D$_3$(0.03%), very weak interaction with the antibody-binding site was observed.

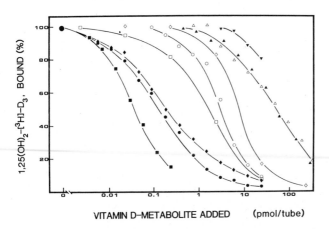

VITAMIN D–METABOLITE ADDED   (pmol/tube)

Fig. 4. Cross-reaction of several metabolites of vitamin D$_3$ in the RIA for 1,25(OH)$_2$D$_3$. ■——■, 1,25(OH)$_2$D$_3$; ●——●, 1,25(OH)$_2$-24-oxo-D$_3$, ◆——◆, 1,24,25(OH)$_3$D$_3$; □——□, 25-OH-D$_3$; ○——○, 25,26(OH)$_2$D$_3$; ◇——◇, 24,25(OH)$_2$D$_3$; △——△, 25-OH-26,23-lactone D$_3$; ▲——▲, 1,25(OH)$_2$-26,23-lactone D$_3$; ▼——▼, 1,23,25(OH)$_3$-24-oxo-D$_3$

Precision and Accuracy

Identical samples from a plasma pool obtained from healthy blood donors were processed in a single assay (10 samples) or in 16 different assays to evaluate the precision of the $1,25(OH)_2D_3$ RIA system. The intraassay coefficient of variation was 12% ($1,25(OH)_2D_3$ level: 113 ± 13.4 pmol/liter, mean $\pm$ SD), interassay coefficient of variation was 16.8% ($1,25(OH)_2D_3$ level: 125 ± 21 pmol/liter, mean $\pm$ SD).

The accuracy of the assay system was evaluated by measuring samples of the plasma pool which were fortified with 120 pmol/liter $1,25(OH)_2D_3$. Recovery of the $1,25(OH)_2D_3$ added was 124.8 ± 21 pmol/liter (mean $\pm$ SD, $n = 12$). To investigate possible blank effects, charcoal-treated sera were checked, and no $1,25(OH)_2D_3$ was detectable in these sera ($n = 12$). Therefore, nonspecific interference by column material or solvents used can be excluded to the best of our knowledge.

Clinical Results

In 30 healthy persons (mean age, 25 years; range, 18–40 years) $1,25(OH)_2D_3$ serum concentrations ranged from 77 to 187 pmol/liter with a mean ($\pm$ SD) of 132 ± 30 pmol/liter. In 35 normal persons employed in a factory with a mean age of 44 years (range, 20–65 years) we found comparable $1,25(OH)_2D_3$ concentrations (145 ± 59 pmol/liter). In this group there was a negative linear correlation ($r = -0.44$) between age and $1,25(OH)_2D_3$ concentration ($P < 0.05$; see Fig. 5).

Fifty-five elderly patients with no sign of kidney disease (mean age, 77 years; range, 60–92 years) revealed low $1,25(OH)_2D_3$ serum levels (77 ± 29 pmol/liter, mean $\pm$ SD). Patients requiring dialysis due to chronic renal failure had strongly reduced serum $1,25(OH)_2D_3$ levels (mean, 13 pmol/liter; range < 8–26.5 pmol/liter, $n = 10$). Three patients with similar disease but receiving

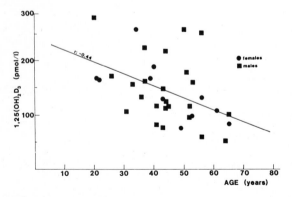

Fig. 5. Serum $1,25(OH)_2D_3$ concentration in 35 unselected employees of a factory: negative correlation with age ($r = -0.44$; $P < 0.05$)

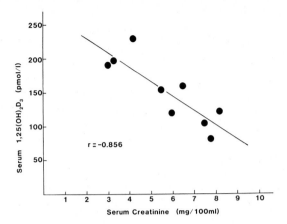

Fig. 6. Correlation of circulating 1,25(OH)$_2$D$_3$ with serum creatinine in a patient with chronic renal failure following kidney transplantation. The values were monitored from the 4th to the 12th day postsurgery

oral 1,25(OH)$_2$D$_3$ treatment had elevated 1,25(OH)$_2$D$_3$ serum concentrations (350 $\pm$ 161 pmol/liter, mean $\pm$ SD). Finally, in a patient with chronic renal failure following kidney transplantation, 1,25(OH)$_2$D$_3$ in serum increased when kidney function improved as indicated by the decreasing serum creatinine concentration ($r = -0.85$; see Fig. 6).

Discussion

Extrelut columns for the prepurification of 1,25(OH)$_2$D$_3$ before HPLC were introduced by Mason et al. [30]. These authors used large Extrelut columns, which therefore required appropriately large volumes of eluant (50 ml dichloromethane/sample). In this paper we propose Extrelut-1 minicolumns (bed volume 3 ml) for the one-step extraction and prepurification of 1,25(OH)$_2$D$_3$ before HPLC. By diisopropylether 1,25(OH)$_2$D$_3$ is eluted from Extrelut-1 minicolumns preferably to less polar compounds such as 25-OH-D$_3$, 24,25(OH)$_2$D$_3$, and 25,26(OH)$_2$D$_3$. Since the extracts are cleared of most of the lipids present in serum, no additional purification step (e.g., by Sephadex LH 20) is required. A prepurification step before HPLC is, in our opinion, obligatory, since otherwise there is a gradual accumulation of lipids, as plasma extracts are chromatographed in succession through the same HPLC column, resulting in decreased separation efficiency and possibly in lipid contamination of the 1,25(OH)$_2$D$_3$ regions collected for RIA. The extraction procedure applying Extrelut-1 minicolumns that we propose in this communication is fairly rapid: one person is able to extract > 100 samples in a single working day.

When establishing this RIA system for $1,25(OH)_2D_3$, we originally added some $1,25(OH)_2[^3H]D_3$ to each serum sample for monitoring recovery of $1,25(OH)_2D_3$ after extraction and HPLC. However, the reproducibility of the amount of $1,25(OH)_2[^3H]D_3$ recovered allowed us to omit the addition of tritiated $1,25(OH)_2D_3$ to each serum sample to monitor recovery. Instead, $1,25(OH)_2[^3H]D_3$ was added solely to the control samples, and its loss through extraction and HPLC was applied to the whole batch processed. Imawari et al. [22] chose this procedure previously. We agree with these authors that improved methodology allowing omission of ^3H-labeled $1,25(OH)_2D_3$ to each serum sample represents an important contribution to the simplification of $1,25(OH)_2D_3$ measurements. Sensitive and specific assays for $1,25(OH)_2D_3$ have been developed by using intestinal mucosal receptor preparations (see Table 1). However, problems in the stability of this protein [12] have sustained efforts in raising antisera against $1,25(OH)_2D_3$. Several RIA systems have appeared in the literature since 1979 [4, 5, 7, 9, 16, 17, 39, 43]. In our RIA for $1,25(OH)_2D_3$ we use an antiserum (supplied by Dr. Bouillon), which was raised against a $1,25(OH)_2D_3$-3-hemisuccinate derivative linked to BSA, thus exposing the side chain of the steroid. Similar antisera raised against this antigen were well characterized by us [33, 34] and others [4, 17]. In this study we provide additional information about the cross-reaction of several more recently identified metabolites of vitamin D_3 with our antiserum. 25-OH-26,23-Lactone D_3, as well as its 1α-hydroxylated analog, was 1250-fold less competitive at the antibody-binding site when compared with $1,25(OH)_2D_3$. This finding is of special importance in the measurement of $1,25(OH)_2D_3$ in the serum of patients on $1,25(OH)_2D_3$ therapy, since the $1,25(OH)_2$-26,23-lactone D_3 serum concentration might here even exceed the $1,25(OH)_2D_3$ level. This assumption is judged from an animal model [37], since data in humans are not available. 25-OH-26,23-lactone D_3 serum concentration in humans was reported to be 34 ng/liter [27]. Therefore, both lactone analogs of vitamin D_3 will not interfere in our $1,25(OH)_2D_3$ assay. Also, they were both separated from $1,25(OH)_2D_3$ by HPLC as were two recently identified metabolites of $1,24,25(OH)_3D_3$, namely $1,25(OH)_2$-24-oxo-D_3 and $1,23,25(OH)_3$-24-oxo-D_3 [35]. The latter was almost not recognized by the antibody, the former strongly competing (25%). $1,25(OH)_2$-24-oxo-D_3 was recently isolated from the sera of $1,25(OH)_2D_3$-treated rats (A.W. Norman, personal communication), but its normal serum concentration is unknown. Its precursor $1,24,25(OH)_3D_3$ has been reported to reach serum levels in normal subjects about three to four times lower than those of $1,25(OH)_2D_3$ [23]. In spite of its interference with the antiserum (20%), it will not influence the $1,25(OH)_2D_3$ level measured, since it is well separated by HPLC. The major circulating metabolites of vitamin D_3, namely 25-OH-D_3 and $24,25(OH)_2D_3$, were 40- and 212-fold less competitive than $1,25(OH)_2D_3$ at the antibody-binding site; their serum concentrations under normal circumstances are about 1000- and 40-fold, respectively, higher when compared with $1,25(OH)_2D_3$, but might even increase by a factor of 20–30 in vitamin D intoxication or in patients with hypoparathyroidism on high-dose vitamin D

Table 1. Methods for the measurement of $1,25(OH)_2D_3$ in human serum and normal ranges

Authors	Year	Extraction	Purification	Volume of serum (ml)	Assay method	Normal range (pmol/liter)
Clemens et al. [7]	1979	Dichloromethane	Sephadex LH 20, HPLC	5–10	RIA[a]	98 ± 6[e]
Shepard et al. [45]	1979	Dichloromethane/methanol	Sephadex LH 20, HPLC	3–5	RRA[b]	75 ± 22[f]
Björkhem et al. [2]	1979	Chloroform/methanol	Sephadex LH 20, HPLC	20	GC-MS[c]	132 ± 24[f]
Taylor et al. [48]	1979	Dichloromethane	Sephadex LH 20, HPLC	5	RRA	78 ± 35[f]
Mason et al. [30]	1980	Extrelut column/dichloromethane	HPLC	5	RRA	86
Peacock et al. [39]	1980	Acetone/dichloromethane	Sephadex LH 20, HPLC	5	RIA	110 ± 29[f]
Bishop et al. [1]	1980	Diethylether	HPLC	2	RRA	101 ± 26[f]
Bouillon et al. [4]	1980	Ethylacetate/cyclohexane	Sephadex LH 20, HPLC	5	RIA	91 ± 29[f]
Mallon et al. [28]	1980	Dichloromethane/methanol	Sephadex LH 20	2	RRA	74 ± 19[f]
Stern et al. [47]	1980	Benzene or isopropylether	HPLC	1–5	Bioassay	79 ± 14[f]
Jongen et al. [24]	1981	n-Hexane/isopropanol/n-butanol	HPLC	5	RRA	125 ± 26[f]
Dokoh et al. [10]	1981	Clin-elute column dichloromethane/acetone	HPLC	0.5	RRA	132 ± 34[f]
Gray et al. [17]	1981	Chloroform/methanol	Sephadex LH 20, HPLC	2	RIA	137 ± 14[e]
Keck et al. [26]	1981	Dichloromethane/methanol	Sephadex LH 20, HPLC	6	RRA	127 ± 67[f]
Dabek et al. [8]	1981	Chloroform/methanol	Sephadex LH 20	2.5–5	RRA	106 ± 36[f]
Manolagas et al. [29]	1982	Clin-elute column, benzene	–	1–2	CRA[d]	82 ± 26[f]
Endres et al. [13]	1982	Diethylether	Sep-Pak C_{18}, HPLC	2	RRA	120 ± 24[f]
Imawari et al. [22]	1982	Ethylacetate/methanol	Sephadex LH 20, HPLC	2	RRA	89 ± 26[f]
Gray and McAdoo [16]	1983	Ethylacetate/cyclohexane	HPLC	3	RIA	82 ± 12[e]
Duncan et al. [11]	1983	Diethylether	HPLC	2–3	RRA	84 ± 26[f]

Table 1. Continued

Authors	Year	Extraction	Purification	Volume of serum (ml)	Assay method	Normal range (pmol/liter)
Reinhardt et al. [41]	1984	Acetonitrile	C-18 Sep-Pak/Silica Sep-Pak	0.2–1	RRA(thymus)	90 ± 5^e
De Leenheer and Bauwens [9]	1985	Benzene	HPLC	1.5	RIA	124 ± 36^f
Hollis [20]	1986	Acetonitrile	Bond Elute C_{18}	0.5–1	RRA(thymus)	68 ± 27^f
Blayau et al. [3]	1986	Methanol/chloroform	Sep-Pak C_{18}, HPLC	2	RRA(Mammary gland)	120 ± 6
Hartwell and Christiansen [18]	1988	Methanol/dichlormethane Extrelut-1 minicolumn,	Sephadex LH 20, HPLC	3–5	RRA(thymus)	91 ± 5^e
Scharla et al.	this report	Diisopropyl ether	HPLC	1	RIA	132 ± 29^f

[a] RIA, Radioimmunoassay
[b] RRA, radioreceptorassay
[c] GC-MS, gas chromatography-mass spectrometry
[d] CRA, cytoreceptorassay
[e] Mean ± SEM
[f] Mean ± SD

treatment. Prepurification on Extrelut-1 minicolumns and final purification by HPLC prevented any influence of 25-OH-D$_3$ and 24,25(OH)$_2$D$_3$ on 1,25(OH)$_2$D$_3$ measurement. Since we have established a practicable HPLC system, which made possible the purification of 4 extracts/h, the small interference by 25,26(OH)$_2$D$_3$ [20% of the 25,26(OH)$_2$D$_3$ contained in the extract] appeared to pose a substantial problem. However, 72% of 25,26(OH)$_2$D$_3$ had already been removed by the initial Extrelut-1 minicolumn step and the interference at the antibody was only 1.1% when compared with 1,25(OH)$_2$D$_3$. Although 25,26(OH)$_2$D$_3$ levels are tenfold higher than those of the serum 1,25(OH)$_2$D$_3$ [27], 25,26(OH)$_2$D$_3$ will not contribute to the serum concentration of 1,25(OH)$_2$D$_3$ measured by our assay.

Since antisera raised against the 3-hemisuccinate derivative of 1,25(OH)$_2$D$_3$ are relatively specific for the side chain of the steroid, metabolites of vitamin D$_2$ will not be recognized [4, 5]. No 1,25(OH)$_2$D$_2$ was available to us to test the cross-reactivity, but we anticipate that it will not be recognized by our antiserum. 1,25(OH)$_2$D$_2$ might contribute to the total 1,25(OH)$_2$D present in serum if vitamin D$_2$ was present in the diet. Therefore, our assay for 1,25(OH)$_2$D$_3$ might underestimate the total 1,25(OH)$_2$D concentration in a similar manner to the RIAs of Gray et al. [16] and Bouillon et al. [4]. However, Hughes et al. [21] showed that > 95% of the vitamin D metabolites occur in the D$_3$ form in humans, unless they are on very high vitamin D$_2$ intake. Therefore, the anticipated low cross-reaction of the antibody with 1,25(OH)$_2$D$_2$ might not be of significance in the measurement of total 1,25(OH)$_2$D. The mean 1,25(OH)$_2$D$_3$ serum concentration measured in 30 healthy adults was 132 pmol/liter, a result which is in close agreement with the values reported by several other laboratories (see Table 1) applying RIA [9, 17], radioreceptor assay [3, 10, 13, 24, 26], or isotope-dilution-mass fragmentography [2]. Several groups, mostly from countries outside Europe, have reported somewhat lower values for 1,25(OH)$_2$D$_3$ (see Table 1). This might reflect a difference in daily calcium intake between the populations and varying fortifications of food with vitamin D. We found slightly lowered serum 1,25(OH)$_2$D$_3$ concentrations in elderly subjects and strongly reduced serum levels of 1,25(OH)$_2$D$_3$ in patients with chronic renal failure. Agreement of these results with earlier reports [15, 19, 29] provides evidence for the validity of the RIA system for 1,25(OH)$_2$D$_3$ which we have developed. In this chapter we propose a sensitive, precise, and accurate RIA for 1,25(OH)$_2$D$_3$ with a rapid prepurification system using Extrelut-1 minicolumns. However, this assay requires HPLC because of the low antiserum specificity.

In conclusion, a sensitive RIA system for 1α,25-dihydroxyvitamin D$_3$ [1,25(OH)$_2$D$_3$] with an improved extraction procedure has been developed. Following one-step extraction and prepurification of 1,25(OH)$_2$D$_3$ by Extrelut-1 minicolumns, final purification was achieved by HPLC using a radial compression separation system equipped with a µPorasil cartridge. The HPLC used allows the purification of 4 extracts/h. Recovery of 1,25(OH)$_2$[^{3}H]D$_3$ after HPLC was 77% ± 2.6% (mean ± SD, $n = 51$) for the manual injection technique and 60% ± 6% (mean ± SD, $n = 26$) using an autosampler system.

Since the recovery of $1,25(OH)_2[^3H]D_3$ was reproducible, addition of labeled steroid to each single serum sample for recovery monitoring was omitted. The sensitivity of the assay was 0.8 pg/tube, resulting in a detection limit of 8 pmol/liter, when 1 ml serum was extracted. Intraassay and interassay coefficients of variation were 12% and 16.8% respectively. Serum $1,25(OH)_2D_3$ concentration in 30 healthy subjects (mean age, 25 years) was 132 ± 30 pmol/liter (mean $\pm$ SD). A group of 35 middle-aged persons (mean age, 44 years) had comparable values of $1,25(OH)_2D_3$ (145 ± 59 pmol/liter), which were negatively correlated with age. Elderly patients (mean age, 77 years, $n = 55$) exhibited lowered concentrations of $1,25(OH)_2D_3$ (77 ± 29 pmol/liter, mean $\pm$ SD). In three patients with renal failure on therapy with $1,25(OH)_2D_3$ (Rocaltrol) a distinct elevation in serum $1,25(OH)_2D_3$ was detected. Patients with chronic renal failure had reduced $1,25(OH)_2D_3$ serum levels (mean 13 pmol/liter, range < 8–26 pmol/ liter, $n = 10$). In one patient with renal failure, following kidney transplantation the serum $1,25(OH)_2D_3$ and creatinine levels were monitored from the 4th to the 12th postsurgical day; a highly significant negative correlation ($r = -0.85$) was found.

References

1. Bishop JE, Norman AW, Coburn JW, Roberts PA, Henry HL (1980) Studies on the metabolism of calciferol XVI. Determination of the concentration of 25-hydroxyvitamin D, 24,25-dihydroxyvitamin D and 1,25-dihydroxyvitamin D in a single two-milliliter plasma sample. Miner Electrolyte Metab 3:181–189
2. Björkhem I, Holmberg I, Kristiansen T, Pedersen JI (1979) Assay of 1,25-dihydroxyvitamin D_3 by isotope dilution-mass fragmentography. Clin Chem 25:584–588
3. Blayau M, Leray G, Prodhomme C, David V, Peron P (1986) An improved source of receptor for 1,25-dihydroxyvitamin D_3 assay. Clin Chim Acta 158:199–206
4. Bouillon R, DeMoor P, Baggiolini EG, Uskokovic MR (1980) A radioimmunoassay for 1,25-dihydroxycholecalciferol. Clin Chem 26:562–567
5. Brown WB, Peacock M (1986) Characteristics of antisera to antigenic forms of 1,25-dihydroxycholecalciferol. Clin Chim Acta 159:111–121
6. Brumbaugh PF, Haussler DH, Bursac KM, Haussler MR (1974) Filter assay for $1\alpha,25$-dihydroxyvitamin D_3. Utilization of the hormone's target tissue chromatin receptor. Biochemistry 13:4091–4097
7. Clemens TL, Hendy GN, Papapoulos SE, Fraher LJ, Care AD, O'Riordan JLH (1979) Measurement of 1,25-dihydroxycholecalciferol in man by radioimmunoassay. Clin Endocrinol 11:225–234
8. Dabek JT, Härkönen M, Adlercreutz H (1981) A sensitive and simplified receptor-assay for $1,25(OH)_2$-vitamin D. Scand J Clin Lab Invest 41:151–158
9. De Leenheer AP, Bauwens RM (1985) Radioimmunoassay for 1,25-dihydroxyvitamin D in serum or plasma. Clin Chem 31:142–146
10. Dokoh S, Pike JW, Chandler JS, Mancini JM, Haussler MR (1981) An improved radioreceptor assay for 1,25-dihydroxyvitamin D in human plasma. Anal Biochem 116:211–222
11. Duncan WE, Aw TC, Walsh PG, Haddad JG (1983) Normal rabbit intestinal cytosol

as a source of binding protein for the 1,25-dihydroxyvitamin D_3 assay. Anal Biochem 132:209–214

12. Eisman JA, Hamstra AJ, Kream BE, DeLuca HF (1976) A sensitive, precise and convenient method for determination of 1,25-dihydroxyvitamin D in human plasma. Arch Biochem Biophys 176:235–243

13. Endres D, Lu J, Mueller J, Adams J, Holick M, Broughton A (1982) Simplified method for the determination of 1,25-dihydroxyvitamin D using automated high pressure liquid chromatography: application to the differential diagnosis of hypercalcemia. In: Norman AW et al. (eds) Vitamin D: chemical, biochemical and clinical endocrinology of calcium metabolism. de Gruyter, New York, pp 813–815

14. Fraher LJ, Adami S, Clemens TL, Jones G, O'Riordan JLH (1983) Radioimmunoassay for 1,25-dihydroxyvitamin D_2: studies on the metabolism of vitamin D_2 in man. Clin Endocrinol 18:151–165

15. Gallagher JC, Riggs BL, Eisman J, Hamstra A, Arnaud SB, DeLuca HF (1979) Intestinal calcium absorption and serum vitamin D metabolites in normal subjects and osteoporotic patients. J Clin Invest 64:729–736

16. Gray TK, McAdoo T (1983) Radioimmunoassay for 1,25-dihydroxycholecalciferol. Clin Chem 29:196–200

17. Gray TK, McAdoo T, Pool D, Lester GE, Williams ME, Jones G (1981) A modified radioimmunoassay for 1,25-dihydroxycholecalciferol. Clin Chem 27:458–463

18. Hartwell D, Christiansen C (1988) Comparisons between two receptor assays for 1,25-dihydroxyvitamin D. Scand J Clin Lab Invest 48:109–114

19. Haussler MR, McCain TA (1977) Basic and clinical concepts related to vitamin D metabolism and action. N Engl J Med 297:1041–1050

20. Hollis BW (1986) Assay of circulating 1,25-dihydroxyvitamin D involving a novel single-cartridge extraction and purification procedure. Clin Chem 32:2060–2063

21. Hughes MR, Baylink DJ, Jones PG, Haussler MR (1976) Radioligand receptor assay for 25-hydroxyvitamins D_2/D_3 and $1\alpha,25$-dihydroxyvitamin D_2/D_3. J Clin Invest 58:61–70

22. Imawari M, Kozawa K, Yoshida T, Osuga T (1982) A simple and sensitive assay for 25-hydroxyvitamin D, 24,25-dihydroxyvitamin D and 1,25-dihydroxyvitamin D in human serum. Clin Chim Acta 124:63–73

23. Ishizuka S, Naruchi T, Hashimoto Y, Orimo H (1981) Radioreceptor assay for $1\alpha,24(R)25$-trihydroxyvitamin D_3 in human serum. J Nutr Sci Vitaminol (Tokyo) 27:71–75

24. Jongen MJM, van der Vijgh WJF, Willems HJJ, Netelenbos JC (1981) Analysis for 1,25-dihydroxyvitamin D in human plasma, after a liquid-chromatographic purification procedure, with a modified competitive protein-binding assay. Clin Chem 27:444–450

25. Jongen MJ, Kuiper S, van der Vijgh WJF, Lips P, Netelenbos JC (1988) Improvements in the simultaneous determination of calcidiol and calcitriol in human serum or plasma. J Clin Chem Clin Biochem 26:25–28

26. Keck E, Krüskemper HL, Von Lilienfeld-Toal H (1981) Protein binding assays for 25-hydroxy, 24,25-dihydroxy and 1,25-dihydroxy metabolites of vitamin D in human plasma. J Clin Chem Clin Biochem 19:1043–1050

27. Lambert PW, DeOreo PB, Hollis BW, Fu IY, Ginsberg DJ, Roos BA (1981) Concurrent measurement of plasma levels of vitamin D_3 and five of its metabolites in normal humans, chronic renal failure patients and anephric subjects. J Lab Clin Med 98:536–548

28. Mallon JP, Hamilton JG, Nauss-Karol C, Karol RJ, Ashley CJ, Matuszewski DS,

Tratnyek CA, Bryce GF, Miller ON (1980) An improved competitive protein binding assay for 1,25-dihydroxyvitamin D. Arch Biochem Biophys 201:277–285

29. Manolagas SC, Howard JE, Abare JM, Culler FL, Brickman AS, Deftos LJ (1982) Cytoreceptorassay for 1,25(OH)$_2$D: a convenient method and its application to clinical studies. In: Norman AW, et al. (eds) Vitamin D: chemical, biochemical and clinical endocrinology of calcium metabolism. de Gruyter, New York pp 769–771

30. Mason RS, Lissner D, Grunstein HS, Posen S (1980) A simplified assay for dihydroxylated vitamin D metabolites in human serum: application to hyper- and hypovitaminosis D. Clin Chem 26:444–450

31. Mawer EB, Berry JL, Bessone J, Shany S, Smith H, White A (1985) Selection of high-affinity and high-specificity monoclonal antibodies for 1α,25-dihydroxyvitamin D. Steroids 46:741-754

32. Mayer E, Schmidt-Gayk H (1984) Interlaboratory comparison of 25-hydroxyvitamin D determination. Clin Chem 30:1199–1204

33. Mayer E, Kadowaki S, Okamura WH, Ohnuma N, Leyes GA, Schmidt-Gayk H, Norman AW (1981) Studies on the mode of action of calciferol XXXV: comparison of the biochemical properties and ligand specificities of receptors and antibodies for 1,25-dihydroxy-vitamin D$_3$. J Steroid Biochem 15:145–151

34. Mayer E, Bouillon R, Norman AW (1982) Studies on the mode of action of calciferol XL: comparison of the biochemical properties of an antiserum and the chick intestinal receptor both specific for 1,25-dihydroxyvitamin D$_3$. Arch Biochem Biophys 217:257–263

35. Mayer E, Bishop JE, Chandraratna RAS, Okamura WH, Kruse JR, Popjak G, Ohnuma N, Norman AW (1983) Isolation and identification of 1,25-dihydroxy-24-oxo-vitamin D$_3$ and 1,23,25-trihydroxy-24-oxo-vitamin D$_3$. J Biol Chem 258:13458–13465

36. Norman AW, Roth J, Orci L (1982) The vitamin D endocrine system: steroid metabolism, hormone receptors, and biological response (calcium binding proteins). Endocr Rev 3:331–366

37. Ohnuma N, Norman AW (1982) Production in vitro of 1,25-dihydroxyvitamin D$_3$-26,23-lactone from 1α,25-dihydroxyvitamin D$_3$ by rat small intestinal mucosa homogenates. Arch Biochem Biophys 213:139–147

38. Ostrem VK, DeLuca HF (1987) The vitamin D-induced differentiation of HL-60 cells: structural requirements. Steroids 49:73–102

39. Peacock M, Taylor GA, Brown W (1980) Plasma 1,25(OH)$_2$ vitamin D measured by radioimmunoassay and cytosol radioreceptor in normal subjects and patients with primary hyperparathyroidism and renal failure. Clin Chim Acta 101:93–101

40. Perry HM III, Chappel JC, Clevinger BL, Haddad JG, Teitelbaum SL (1983) Monoclonal antibody with high affinity for 1,25-dihydroxycholecalciferol. Biochem Biophys Res Commun 112:431–436

41. Reinhardt TA, Horst RL, Orf JW, Hollis BW (1984) A microassay for 1,25-dihydroxyvitamin D not requiring high performance liquid chromatography: application to clinical studies. J Clin Endocrinol Metab 58:91–98

42. Rigby WFC, Noelle RJ, Krause K, Fanger MW (1985) The effects of 1,25-dihydroxyvitamin D$_3$ on human T lymphocyte activation and proliferation: a cell cycle analysis. J Immunol 135:2279–2285

43. Scharla S, Schmidt-Gayk H, Reichel H, Mayer E (1984) A sensitive and simplified radioimmunoassay for 1,25-dihydroxyvitamin D$_3$. Clin Chim Acta 142:325–338

44. Schilling M, Armbruster FP, Schmidt-Gayk H (1987) Rapid selective separation of

1α,25-dihydroxy-vitamin D$_3$ from serum with Extrelut-1 columns. Clin Chem 33:187

45. Shepard RM, Horst RL, Hamstra AJ, DeLuca HF (1979) Determination of vitamin D and its metabolites in plasma from normal and anephric man. Biochem J 182:55–69

46. Smith EL, Holick MF (1987) The skin: the site of vitamin D$_3$ synthesis and a target tissue for its metabolite 1,25-dihydroxyvitamin D$_3$. Steroids 49:103–131

47. Stern PH, Phillips TE, Mavreas T (1980) Bioassay of 1,25-dihydroxyvitamin D in human plasma purified by partition, alkaline extraction and high-pressure chromatography. Anal Biochem 102:22–30

48. Taylor CM, Hann J, St John J, Wallace JE, Mawer EB (1979) 1,25-Dihydroxycholecalciferol in human serum and its relationship with other metabolites of vitamin D$_3$. Clin Chim Acta 96:1–8

A Double Antibody Radioimmunoassay for Measurement of 1α,25-Dihydroxyvitamin D in Serum

F.P. Armbruster, H. Reichel and H. Schmidt-Gayk

Introduction

The biologically active vitamin D_3 metabolite 1α,25-dihydroxyvitamin D_3 [1α,25$(OH)_2D_3$] is one of the major hormonal regulators of calcium metabolism in man [23, 26]. Measurement of 1α,25$(OH)_2D$ plasma levels is indicated in a variety of disorders which lead to alterations in the concentrations of circulating hormone. These disorders include chronic renal failure [13, 15], hyperparathyroidism [5, 13, 16] and hypoparathyroidism [16], rickets syndromes [6, 14], sarcoidosis [1, 24], and tumor-associated hypercalcemia [28, 34].

Various assays for quantitation of 1α,25$(OH)_2D$ in serum or plasma have been described. The assays differ considerably in methodology, technical requirements and assay time. Techniques which have been used for 1α,25$(OH)_2D$ measurements include dilution-mass fragmentography [2], bioassay [21, 33], competitive protein binding assay [3, 8, 12, 27], cytoreceptor assay [19, 22], and radioimmunoassay (RIA) [4, 9–11, 18, 20, 25, 31].

The standard method to separate free from bound antigen in 1α,25$(OH)_2D$ assays was separation by dextran coated charcoal (DCC) or hydroxylapatite. Double antibody separation (DAB) techniques in competitive binding assays are usually associated with a more specific separation of bound from free antigen. The utilization of DAB separation for the quantitation of steroid hormones has been problematic because of high nonspecific binding (NSB) and low maximal binding (Bmax) of the antigen to antibody. In this chapter we describe a DAB-RIA for 1α,25$(OH)_2D$ and compare the properties of two antibodies against 1α,25$(OH)_2D_3$ in the DAB-RIA.

Materials and Methods

Chemicals

Bovine serum albumin (BSA) and Norit A (activated charcoal) were obtained from Serva, Heidelberg, FRG. Gelatin, Brij-35, dextran T 70 and buffer reagents were obtained from Merck, Darmstadt, FRG. The following buffers were used:

BSA buffer: phosphate buffer (pH 7.4; 0.06 mol/l) with 1 g/l BSA, 1 g/l sodium azide and 0.4 g/l EDTA; gelatin buffer [29]: phosphate buffer (pH 7.4; 0.06 mol/l) with 2 g/l gelatin, 1 g/l sodium azide and 0.4 g/l EDTA; rinsing buffer: 9 g/l NaCl with 1 ml/l Brij-35 (= 300 mg/l).

Vitamin D Metabolites

$1\alpha,25(OH)_2D_3$, 25-hydroxyvitamin D_3 [$25(OH)D_3$] and 24(R),25-dihydroxyvitamin D_3 [$24(R),25(OH)_2D_3$] were from Duphar B.V., Amsterdam, Netherlands. Vitamin D_2, vitamin D_3, 1α-hydroxyvitamin D_3 [$1\alpha(OH)D_3$], $24(S),25(OH)_2D_3$, $1\alpha,24(R),25$-trihydroxyvitamin D_3 [$1\alpha,24(R),25(OH)_3D_3$], 25(S),26-dihydroxyvitamin D_3 [$25(S),26(OH)_2D_3$] 23(S),25(R)-25-hydroxyvitamin D_3-26,23-lactone [$23(S),25(R)-25(OH)D_3$-26,23 lactone] and $23(R),25(S)-25(OH)D_3$-26,23-lactone were kindly provided by Dr. A.W. Norman, University of California, Riverside, CA, USA. $1\alpha,25(OH)_2[23,24(n)-^3H]D_3$ (specific activity 180 Ci/mmol), $25(OH)[23,24(n)-^3H]D_3$ (specific activity 102 Ci/mmol) and $24,25(OH)_2[23,24(n)-^3H]D_3$ (specific activity 90 Ci/mmol) were from Amersham Buchler, Braunschweig, FRG. The purity of all vitamin D metabolites was verified by HPLC. All metabolites were dissolved in absolute ethanol and stored at $-20\,°C$. The radioinert metabolites were quantitated by UV spectrophotometry and used at the indicated concentrations.

Antisera

Two antisera directed against $1\alpha,25(OH)_2D_3$ were compared in our studies. One antiserum (code: KH 090478) was raised in rabbits against a 3-hemisuccinate derivative of $1\alpha,25(OH)_2D_3$ bound to BSA [4]. The antiserum was kindly provided by Dr. R. Bouillon, Louvain, Belgium. The other antiserum was obtained by immunization of sheep with a $1\alpha,25(OH)_2D_3$-25-hemisuccinate conjugated to BSA [code: S7 (7-12-81)] [10]. The antiserum was kindly made available by Dr. J.L.H. O'Riordan, Middlesex, UK. Donkey-anti-rabbit-IgG (from our own production or from Dako Inc., Hamburg, FRG) was used as the precipitating antiserum for the double antibody separation. Both the first antibody (directed against $1\alpha,25(OH)_2D_3$) and the second antibody (anti-rabbit-IgG) were diluted as whole serum and as gamma globulin fractions [17]. The BSA and gelatin buffers were used as dilution media. Unless indicated otherwise, the first antibody (Ab) was used at a 1:64 000 dilution. The second was used at a 1:11 dilution. Normal rabbit serum or normal rabbit IgG (Dako) were added to the first Ab solution at the indicated concentrations.

$1\alpha,25(OH)_2D$-RIA

The extraction of $1\alpha,25(OH)_2D$ from 1 ml serum or plasma by Extrelut columns and high performance liquid chromatography (HPLC) was carried out as described [31]. The tests were performed in duplicate in immunoassay vials [32] (see chapter 1.4, 600 µl total volume, Sarstedt, Nümbrecht, FRG) in an ice water bath at 4 °C. The $1\alpha,25(OH)_2D$ fractions from HPLC were dried down and taken up in ethanol. The HPLC fractions or vitamin D-metabolite standards were transferred to immunoassay vials, evaporated under nitrogen and re-dissolved in 300 µl BSA buffer or gelatin buffer. Approximately 5500 cpm $1\alpha,25(OH)_2[^3H]D_3$ dissolved in 20 µl ethanol were added. After first addition of 100 µl Ab, the assay was incubated for 12 h at 4 °C.

Double Antibody Separation

After addition of 100 µl second Ab solution, the assay was incubated at 4 °C for 1 h. The bound fraction was pelleted by centrifugation (10 min × 1800 g). The supernatant was removed by suction and discarded. The sediment was rinsed with 500 µl rinsing buffer and spun again (10 min × 1800 g). The supernatant was discarded, the protein precipitate was dissolved in 10 µl 1 N NaOH and 250 µl scintillation fluid (Pico-Fluor 15, Packard Instruments, Frankfurt, FRG) were added to the RIA vials. After vigorous mixing, the radioactivity was measured in a liquid scintillation counter (Model LS 7000, Beckman Instruments Inc., Fullerton, CA, USA).

Charcoal Separation

The charcoal-based RIA was carried out as described [31]. For separation of bound from free antigen, 100 µl of charcoal suspension (1.25 g Norit A and 0.125 g Dextran T 70 per 100 ml distilled water) were added, incubated for 2 min at 4 °C and then centrifuged for 10 min at 1800 g. A total of 400 µl clear supernatant was transferred to Pico plastic vials (Packard Instruments) and mixed with 3 ml scintillation fluid. The tritium contents of the samples were measured by liquid scintillation counting.

Assay Conditions

The experiments to determine the optimal rinsing solution for the pellet were carried out with the following reagents: (i) whole first antiserum, diluted to 1:40000 with BSA buffer; (ii) normal rabbit serum as precipitation adjuvant; (iii) BSA buffer; (iv) whole second antiserum, diluted to 1:11. To determine the effect of DBP on the assay, 4 ml of normal rabbit serum or 40 mg rabbit IgG were added to 1 liter of the first Ab solution. For the binding experiments, approximately 20 fmol of $1\alpha,25(OH)_2[^3H]D_3$, $25(OH)[^3H]D_3$ or $24,25(OH)_2$ $[^3H]D_3$ were used. The affinity constants (Ka) for the antibody were calculated according to Scatchard [30].

Results

Nonspecific Binding

DAB separation was initially performed with reagents routinely used in a charcoal-based RIA [31]. The $1\alpha,25(OH)_2D_3$-antiserum was KH 090478. We found that these conditions led to high NSB of $1\alpha,25(OH)_2[^3H]D_3$ ($> 30\%$ of Bmax). We then tried to reduce the NSB by testing various conditions for washing the sediment. The results are shown in Fig. 1. The best conditions were obtained with a 9 g/l NaCl solution containing 1 ml/l Brij-35. Unspecific binding was, on average, 60–80 cpm, and the maximum binding was 1000–1100 cpm. The unspecific binding was clearly lower than specific binding under conditions of maximal displacement of tracer by 1 ng $1\alpha,25(OH)_2D_3$. For all further experiments, the sediment was rinsed after double antibody separation with 500 µl NaCl solution containing 1 ml/l Brij-35.

Incubation Time

To determine the incubation period required until equilibrium of the antigen–antibody reaction, $25(OH)[^3H]D_3$ or $1\alpha,25(OH)_2[^3H]D_3$ (about 5000 cpm/tube) were added to the first Ab (KH 090478). The experiments were performed either under DBP-free conditions or with buffers containing DBP.

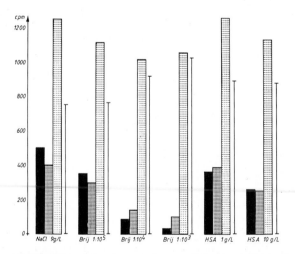

Fig. 1. Effects of various rinsing conditions on NSB in the DAB-RIA. The assay reagents contained DBP. The first Ab (KH 090478) was used at a 1:40 000 dilution. The incubation times were 12 h for the first and 1 h for the second Ab. Rinsing solutions contained NaCl (9 g/l) and the indicated additives. The results are the means of 2 experiments, each performed in duplicate, NSB, nonspecific binding; *125D₃*, $1\alpha,25$-dihydroxyvitamin D_3; *Bo*, maximal binding; *HSA*, human serum albumin.

After various incubation times the reactions were stopped by charcoal separation. An incubation time of approximately 10 h was sufficient for the antigen–antibody reaction to reach equilibrium (data not shown). DBP had no effects on this point. For all further experiments we chose a 12 h incubation time for the first Ab. Comparable results were obtained for the antiserum S7 (7-2-81).

Influence of DBP on Maximal Binding

The effects of DBP on assay binding conditions were examined by successively removing DBP from the first antibody, normal rabbit serum, second antibody, and buffer. The experiments were carried out with antiserum KH 090478. The

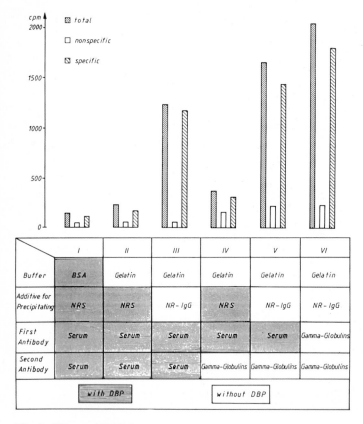

Fig. 2. Effects of DBP in assay reagents on Bmax of the $1\alpha,25(OH)_2D$ DAB-RIA. The experiments were carried out with antiserum KH 090478. Reagents with DBP (*shaded areas*) were replaced by DBP-free reagents (*white areas*) as indicated under "Materials and Methods". The results are the means of two experiments, each performed in duplicate. *BSA*, bovine serum albumin; *NRS*, normal rabbit serum; *NR-IgG*, normal rabbit IgG.

albumin in the buffer (dilution reagent for the first and second Ab) was replaced by gelatin since the crude albumin preparation used contained trace amounts of DBP. Gamma globulin fractions of first and second antisera were prepared and used in the assay. Normal rabbit serum (4 ml/l) for precipitation was replaced by pure rabbit IgG (40 mg/l).

Six different combinations of DBP-containing and DBP-free assay reagents were tested. The results are shown in Fig. 2. The lowest binding of $1\alpha,25(OH)_2D_3$ to antibody (2.0% of total activity) occurred with normal rabbit serum as precipitation adjuvant. When rabbit IgG was used for precipitation, Bmax rose markedly to 22.5%. Similarly, the use of whole antisera instead of gamma globulin fractions markedly impaired Bmax (Fig. 2). Use of the first Ab

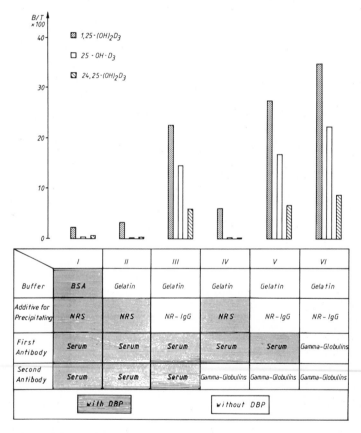

Fig. 3. Effects of DBP in assay reagents on binding of $1\alpha,25(OH)_2D_3$, $25(OH)D_3$ and $24,25(OH)_2D_3$ in the DAB-RIA. The experiments were carried out with antiserum KH 090478. Conditions were as described in the legend to Fig. 2. The results are the means of 2 experiments, each performed in duplicate. *BSA*, bovine serum albumin; *NRS*, normal rabbit serum; *NR-IgG*, normal rabbit IgG; *B/T*, bound vitamin D_3 metabolite/total activity.

as a gamma globulin fraction increased Bmax from 27.5% to 34.6%. When whole second antiserum was replaced by the gamma globulin fraction, Bmax increased from 22.5% to 27.5%. The effect of DBP in the BSA buffer was less pronounced (Fig. 2). Replacement of albumin in the buffer by gelatin increased Bmax from 2.0% to 3.2%.

As shown in Fig. 3, the specificity of the assay for $1\alpha,25\text{-}(OH)_2D_3$ was decreased under DBP-free conditions. After elimination of DBP from the assay, the binding of $25(OH)D_3$ and $24,25(OH)_2D_3$ to the first Ab rose from less than 1% of total activity to 22.2% and 8.6%, respectively. When binding of $1\alpha,25(OH)_2D_3$ to the antibody was set as 100%, the specific binding of $25(OH)D_3$ and $24,25(OH)_2D_3$ was 8% and 18%, respectively, when assay reagents contained DBP. Under DBP-free conditions the relative binding of $25(OH)D_3$ and $24,25(OH)_2D_3$ increased to 62% and 24%, respectively.

The experiments described above demonstrated that maximal binding of $1\alpha,25(OH)_2D_3$ to the antibody could be achieved with DBP-free assay reagents. In all further experiments, the first AB was used as gamma globulin fraction and diluted 1:64000 in gelatin buffer, working dilution. Under these conditions, the binding of $1\alpha,25(OH)_2D_3$ was approximately 35% of total activity.

Affinity

The affinity constants of the two first Ab [(KH 090478 and S7 (7-12-81)] for $1\alpha,25(OH)_2D_3$, $25(OH)D_3$ and $24,25(OH)_2D_3$ were determined according to the method of Scatchard [30]. All tests were done with DBP-free reagents. The results are shown in Table 1. Under these conditions, the S7 (7-12-81) Ab bound $1\alpha,25(OH)_2D_3$ with an approximately five-fold higher affinity and with higher specificity than KH 090478.

Table 1. Affinity constants of antibodies directed against $1\alpha,25(OH)_2D_3$ for vitamin D metabolites.

| | Affinity Constant [l/mol] | |
	KH 090478	S7 (7–12–81)
Metabolite		
$1\alpha,25(OH)_2D_3$	2.70×10^{-10}	1.36×10^{-11}
$25(OH)D_3$	1.20×10^{-10}	4.14×10^{-10}
$24,25(OH)_2D_3$	2.80×10^{-10}	4.29×10^{-10}

The affinity constants of the antisera KH 090478 and S7 (7-12-81) for vitamin D metabolites were determined by the method of Scatchard [30] under DBP-free conditions. Both antisera were diluted 1:64,000.

Cross-reactivity

The assay was further characterized by determining the cross-reactivity of the Ab with other vitamin D metabolites (Fig. 4). The indicated amounts of radioinert metabolites were added to the first antibodies [KH 090478 or S7 (7-12-81)] and $1\alpha,25(OH)_2[^3H]D_3$.

The results for KH 090478 are shown in Fig. 4. Assay conditions were either with DBP (Fig. 4a) or without DBP (Fig. 4b). Cross-reactivity was calculated at the point of 50% competition. $1\alpha,25(OH)_2D_3$ displaced the tracer in assays containing DBP with a potency that was 20-fold higher than $25(OH)D_3$. Under DBP-free conditions, $1\alpha,25(OH)_2D_3$ was 3.8 times more effective than $25(OH)D_3$. Similar results as with $25(OH)D_3$ were obtained with $24,25(OH)_2D_3$. The cross-reactivity of other vitamin D metabolites was negligible under conditions with DBP. As shown in Fig. 4, elimination of DBP from the assay also led to a higher interference by the other metabolites.

A comparison of KH 090478 and S7 (7-12-81) under DBP-free conditions is shown in Fig. 5. At the point of 50% competition, the specificity of KH 090478 for $1\alpha,25(OH)_2D_3$ is approximately fourfold higher than for $25(OH)D_3$. In contrast, S7 (7-12-81) has an approximately 100-fold higher specificity for $1\alpha,25(OH)_2D_3$ as compared to $25(OH)D_3$.

Precision

The precision of the DAB-RIA was examined by measuring serum samples containing $1\alpha,25(OH)_2D_3$ concentrations of 54 ng/l, 130 ng/l or below the detection limit. The results are shown in Table 2. Aliquots of each sample were measured 12 times in one assay. The intraassay variation coefficients for the samples with 54 and 130 ng/l were 15.9% and 10.5%, respectively. All aliquots of the sample with low $1\alpha,25-(OH)_2D$ were below the detection limit.

The plasma samples were also measured in nine consecutive assays. The variation coefficients for interassay variance were 18.0% and 16.7% for the 54 ng/l and 130 ng/l samples, respectively. In all nine tests, no $1\alpha,25(OH)_2D$ was found in the samples below the detection limit.

Clinical Studies

$1\alpha,25(OH)_2D$ was quantitated in sera from 40 healthy subjects (age 20 to 34), from 21 patients with preterminal renal failure, from 20 patients on chronic hemodialysis, and from 7 patients with primary hyperparathyroidism. The assays were carried out with the antibody KH 090478. The results are shown in Fig. 6. The mean concentration of $1\alpha,25(OH)_2D$ in normal subjects was 62.8 ng/l (SD 22.2, range 23.0–118.5, median 64.2). One sample from an apparently healthy donor which yielded $1\alpha,25(OH)_2D$ concentrations above 150 pg/ml both in the DAK-RIA and the charcoal-based reference assay was excluded.

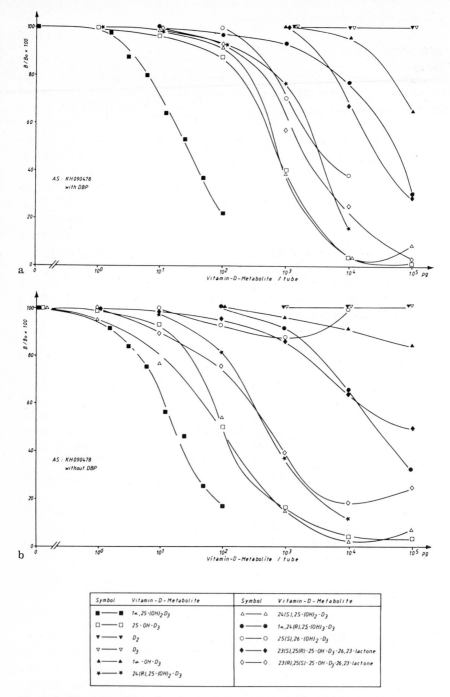

Fig. 4a,b. Cross-reactivity of various vitamin D metabolites in the $1\alpha,25(OH)_2D$ RIA. The antiserum was KH 090478. **a** The RIA was carried out with charcoal-separation of bound from free antigen exactly as described by Scharla et al. [31]. **b** The RIA was carried out with DAB separation under DBP-free conditions. B/Bo, bound antigen/Bmax.

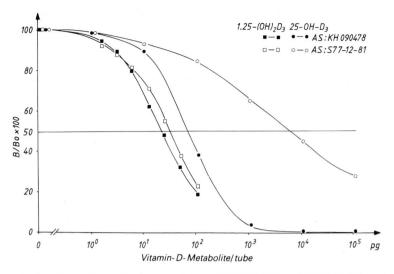

Fig. 5. Comparison of cross-reactivity of KH 090478 and S7 (7-12-81) under DBP-free conditions. Dilution of antisera was 1:64 000. B/Bo, bound antigen/Bmax.

Table 2. Precision of the $1\alpha, 25\,(OH)_2D_3$-DAB RIA.

A) *Intraassay variance* Sample concentration	Sample number	Variation coefficient [%]
< 6 ng/l	12	a)
54 ng/l	12	15.9
130 ng/l	12	10.5

B) *Interassay variance* Sample concentration	Sample number	Variation coefficient [%]
< 6 ng/l	9	a)
54 ng/l	9	18.0
130 ng/l	9	16.7

Inter- and intra-assay variance of the $1\alpha,25(OH)_2D_3$-DAB RIA were determined with antiserum KH 090478. a) in all experiments below detection limit.

The mean concentration of $1\alpha,25(OH)_2D$ in the 21 patients with preterminal renal failure was 17.4 ng/l (SD 10.6, range 4.4–42.9, median 15.0). The mean creatinine clearance of these patients was 14.3 ml/min (SD 7.3, range 6.0–35.0, median 13.5). None of the patients had been treated with vitamin D metabolites.

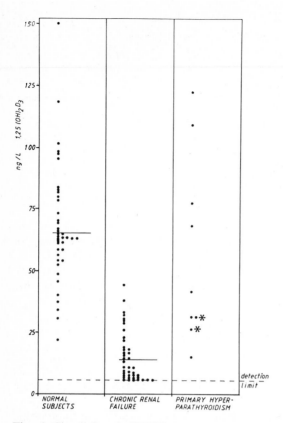

Fig. 6. Circulating 1α,25(OH)₂D of normal subjects, patients with chronic renal failure and patients with primary hyperparathyroidism. The samples were measured by the DAB-RIA with antiserum KH 090478 under standard conditions. ∗, after parathyroidectomy.

Patients on hemodialysis who did not receive vitamin D metabolites ($n = 17$) had a mean 1α,25(OH)₂D serum concentration of 6.3 ng/l (SD 2.7, range < 3.8–13.7, p < 0.001 vs. preterminal renal failure by Student's t-test). Two hemodialysis patients who received 0.25 µg 1α,25(OH)₂D₃/day had 1α,25(OH)₂D levels of 20.1 ng/l and 28.0 ng/l, respectively; one patient on 0.5 µg 1α,25(OH)₂D₃/day had a 1α,25(OH)₂D level of 27.7 ng/l. 1α,25(OH)₂D serum levels in the patient group with primary hyperparathyroidism ($n = 7$) varied over a range of 14.8–122.9 ng/l. The mean 1α,25(OH)₂D concentration was 66.5 ng/l (SD 35.8). Circulating 1,25(OH)₂D was measured in 2 patients before and after subtotal parathyroidectomy. The respective values were 109.2 ng/ml (one day before surgery) and, 26.2 ng/ml (7 days after surgery), and 77.9 ng/ml (3 days before surgery) and 31.8 ng/ml (10 days after surgery).

The results of the DAB-RIA were directly compared with a standard RIA [31] using the same extraction steps and charcoal-based separation of bound from free $1,25(OH)_2D$. Serum samples from normal subjects, patients with chronic renal failure and primary hyperparathyroidism ($n = 65$) were assayed by both methods. When DCC-RIA data were plotted on the abscissa and DAB-RIA on the ordinate, the correlation coefficient for this comparison was 0.843, with a slope of 1.19 and an intercept of -12.7.

Discussion

In this chapter we describe the development of a $1\alpha,25(OH)_2D_3$-RIA which utilizes a double antibody (DAB) technique to separate bound from free antigen. When DAB separation was initially done with reagents from a charcoal-based assay, two main problems became apparent: (i) high nonspecific binding (NSB) of $1\alpha,25(OH)_2[^3H]D_3$ to vials and sediments and (ii) low Bmax of $1\alpha,25(OH)_2D_3$.

The first problem of high NSB was overcome by washing the sediment after the DAB separation with 500 µl NaCl solution (9 g/l) containing 1 ml/l Brij-35. Brij-35 proved to be an optimal reagent for removing nonspecifically bound antigen without impairing the antigen-antibody binding. Thus, NSB could be reduced from formerly 30%–40% to less than 10% of Bmax.

The DBP in the $1\alpha,25(OH)_2D$ RIA might reduce the $1\alpha,25(OH)_2[^3H]D_3$ available for binding to the antibody and therefore result in decreased Bmax. To solve this second problem, DBP was systematically removed from all 4 DBP sources in the assay (first Ab, normal rabbit serum, second Ab and buffer). The first and second Ab were added as gamma globulin fractions. Normal rabbit serum (precipitation adjuvant) was replaced by normal rabbit IgG, and the albumin in the BSA buffer was replaced by gelatin. We found that DBP in the normal rabbit serum strongly interfered with the assay by reducing Bmax. Similarly, whole first and second antisera markedly decreased Bmax as compared to conditions where gamma globulin fractions were used. In contrast, the effect of BSA buffer which contained only trace amounts of DBP was less pronounced. Altogether, the elimination of DBP from the assay enhanced Bmax of $1\alpha,25(OH)_2D_3$ from 2% to approximately 35%.

The sensitivity and precision of the DAB-RIA were comparable to those of previously described assays which relied on charcoal separation [31]. The variation coefficients of intra- and interassay variance were between 10% and 18%. Since the DAB technique in our RIA vials gave a variation coefficient of less than 5%, the higher variation in the whole assay was due to sample extraction with Extrelut columns and subsequent HPLC separation.

Brown and Peacock [7] and Bouillon et al. [4] found that the presence of DBP in $1\alpha,25(OH)_2D$-RIAs increased specificity but decreased sensitivity. These observations were confirmed by our studies. Under DBP-free conditions, both $25(OH)D_3$ and $24,25(OH)_2D_3$ bound markedly higher to the antibody than in the presence of DBP. Therefore the DAB-RIA required adequate preparation of samples with complete separation of $1\alpha,25(OH)_2D$ from other vitamin D metabolites.

In addition we compared the properties of two antisera in the $1\alpha,25(OH)_2D_3$-DAB RIA. Antiserum KH 090478 was raised against a $1\alpha,25(OH)_2D_3$-3-hemisuccinate, while antiserum S7 (7-12-81) was raised against a $1\alpha,25(OH)_2D_3$-25-hemisuccinate. We found that S7 (7-12-81) had an approximately fivefold higher affinity for $1\alpha,25(OH)_2D_3$ than KH 090478. Moreover, the specificity of S7 (7-12-81) for $1\alpha,25(OH)_2D_3$ at 50% competition was markedly higher than KH 090478 (Fig. 5). Therefore our data suggest that production of antibodies against $1\alpha,25(OH)_2D_3$ is facilitated by coupling the hemisuccinate to the side-chain rather than to the A-ring of the $1\alpha,25(OH)_2D_3$-molecule.

The DAB-RIA was validated by quantitating $1\alpha,25(OH)_2D$ in samples from normal individuals and from patients with several clinical disorders. The mean serum $1\alpha,25(OH)_2D$ of normal subjects was within the range of previously published values. The DAB-RIA was further tested by measuring samples from patients with reduced kidney function. In accordance with the literature, circulating $1\alpha,25(OH)_2D$ was markedly lower in these patients. The assay also distinguished between hemodialysis patients and patients with preterminal renal failure in that chronic dialysis patients had lower $1\alpha,25(OH)_2D$ values than patients with preterminal renal failure (mean creatinine clearance 14.3 ml/min). While most previous reports have quoted elevated mean $1\alpha,25(OH)_2D$ in primary hyperparathyroidism, a considerable overlap between normal individuals and hyperparathyroid patients (up to 80%) has been found [19, 25]. The average $1\alpha,25(OH)_2D$ value for the seven patients with primary hyperparathyroidism was higher than the average for normal subjects; however, there was wide variation of circulating $1\alpha,25(OH)_2D$. $1\alpha,25(OH)_2D$ concentrations were markedly decreased in two patients whose serum was evaluated several days after subtotal parathyroidectomy.

DAB separation is faster and easier to perform than charcoal separation. The use of immunoassay vials with only 250 µl scintillation fluid/tube is economical and reduces the amount of radioactive waste. Possibly our method will also be useful for the development of DAB-RIAs for other steroid hormones which are bound to carrier proteins.

Conclusion

A sensitive radioimmunoassay (RIA) for $1\alpha,25$-dihydroxyvitamin D [$1\alpha,25(OH)_2D$] with a double antibody (DAB) separation technique to separate free from bound antigen has been developed. The hormone was extracted from 1 ml serum or plasma by Extrelut columns and normal phase high performance liquid chromatography and quantitated in the DAB-RIA. The separation of bound from free antigen was based on the following modifications of our previous charcoal-separation method: (i) Utilization of the IgG fraction instead of whole serum for first Ab (rabbit anti-1α,25(OH)$_2$D$_3$-3-hemisuccinate) and second Ab (donkey anti-rabbit IgG); (ii) addition of gelatin instead of albumin to the assay buffer; (iii) utilization of unspecific IgG instead of whole serum as the inactive ingredient for precipitation of antigen-antibody complexes. The elimination of serum vitamin D-binding protein (DBP) led to an increase in the maximal binding of antigen to 35% of total activity as compared to 2% with reagents that contained DBP. The incubation times for the equilibrium RIA were 12 h for the first Ab and 1 h for the second Ab. The detection limit of the assay was 3.75 ng/l. The intraassay variation coefficients were 15.9% and 10.5% for samples with 1α,25(OH)$_2$D$_3$ concentrations of 54 ng/l and 130 ng/l, respectively. The interassay variation coefficients were 18.0% and 16.7% for these two concentrations. Mean (and SD) values for 1,25(OH)$_2$D in serum of 40 normal subjects and 38 patients with chronic renal failure who did not receive 1,25(OH)$_2$D$_3$ were 62.8 ng/ml (22.2) and 12.4 ng/ml (9.8), respectively. The mean value for seven patients with primary hyperparathyroidism was 66.5 ng/ml (35.8) before surgery. These results compared well with those of an established charcoal-based RIA. A 1α,25(OH)$_2$D antiserum raised against a 1α,25(OH)$_2$D$_3$-25 hemisuccinate had an approximately fivefold higher affinity for 1α,25(OH)$_2$D$_3$ and an approximately 20-fold higher specificity for 1α,25(OH)$_2$D$_3$ than a 1α,25(OH)$_2$D$_3$-antiserum raised against a 1α,25(OH)$_2$D$_3$-3-hemisuccinate. Compared to charcoal-based RIAs, the DAB-RIA is faster and requires less laborious assay procedures.

References

1. Bell NH, Stern PH, Pantzer E, Sinha TK, DeLuca HF (1979) Evidence that increased circulating 1α,25-dihydroxyvitamin D is the probable cause for abnormal calcium metabolism in sarcoidosis. J Clin Invest 64:218–225
2. Björkhem I, Holmberg I, Kristiansen T, Pedersen JI (1979) Assay of 1,25-dihydroxyvitamin D$_3$ by isotope dilution-mass fragmentography. Clin Chem 25:584–588
3. Blayau M, Leray G, Prodhomme C, David V, Peron P (1986) An improved source of receptor for 1,25-dihydroxyvitamin D$_3$ assay. Clin Chim Acta 158:199–206
4. Bouillon R, De Moor P, Baggiolini EG, Uskokovic MR (1980) A radioimmunoassay for 1,25-dihydroxycholecalciferol. Clin Chem 26:562–567
5. Broadus AE, Horst RL, Lang R, Littledike TE, Rasmussen H (1980) The importance of circulating 1,25-dihydroxyvitamin D in the pathogenesis of hypercalciuria and renal-stone formation in primary hyperparathyroidism. N Engl J Med 302:421–426
6. Brooks MH, Bell NH, Love L (1978) Vitamin-D-dependent rickets type II. Resistance of target organs to 1,25-dihydroxyvitamin D. N Engl J Med 298:996–999
7. Brown WB, Peacock M (1986) Characteristics of antisera to antigenic forms of 1,25-dihydroxycholecalciferol. Clin Chim Acta 159:111–121
8. Brumbaugh PF, Haussler DH, Bressler R, Haussler MR (1974) Radioreceptor assay for 1,25-dihydroxyvitamin D. Science 183:1089–1091

9. Clemens TL, Hendy GN, Graham RF, Baggiolini EG, Uskokovic MR, O'Riordan JLH (1978) A radioimmunoassay for 1,25-dihydroxycholecalciferol. Clin Sci 54: 329–332

10. Clemens TL, Hendy GN, Papapoulos SE, Fraher LJ, Care AD, O'Riordan JLH (1979) Measurement of 1,25-dihydroxycholecalciferol in man by radioimmunoassay. Clin Endocrinol 11:225–234

11. De Leenheer AP, Bauwens RM (1985) Radioimmunoassay for 1,25-dihydroxy-vitamin D in serum or plasma. Clin Chem 31:142–146

12. Eisman JA, Hamstra AJ, Kream BE, DeLuca HF (1976) A sensitive, precise, and convenient method for determination of 1,25-dihydroxyvitamin D in human plasma. Arch Biochem Biophys 176:235–243

13. Feinfeld DA, Sherwood LM (1988) Parathyroid hormone and 1,25(OH)$_2$D$_3$ in chronic renal failure. Kidney Int 33:1049–1058

14. Fraser D, Kooh SW, Kind HP, Holick MF, Tanaka Y, DeLuca HF (1973) Pathogenesis of hereditary vitamin-D-dependent rickets. An inborn error of vitamin D metabolism involving defective conversion of 25-hydroxyvitamin D to 1α,25-dihydroxyvitamin D. N Engl J Med 289:817–822

15. Haussler MR, McCain TA (1977) Basic and clinical concepts related to vitamin D metabolism and action. N Engl J Med 297:974–983, 1041–1050

16. Haussler MR, Baylink DJ, Hughes MR (1976) The assay of 1α,25-dihydroxyvitamin D$_3$: physiologic and pathologic modulation of circulating hormone levels. Clin Endocrinol 5:151s–165s

17. Hebert GA, Pelham PL, Pittman P (1972) Determination of the optimal ammonium sulfate concentration of rabbit, sheep, horse and goat antisera. Appl Microbiol 25:26–36

18. Hummer L, Christiansen C, Tjellesen L (1985) Discrepancy between serum 1,25-dihydroxycholecalciferol measured by radioimmunoassay and cytosol radioreceptor assay. Scand J Clin Lab Invest 45:725–733

19. Manolagas SC, Culler FL, Howard JE, Brickman AS, Deftos LJ (1983) The cytoreceptor assay for 1,25-dihydroxyvitamin D and its application to clinical studies. J Clin Endocrinol Metab 56:751–760

20. Mason RS, Lissner D, Grunstein HS, Posen S (1980) A simplified assay for dihydroxylated vitamin D metabolites in human serum: application to hyper- and hypovitaminosis D. Clin Chem 26:444–450

21. McCollum EV, Simmonds N, Shipley PG, Park EA (1922) Studies on experimental rickets. A delicate biological test for calcium-depositing substances. J Biol Chem 51:41–49

22. Nicholson GC, Kent JC, Gutteridge DH, Retallack RW (1985) Estimation of 1,25-dihydroxyvitamin D by cytoreceptor and competitive protein binding assays without high pressure liquid chromatography. Clin Endocrinol 22:597–609

23. Norman AW, Roth J, Orci L (1982) The vitamin D endocrine system: steroid metabolism, hormone receptors, and biological response (calcium binding proteins). Endocr Rev 3:331–366

24. Papapoulos SE, Clemens TL, Fraher LJ, Lewin IG, Sandler LM, O'Riordan JLH (1979) 1,25-Dihydroxycholecalciferol in the pathogenesis of the hypercalcemia of sarcoidosis. Lancet i:627–630

25. Peacock M, Taylor GA, Brown W (1980) Plasma 1,25(OH)$_2$ vitamin D measured by radioimmunoassay and cytosol radioreceptor assay in normal subjects and patients with primary hyperparathyroidism and renal failure. Clin Chim Acta 101:93–101

26. Reichel H, Koeffler HP, Norman AW (1989) The role of the vitamin D endocrine system in health and disease. N Engl J Med 320:980–991
27. Reinhardt TA, Horst RL, Orf JW, Hollis BW (1984) A microassay for 1,25-dihydroxyvitamin D not requiring high performance liquid chromatography: application to clinical studies. J Clin Endocrinol Metab 58:91–98
28. Rosenthal N, Insogna KL, Godsall JW, Smaldone L, Waldron JA, Stewart AF (1985) Elevations in circulating 1,25-dihydroxyvitamin D in three patients with lymphoma-associated hypercalcemia. J Clin Endocrinol Metab 60:29–33
29. Samaké H, Rajkowski KM, Cittanova N (1983) The choice of buffer protein in steroid (enzyme-) immunoassay. Clin Chim Acta 130:129–135
30. Scatchard G (1949) The attractions of proteins for small molecules and ions. Ann NY Acad Sci 51:66
31. Scharla S, Schmidt-Gayk H, Reichel H, Mayer E (1984) A sensitive and simplified radioimmunoassay for 1,25-dihydroxyvitamin D_3. Clin Chim Acta 142:325–338
32. Schmidt-Gayk H, Wahl M, Limbach HJ, Walch S (1979) Ein spezielles Gefäß zur Durchführung des Radioimmunoassay (RIA). Medizintechnik 99:103–104
33. Stern PH, Hamstra AJ, DeLuca HF, Bell NH (1979) A bioassay capable of measuring one picogram of 1,25-dihydroxyvitamin D_3. J Clin Endocrinol Metab 146:891–896
34. Stewart AF, Horst R, Deftos LJ, Cadman EC, Lang R, Broadus AE (1980) Biochemical evaluation of patients with cancer-associated hypercalcemia: evidence for humoral and non-humoral groups. N Engl J Med 303:1377–1383

Chapter 5.7

Competitive Protein-Binding Assay of Calcitriol with an Advanced Preparation of Bovine Calf Thymus Cytosol

T.A. Reinhardt and R.L. Horst

Introduction

Our laboratory has previously published comprehensive procedures for the accurate determination of vitamin D_2, vitamin D_3, and their many metabolites. The measurement of these metabolites required extensive purification by high-performance liquid chromatography (HPLC) [1, 2], and assays for many of these metabolites of vitamin D were of only academic interest. The most useful vitamin D metabolite assays, in the majority of clinical and experimental settings, are those for 25-(OH)D and 1,25-(OH)$_2$D. The assay of 25-(OH)D is useful in detecting states of vitamin D deficiency and excess. The assay of 1,25-(OH)$_2$D is useful in diagnosing states of inadequate (e.g., pseudohyper-parathyroidism, diabetes) or excessive (e.g., hyperparathyroidism, sarcoidosis) vitamin D activation. Another metabolite of vitamin D, namely, 24,25-(OH)$_2$D, has also been proposed as an active form of vitamin D important in normal bone formation.

Recently, we developed simplified procedures for assay of 1,25-(OH)$_2$D and 25-OHD which do not require HPLC [2, 5]. The simplified assay for 1,25-(OH)$_2$D utilizes crude 1,25-(OH)$_2$D receptor prepared from calf thymus glands [3–5]. To further optimize the preparation of a high-quality and stable receptor-binding protein, we have made several modifications in the published procedures for the preparation of calf thymus cytosol. These modifications will be presented, as will modifications in Sep-Pak chromatography procedures (Waters Associates, Inc., Milford, MA, United States) which form the basis for an assay of 24,25-(OH)$_2$D in addition to 1,25-(OH)$_2$D and 25-OHD.

Reagents

Synthetic 1,25-(OH)$_2$D$_3$ and 1,25-(OH)$_2$D$_2$ were generous gifts from Dr. Milan Uskokovic and Dr. John Partridge of Hoffmann-La Roche, Inc. (Nutley, NJ, United States). 1,25-Dihydroxy[26,27-^{3}H]vitamin D$_3$ (80 Ci/mmol) and 1,25-(OH)$_2$[26,27-^{3}H]D$_2$ (80 Ci/mmol) were prepared in our laboratory by C[^{3}H]$_3$MgI reduction of 27-nor-25-keto-1-OHD$_3$ and 27-nor-25-keto-1-

OHD_2, respectively. The purity and concentrations of 1,25-$(OH)_2D_3$ and 1,25-$(OH)_2D_2$ were confirmed by UV spectroscopy using an extinction coefficient (E_{264}) of 18 200/M per centimeter for 1,25-$(OH)_2D_3$ and an E_{264} of 19 400/M per centimeter for 1,25-$(OH)_2D_2$. All solvents used were HPLC grade and, unless noted, all other reagents were reagent grade.

Collection and Storage of Calf Thymus Tissue

Thymus glands are removed from 1- to 12-month-old calves at euthanasia or slaughter. The tissue is immediately cut into moderate-sized pieces ($\sim 4\,cm^3$ to facilitate tissue cooling) and placed in ice-cold phosphate buffer saline (PBS) for transport to the laboratory. On ice, the tissue is trimmed to remove blood and connective tissue and cut into small pieces ($\sim 1\,cm^3$). The cubed thymus is washed extensively with ice-cold PBS. At this point, the tissue may either be processed immediately to cytosol or quick frozen in liquid nitrogen. Frozen tissue is stored at $-70\,°C$ and is stable for up to 1 year.

Preparation of Thymus Cytosol

Frozen or fresh tissue is processed for cytosol as follows (all steps are carried out at 4 °C). Thymus tissue is minced (we use a meat grinder) and homogenized (20% w/v) in a *modified* buffer containing 50 mM K_2HPO_4, 5 mM dithiothreitol, 1 mM ethylenediaminetetraacetic acid (EDTA), and 400 mM KCl, pH 7.5. [Note: This modified buffer provides better pH control during the $(NH_4)_2SO_4$ precipitation step and eliminates the occasional homogenate gelling seen when using the previous buffer system.] The tissues are homogenized by five 30-bursts of a Polytron PT-20 tissue disrupter using power setting 7 (Brinkman Instruments, Westburg, NY, United States). Tissue is cooled on ice between homogenization steps. The homogenate is then centrifuged for 15 min at 15 000–20 000 g to remove large particulates. The resulting supernatant is then centrifuged at 100 000 g for 1 h, and the cytosol is collected (minus pellet and floating lipid layer). This cytosol is then fractionated by the slow addition of solid $(NH_4)_2SO_4$ to 35% saturation (enzyme grade Schwarz-Mann, Orangeburg, NY, United States). The cytosol $(NH_4)_2SO_4$ mixture is stirred for 30 min while maintaining temperature at 4 °C. [Note: Maintenance of pH at ~ 7.5 during the $(NH_4)_2SO_4$ step is critical and becomes a greater problem if nonenzyme grade $(NH_4)_2SO_4$ is used.] The mixture is then aliquoted into 15-ml centrifuge tubes 7–10 ml/tube) and centrifuged at 20 000 g for 20 min. The supernatant is discarded and tubes are allowed to drain for 5 min. The pelleted receptor is lyophilized and stored under argon or nitrogen at $-70\,°C$. Receptor prepared in this manner is stable for up to 60 h at room temperature.

Reconstitution of Thymus Cytosol

Prior to assay, the pellet-containing receptor is reconstituted to its original volume (7–10 ml/tube) with assay buffer. The assay buffer contains 50 mM K_2HPO_4, 5 mM dithiothreitol, 1.0 mM EDTA, and 150 mM KCl at pH 7.5. The receptor pellet is redissolved by gently stirring on ice using a magnetic stir bar. [Note: Vortexing or shaking are to be avoided, as these methods generate foaming, which denatures the receptor.] Allow the receptor solution to mix for 20–30 min. Typically, a small portion of the protein pellet resists solubilization. This insoluble protein is removed by centrifugation at 3000 rpm for 10 min. The receptor solution is then diluted one-third to one-ninth with assay buffer and used in the assay at 450 μl/tube. The correct dilution of reconstituted receptor used in the assay is determined empirically for each new batch of receptor. In our laboratory, we determine the correct dilution for a new batch of receptor by comparing standard curves generated for various dilutions of receptor. At the appropriate dilution for assay use, specific binding in the absence of cold 1,25-$(OH)_2D$ is 900–1200 cpm, nonspecific binding is 200–300 cpm, and an 8-pg standard results in ~ 40%–45% displacement of labeled 1,25-$(OH)_2D$. These results assume a specific activity of 80–90 Ci/mmol for [^{3}H]1,25-$(OH)_2D$ and a 40% counting efficiency for tritium.

Troubleshooting Guide for Thymic Receptor Preparation

Low or absence of receptor-binding activity

1. Inadequate cooling at all steps of preparation.
2. Incomplete homogenization (mince tissue prior to homogenization).
3.[1] Inadequate pH control, especially during $(NH_4)_2SO_4$ precipitation step.
4.[1] Excessive foaming during reconstitution of receptor prior to assay.
5. Substantial degradation of labeled 1,25-$(OH)_2D_3$ used in the binding assay. (This also results in elevated nonspecific binding.)
6. Receptor excessively diluted (the receptor concentration in calf thymus is ~ 1/5–1/15 of that present in chick intestine).

Sep-Pak Preparation

Both new and used Sep-Paks or equivalent are prepared as follows before use. C_{18} Sep-Paks are washed by the sequential addition of 5 ml hexane, 5 ml chloroform, 5 ml methanol, and 5 ml distilled water. Silica Sep-Paks are washed

---

[1] Most common reasons leading to low receptor binding.

by sequential additions of 5 ml methanol, 5 ml chloroform, 5 ml hexane, and 5 ml hexane:isopropanol (96:4). This conditioning procedure allows reuse of Sep-Pak cartridges at least four times without significant loss of capacity of changes in elution patterns.

Sample Preparation for Assay of 25-OHD and 1,25-(OH)₂D

A flow diagram depicting the steps required for sample extraction and purification is presented in Fig. 1. Plasma (0.2–1.0 ml) is added to 12 × 75-mm borosilicate glass tubes and brought up to 1 ml total volume with saline. Eight hundred counts per minute of [³H]1,25-(OH)₂D₃ in 20μl ethanol is added to each plasma sample and to a counting vial for the estimation of recoveries. The samples are then vortexed and allowed to stand for 10 min. One volume of acetonitrile is then added to each plasma sample. The samples are vortexed vigorously for 20 s and then centrifuged for 10 min at 1500 g. Following centrifugation, the supernatant is decanted into a tube containing 0.5 volume 0.4 M K₂HPO₄, pH 10.6, and vortexed. This extract is then applied directly to a prewashed C₁₈ Sep-Pak. Excess salt is removed by washing the cartridge with 5 ml distilled water, and polar lipids are eluted by washing the cartridge with 3 ml methanol:water (70:30). The vitamin D metabolites are then eluted in 4 ml acetonitrile. The acetonitrile fraction is then dried under a stream of nitrogen. The vitamin D

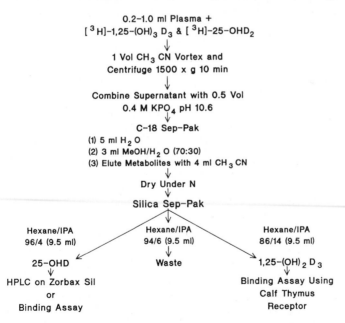

Fig. 1. Flow diagram presenting the purification step prior to the assay of 25-OHD and 1,25-(OH)₂D

metabolite extract is then applied to a silica Sep-Pak cartridge in 0.5 ml hexane:isopropanol (99:1), and the tube is washed with an additional 0.5 ml solvent, which was applied to the cartridge. The cartridge is then washed with 10 ml of the starting solvent, followed by 9.5 ml (96:4) hexane:isopropanol, which results in the elution of 25-OHD. The cartridge is then washed with 8 ml hexane:isopropanol (94:6), which elutes 60% of the 24,25-$(OH)_2$D. The 1,25-$(OH)_2$D is then eluted with 9.5 ml hexane:isopropanol (86:14) and dried under a stream of nitrogen. The 25-OHD fraction is prepared for analysis by HPLC or binding assay as described previously [1, 2]. The 1,25-$(OH)_2$D fraction is redissolved in 100 µl absolute ethanol. From this volume, 25 µl is used to determine recovery of tracer and two 25-µl aliquots are used for assay of 1,25-$(OH)_2$D in duplicate.

Alternate Sample Preparation Method Used for the Assay of 24,25-$(OH)_2$D

A flow diagram depicting the steps required for this alternate sample preparation procedure is presented in Fig. 2. One volume of saturated ammonium sulfate is added to each sample containing [^{3}H]-metabolites for recovery estimation. After vortexing, two volumes of acetonitrile are added and the sample is vortexed until an emulsion is formed. The emulsion is broken by the addition of 0.5 volumes of methanol and the sample is then centrifuged. The supernatant is transferred to a tube containing one volume of 0.4 M K_2HPO_4, pH 10.6, and vortexed. This extract is then applied to an all-glass, 1-cm ID minicolumn fitted with a 1-cm disk of Watmann #1 filter paper at the affluent end to prevent leakage of the column bed. The column bed contains 0.4 g ODS from Waters Associates. Following sample application, the column is washed with 3 ml methanol:water (60:40). The vitamin D metabolites are then eluted with 8 ml acetonitrile and this fraction is dried under a stream of nitrogen. This fraction is applied to a Baker silica column in 0.5 ml 99:1 hexane:isopropanol followed by a 0.5-ml wash. The cartridge is washed with 10 ml starting solvent followed by 9.5 ml (96:4) hexane isopropanol to elute 25-OHD. The cartridge is then washed with 8 ml methylene chloride:acetonitrile:isopropanol, which elutes 24,25-$(OH)_2$D. The 1,25-$(OH)_2$D is eluted with 8 ml 86:14 hexane:isopropanol. The 25-OHD fraction is prepared for analysis by HPLC or binding assay as described [1,2]. The 24,25-$(OH)_2$D fraction is applied to an HPLC column developed in methanol:acetonitrile:isopropanol (180/20/1) for separation of the 24,25-$(OH)_2$D from contaminates. The 24,25-$(OH)_2$D is collected and assayed in a competitive binding assay as described [1, 2]. The 1,25-$(OH)_2$D fraction is reapplied to a Baker silica column and the 1,25-$(OH)_2$D repurified as described above to remove [^{3}H]24,25-$(OH)_2$D contamination which would otherwise result in overestimation of 1,25-$(OH)_2$D recoveries. The 1,25-$(OH)_2$D fraction is collected and assayed in the thymus-binding assay as described.

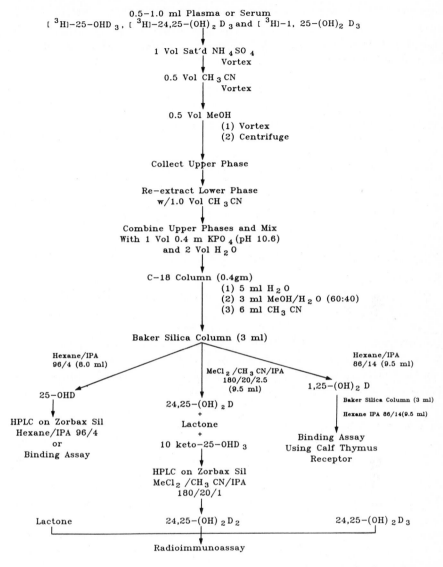

Fig. 2. Flow diagram presenting an alternate purification scheme which allows the assay of 24,25-(OH)$_2$D in addition to that of 25-OHD and 1,25-(OH)$_2$D

Preparation of Dextran-Coated Charcoal

Six grams of charcoal (Norit-A, Sigma Chemical Co., St. Louis, MO, United States) and 0.6 g dextran T70 (Pharmacia Fine Chemicals, Piscataway, NJ, United States) are suspended in 500 ml of a buffer containing 0.1 M boric acid and 0.05% BSA, pH 8.6, and stirred overnight at 4 °C. The next morning, the suspension is centrifuged at 1500 g for 15–20 min, and the supernatant is carefully decanted and discarded. The pelleted dextran-coated charcoal is then resuspended in 500 ml of the buffer described. This charcoal suspension is stable for at least 2 weeks at 4 °C.

Nonequilibrium Radioreceptor Assay for 1,25-(OH)$_2$D

Standards (1–64 and 800 pg for nonspecific binding determination in 25 μl ethanol) and samples are added to 12 × 75-mm glass tubes on ice. An aliquot of stock receptor sufficient for the number of tubes to be assayed is diluted as described above, and 450 μl receptor solution is added to the standards and samples on ice and vortexed. The samples and standards are incubated for 45 min with gentle shaking at 25 °C. At the end of 45 min, the tubes are transferred to an ice bath to cool for 5 min, and then each tube receives 5000 cpm [^{3}H]1,25-(OH)$_2$D (80 Ci/mmol) in 25 μl ethanol. The tubes are vortexed and incubated for 30 additional minutes at 25 °C. The tubes are then cooled for 5 min in an ice bath, and 200 μl dextran-coated charcoal suspension is added to each, followed by vortexing. The tubes are vortexed again after 10 min, and after 20 min of charcoal treatment, bound and free hormone are separated by centrifugation. Tubes are centrifuged at 2000 g for 10 min, and the supernatant containing bound hormone is decanted into a scintillation vial and counted. A typical standard curve is shown in Fig. 3.

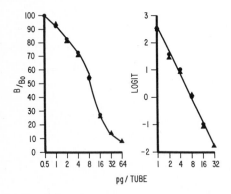

Fig. 3A,B. A typical standard curve obtained for 1,25-(OH)$_2$D using thymus 1,25-(OH)$_2$D receptor and nonequilibrium incubation conditions is depicted in **A**. **B** shows the linearization of the curve afforded by a logit-log transformation. ●, 1,25-(OH)$_2$D$_3$; ▲, 1,25-(OH)$_2$D$_2$

Calculations

The 1,25-(OH)$_2$D values (picograms/tube) are calculated using a logit/log plot of the binding assay data.

$$\text{logit} = In\ \frac{B/B_0}{1 - B/B_0}$$

For our purposes, this is done using a Hewlett–Packard HP41CV calculator and the RIA program contained in their Clinical Lab and Nuclear Medicine Program Pak (Hewlett–Packard, Palo Alto, CA, United States). This procedure provides optimal linearization of the standard curve. The 1,25-(OH)$_2$D concentrations (picograms per milliliter) of plasma or serum are then obtained by correcting picogram per tube data for recovery and plasma volume equivalent/assay tube.

Quality Control

Every assay should include control sera or plasma to assure assay repeatability and validity. We typically run two controls which are the first and last samples in every assay. An acceptable range for the control samples is determined following repeated assay of control sera in 10–20 separate assays. An acceptable range for the control serums is the mean $\pm$ 2 SD of previously assayed controls.

We have found that the optimal assay size using this procedure is 68 tubes. This represents 24 samples and 10 standards, all done in duplicate. It has been our experience that large assays lead to systematic errors due to large differences in time between the first tube being treated with charcoal and the last tube

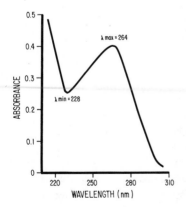

Fig. 4. Ultraviolet spectra of a pure vitamin D compound

treated. Therefore, in order to maintain a high degree of quality control, one should not exceed these assay size constraints without first testing them in one's own laboratory.

Standards should be prepared regularly from a stock metabolite solution whose concentration and purity is checked by ultraviolet spectroscopy prior to standard preparation. As a general guide, stock solutions of metabolites are suitable for standard preparation if the ratio of absorbance at 264–228 nM is ≥ 1.5. A typical UV spectra for a vitamin D metabolite is presented in Fig. 4. A shift of the 228-nM valley of spectra upfield and/or a drop in the ratio of absorbance at 264–228 nM below 1.5 indicates significant degradation or contamination of the metabolites. Stock solution concentrations are determined using a molar extinction coefficient (E_{264}) of 18 200/M per centimeter for vitamin D_3 metabolites and an E_{264} of 19 300/M per centimeter for vitamin D_2 metabolites. The formula for determining the concentration of vitamin D metabolites in ethanol solutions is therefore as follows:

$$\frac{\text{Absorbance}_{264}}{E} \times \text{mol. wt.} = \text{ng}/\mu\text{l}$$

$E = 18.2$ for vitamin D_3 metabolites or 19.3 for vitamin D_2 metabolites.

Purity of the [^{3}H]-metabolites used for recovery estimation is of paramount importance in these assays. Significant degradation of these labeled compounds will lead to artificially low recovery estimates and will consequently result in an overestimation of assay results. Therefore, the [^{3}H]-metabolites used for recovery estimates must be rigorously monitored for purity and repurified as needed in order accurately to assay these vitamin D metabolites.

General Troubleshooting Guide for Assays

1. Assay results overestimate true vitamin D metabolite concentrations.
   a)[1] Labeled vitamin D metabolite used to estimate extraction and chromatographic losses have degraded.
   b)[2] Standard concentrations are lower than expected due to degradation or incorrect preparation.
2. Assay results underestimate true vitamin D metabolite concentrations.
   a) Standard concentrations are higher than expected due to incorrect preparation.
3. Excessively low recoveries of vitamin D metabolite following extraction and chromatography.
   a) Incorrect column solvent composition.
   b) Labeled vitamin D metabolites used to estimate recovery have degraded.

---

[1] Most common reasons leading to low receptor binding.
[2] Most common reasons for inaccurate assays

4. Assay results drift from beginning to end of assay.
   a) Too many samples run/assay; we limit assay size to 24 samples in duplicate/assay.

Assay Characteristics and Validation

Extraction and purification of 1,25-$(OH)_2$D from plasma or serum samples is accomplished by protein precipitation with acetonitrile followed by solid-phase extraction of the 1,25-$(OH)_2$D from the acetonitrile-K_2HPO_4-treated supernatant on a C_{18} Sep-Pak. Polar lipids, pigments, and salts are removed by the water and methanol:water (70:30) washes. Approximately 85%–90% of the sample 1,25-$(OH)_2$D is recovered in the 4 ml acetonitrile used for the final elution of the C_{18} Sep-Pak. The addition of basic K_2HPO_4 greatly enhances the removal of lipids from the 1,25-$(OH)_2$D fraction which might otherwise interfere in the assay.

Following solid-phase extraction, nonpolar lipids, 25-OHD, and 24,25-$(OH)_2$D are removed from the 1,25-$(OH)_2$D fraction using silica Sep-Paks. The 25-OHD is completely removed in the first 9–10 ml elution with hexane:isopropanol (96:4). The majority of 24,25-$(OH)_2$D remaining in the sample is then eluted with 8 ml hexane:isopropanol (94:6) followed by the elution of both 1,25-$(OH)_2D_3$ and 1,25-$(OH)_2D_2$ with 9 ml hexane:isopropanol (84:16). An average of 70%-80% of the sample 1,25-$(OH)_2$D is recovered.

The sensitivity of the thymus-based radioreceptor assay is optimized using a nonequilibrium incubation technique. Using this technique, the sensitivity of the assay, defined at 2 SD of the zero tube, is 1.5 pg/tube. Fifty percent displacement of bound trace occurs approximately at 8–9 pg/tube (Fig. 2). The unique character of the thymus 1,25-$(OH)_2$D receptor used in this assay is that it recognizes both 1,25-$(OH)_2D_3$ and 1,25-$(OH)_2D_2$ equally, while it detects other vitamin D metabolites poorly. Cross-reactivities compared with 1,25-$(OH)_2$D are 0.1% for 25-OHD, 0.02% for 24,25-$(OH)_2$D, and 0.008% for 25,26-$(OH)_2D_3$. Because of the low recoveries of these metabolites in the 1,25-$(OH)_2$D fraction, low cross-reactivities, and a maximum of 0.33 ml plasma equivalent/assay tube, we have determined that normal and above normal circulating concentrations of 25-OHD, 24,25-$(OH)_2$D, and 25,26-$(OH)_2$D do not interfere with 1,25-$(OH)_2$D measurement. Experiments in which normal human plasma samples were spiked with 24,25-$(OH)_2$D or 25,26-$(OH)_2$D at five times normal levels and assayed for 1,25-$(OH)_2$D showed no difference between the values obtained for 1,25-$(OH)_2$D between spikes and control samples.

In validating our assay method, we have determined that the analytical recovery of 1,25-$(OH)_2D_2$ and 1,25-$(OH)_2D_3$ added to plasma samples (8–64 pg 1,25-$(OH)_2$D added/ml plasma) averaged 99.0% $\pm$ 6.2% for added 1,25-$(OH)_2D_2$ and 93.3% $\pm$ 7.9% [mean $\pm$ SEM for added 1,25-$(OH)_2D_3$], thus indicating that our assay accurately measures total 1,25-$(OH)_2$D and that 1,25-

$(OH)_2[^3H]D_3$ accurately estimates extraction and purification recoveries for both $1,25\text{-}(OH)_2D_2$ and $1,25\text{-}(OH)_2D_3$. In light of our recent finding that $25\text{-}OHD_2$ constitutes as much as 39% of the total 25-OHD circulating in patients in which $1,25\text{-}(OH)_2D$ assays are often applied, it is clear that it is important to obtain accurate total $1,25\text{-}(OH)_2D$ measurements as are obtained by this assay [3].

The ultimate validation of this simplified method for $1,25\text{-}(OH)_2D$ assay was obtained by direct comparison of the results obtained with this assay with a well-established assay employing rigorous purification of sample $1,25\text{-}(OH)_2D$ using Sephadex LH-20 and HPLC chromatography prior to assay. Human plasma samples from patients with a wide variety of clinical problems were assayed by both methods. There was an excellent correlation between the results obtained by the established method and our simplified method. The correlation coefficient for this comparison was 0.96, with a slope of 1.05 and an intercept of -0.19.

The reproducibility of the assay was confirmed by its low intra-(8.8%) and interassay (12.8%) coefficients of variations. Table 1 summarizes the results obtained by the application of this assay to human samples. The mean values for $1,25\text{-}(OH)_2D$ obtained with this simplified methodology are in excellent agreement with $1,25\text{-}(OH)_2D$ values obtained using more technically demanding methodology.

In summary, the radioreceptor assay for $1,25\text{-}(OH)_2D$ described here simplifies the quantitation of $1,25\text{-}(OH)_2D$. The unique features of the assay are a widely available, inexpensive, and stable receptor protein which is resistant to lipid interference. This assay processes the characteristics of high sensitivity and specificity: small sample requirements and simultaneous measurements of both $1,25\text{-}(OH)_2D_2$ and $1,25\text{-}(OH)_2D_3$. It eliminates the need for HPLC. The assays presented are rapid and useful for quantitation of $1,25\text{-}(OH)_2D$, 25-OHD, and $24,25\text{-}(OH)_2D$ in human and experimental animal samples.

Table 1. Concentrations of $1,25\text{-}(OH)_2D$ determined for normal subjects and patients[a]

| Sample | Normals | Concentration of $1,25\text{-}(OH)_2D$ (pg/ml) | | | |
		Children	Primary hyperpara-thyroidism	Chronic renal failure	Anephrics
Mean	35.2	50.2	68.9	10.6	ND[b]
SEM	± 2.5	± 5.5	± 6.5	± 1.5	–
Range	18–65	29–92	39–115	< 5–16	–
n	30	14	13	7	10

[a] Detection limit is 5 pg of $1,25\text{-}(OH)_2D$/ml plasma
[b] ND, nondetectable

References

1. Horst RL, Littledike ET, Riley JL, Napoli JL (1981) Quantitation of vitamin D and its metabolites and their plasma concentrations in five species of animals. Anal Biochem 116:189–203
2. Horst RL, Reinhardt TA, Hollis BW, Napoli JL (1985) Assays for vitamin D metabolites. In: Norman AW, Schaefer K, Grigoleit H-G, Herrath DV (eds) Vitamin D: chemical, biochemical and clinical update. de Gruyter, New York: 807–816
3. Reinhardt TA, Horst RL, Orf JW, Hollis BW (1984) A microassay for 1,25-dihydroxyvitamin D_3 not requiring HPLC: application to clinical studies. J Clin Endocrinol Metab 58:91–98
4. Reinhardt TA, Horst RL, Littledike ET, Beitz DC (1982) 1,25-dihydroxyvitamin D receptor in bovine thymus gland. Biochem Biophys Res Commun 106:1012–1018
5. Reinhardt TA, Hollis BW (1986) 1,25-Dihydroxyvitamin D microassay employing radioreceptor techniques. Methods Enzymol 123:176–185

6 Assay of Calcitonin and Related Peptides

Design of New Methods for Measuring Calcitonin and Related Peptides Using Monoclonal Antipeptide Antibodies

P. Motté, P. Ghillani, F. Troalen, C. Bohuon, and D. Bellet

Introduction

Calcitonin (CT) is a small hypocalcemic peptide hormone secreted by thyroid C cells [14, 35]. Its physiological role, still a matter of discussion, appears to be that of a hypocalcemic hormone. The ability to measure the circulating level of this hormone may be important in understanding the regulation of calcemia; an additional reason for developing reliable methods for CT measurement stems from the demonstration of its usefulness as a tumor marker in the diagnosis and follow-up of medullary carcinoma of the thyroid (MCT) [40], a neoplastic proliferation of C cells [21, 42], which is transmitted in a familial pattern in 25%–30% of cases [38]. The genetic alteration associated with multiple endocrine neoplasia type 2A has recently been identified [25, 37]. Hyperplasia of the C cells is considered to be a pretumoral stage. Screening of subjects from at-risk families is performed by measuring serum CT level. Diagnosis is usually based either on elevation of the basal level or on a dramatic rise after pentagastrin stimulation. The ability to diagnose MCT in early childhood is essential; indeed, if the tumor is diagnosed when the patient is young, it is likely to be small and without metastasis, in which case surgery (total thyroidectomy) is the treatment of choice [16, 17].

Beginning with the first description of a competitive radioimmunoassay (RIA) for CT, several investigators have emphasized problems associated with such technology (for review, see [7]). First, competitive RIAs utilize iodinated CT as a tracer; the latter is highly sensitive to oxidizing conditions used during labeling, and the labeled product is unstable and must be utilized immediately. Second, physiological circulating CT levels are extremely low, and nonequilibrium RIAs or concentration methods are needed to attain sensitivity which will provide clinically useful information. Third, and most important, several groups have emphasized the presence of multiple immunoreactive forms of CT in plasma and other biological fluids [19]. Major discrepancies in the definition of CT-immunoreactive species in plasma have arisen among laboratories; even within a given laboratory, differences exist concerning antisera. It must be emphasized that the latter studies were performed using polyclonal antiserum-based RIAs; such antisera were raised using various immunogens (CT, either conjugated to carriers or unconjugated, or extracts from medullary thyroid carcinoma), and a partial explanation of these results might be the heterogeneity of the population of immunoglobulins present in a given antiserum in terms of both the affinity constant and the epitope of each antibody. Strikingly, the normal upper limit range for CT has decreased from hundreds of nanograms per milliliter to picograms per milliliter over the past decade [11, 26], reflecting the evolution in the immunochemical characteristics of the antisera used as well as technical improvements in RIAs.

We were interested in determining whether monoclonal antibodies (mAbs) of predetermined specificities might help to meet the challenge of developing accurate, sensitive techniques for the measurement of CT. We felt that mAbs could be useful tools for precisely defining the CT-like immunoreactive species present in biological fluids and for circumventing some of the technical drawbacks linked to the technology of competitive RIAs. For this purpose, we undertook a detailed immunochemical mapping of the antigenic determinants expressed by CT and other peptides encoded by the CT gene.

The biosynthetic pathway of CT has been extensively studied, and a schematic summary is shown in Fig. 1. CT is a 32-amino-acid-long polypeptide hormone which, in its mature form, is derived from the posttranslational processing of a larger precursor (designated preprocalcitonin). Transcription of the CT gene leads to a large RNA, which is alternatively spliced and poly-adenylated into either a CT- or a Calcitonin gene-related peptide (CGRP) encoding messenger RNA, probably under the influence of tissue-specific factors [22]. The CT-encoding messenger RNA is then translated into a preprocalci-tonin. The complete sequence of this molecule has been deduced from the nucleotide sequence of cloned cDNAs encoding the peptide [23]. The CT molecule is situated internally within the precursor molecule: the hormone is preceded by an 84-amino-acid-long terminal region which terminates in a Lys-Arg cleavage signal; downstream, the cleavage-amidation signal Gly-Lys-Lys-Arg separates the CT sequence from the 21-amino-acid residues of katacalcin

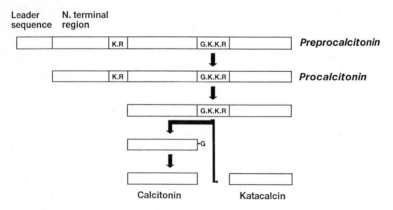

Fig. 1. Schematic representation of the biosynthetic pathway of CT in thyroid C-cells (the one-letter code was used to represent amino acid residues)

(KC). The biosynthesis of CT involves successive proteolytic events affecting preprocalcitonin. The signal peptide is removed as preprocalcitonin enters the endoplasmic reticulum and the resulting molecule, designated as procalcitonin, is processed by removing the N-terminal region. The resulting 57-amino-acid-long peptide is composed of the CT sequence linked to the KC sequence. Finally, the CT molecule is released by amidating cleavage at the Gly-Lys-Lys-Arg site. In fact, experimental results suggest that proteolytic enzymes might act first to liberate a "glycine-extended" CT (CT-Gly), which would subsequently serve as a substrate for conversion to the C-terminal prolinamide mature CT [10].

We produced monoclonal antipeptide antibodies by immunizing mice with different tetanus-toxoid-conjugated synthetic peptides having sequences analogous to various regions of procalcitonin and its cleavage products. High-affinity antibodies were subsequently selected and the epitope recognized by these mAbs was identified. Then, using this library of high-affinity mAbs of predetermined specificity, we developed a series of monoclonal immunoradiometric assays specific to either the biosynthetic intermediates of CT or the mature hormone. New insights into the identification and measurement of CT-like circulating products and the serum values of CT have been gained from these studies, as will be discussed in this chapter.

Generation and Characterization of Monoclonal Antipeptide Antibodies

Selection of Synthetic Peptides Used as Haptens, and Production of mAbs

As haptens, synthetic peptides mimicking sequences analogous to different regions of CT and CT-related biosynthetic intermediates were used. We found that the selection of these "synthetic analogs" of natural molecules was of dramatic importance in the orientation of the immune response. Numerous rules have been edicted for guiding the choice of peptide sequences analogous to various portions of a protein, and those most likely to raise antibodies capable of binding to the cognate protein [5]. Such rules are derived from the computerized prediction of the hydrophilicity of the sequences, their native conformation, their mobility inside the protein, and their exposure at the surface of the molecule. Other parameters which influence the immunogenicity of the peptide used as a hapten include the method used for conjugation of the peptide to a protein carrier and the presence of a particular chemical group [1]. It is generally accepted that the best results are obtained using hydrophilic peptides which can adopt a folded conformation (β-turn) and correspond to regions of high atomic mobility in the protein. In this respect, the structure of CT (Fig. 2) is remarkable. First, a disulfide bridge links amino acids one and seven. Five out of

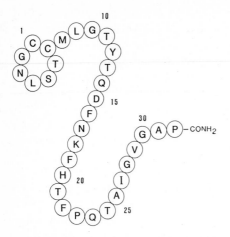

Fig. 2. Primary structure of human CT (the one-letter code was used to represent amino acid residues)

these seven amino acids are hydrophobic (Cys, Gly, Asn, Leu, and Cys), and this sequence is engaged in a ring of constrained conformation. This conjunction defines a region of poor immunogenic potential; indeed, the production of antibodies directed against the 1-10 sequence has not yet been reported. Second, the central portion of the molecule (residues 8–22) adopts an amphiphilic helical conformation: one side of the α-helix bears hydrophilic amino acid side chains, whereas the other bears hydrophobic residues [26]. Third, the mature hormone bears a prolinamide at the C-terminal residue, and this region of the molecule is what distinguishes CT from its precursors, as in the case of other peptide hormones [13].

We have generated a library of synthetic peptides encompassing different regions of CT and its precursors, and bearing various chemical modifications. Figure 3 depicts these peptides, which were assembled by the solid-phase method [27] using an "Applied Biosystems Model 430A" peptide synthesizer and t-Boc strategy. Two solid-phase resins were used for obtaining either $CONH_2$ peptides or COOH peptides. After synthesis, the peptides were deprotected, cleaved, and purified. A detailed description of the corresponding steps has been published elsewhere [6, 30]. The sequences of these peptides corresponded to the following: (1) CT and subfragments of CT designated as PCG-10, PTP-13, PNP-16, PQP-9, PAP-7, and PIP-6; (2) glycine-extended fragments of CT designated as PAG-8, PKG-16, and PTG-23; (3) KC (PDN-21) and subfragments of KC identified as PDR-11 and PPN-10; a tyrosine residue was also added at the N-terminus of KC to facilitate the iodination of the peptide; this peptide was designated PYN-22; and (4) the 34, 47, and 57 C-terminal amino acid regions of procalcitonin, designated as PQN-34, PTN-47, and PCN-57, respectively. The identity and purity of the peptides was carefully checked by performing amino acid analysis and high-performance liquid chro-

	Designation
CGNLSTCMLGTYTQDFNKFHTFPQTAIGVGAP*	CT
CGNLSTCMLG	PCG-10
TYTQDFNKFHTFP	PTP-13
TYTQDFNKFHTFPQTAIGVGAPG	PTG-23
NKFHTFPQTAIGVGAP*	PNP-16
KFHTFPQTAIGVGAPG	PKG-16
QTAIGVGAP*	PQP-9
AIGVGAP*	PAP-7(*)
AIGVGAP	PAP-7
IGVGAP*	PIP-6
AIGVGAPG	PAG-8
QTAIGVGAPGKKRDMSSDLERDHRPHVSMPQNAN	PQN-34
TYTQDFNKFHTFPQTAIGVGAPGKKRDMSSDLERDHRPHVSMPQNAN	PTN-47
CGNLSTCMLGTYTQDFNKFHTFPQTAIGVGAPGKKRDMSSDLERDHRPHVSMPQNAN	PCN-57
YDMSSDLERDHRPHVSMPQNAN	PYN-22
DMSSDLERDHRPHVSMPQNAN	PDN-21
DMSSDLERDHR	PDR-11
PHVSMPQNAN	PPN-10

Fig. 3. Amino acid sequence of synthetic peptides used in this study (the one-letter code was used to represent amino acid residues). *Asterisk* identifies peptides bearing a carboxamide function at the C-terminus

matography (HPLC); in addition, fast-atom bombardment mass spectrometry was used when the peptide was of suitable size.

We prepared four distinct immunogens by separately linking CT, KC, PQN-34, and PKG-16 to tetanus toxoid (TT) using glutaraldehyde as a coupling agent [2]. The CT-TT conjugate was used for obtaining monoclonal anti-CT antibodies; KC-TT and PQN-34-TT conjugates were used for obtaining monoclonal anti-KC antibodies and, finally, the PKG-16-TT conjugate was used for the generation of anti-PKG-16 antibodies. Antibodies were obtained by immunizing Biozzi high-responder mice [8] with the conjugates according to a procedure involving four injections, of 15, 20, or 50 µg peptide each, by the following consecutive routes: subcutaneous (s.c.) in Freund's complete adjuvant (FCA), s.c. in Freund's incomplete adjuvant (FIA), intraperitoneal (i.p.) in FIA, and then intravenous (i.v.) in saline. The immunization schedules used for PKG-16-TT, KC-TT, PQN-34-TT, and CT-TT spanned 19, 28, 35, and 90 weeks, respectively. As with other immunogens [3, 4, 39], it was considered important to use a long interval between the primary and booster immunizations in order to select for high-affinity antibodies. Three days after the last i.v. injection of conjugate, splenocytes from immunized mice were fused with the NS1 mouse

Table 1. Immunochemical characteristics of monoclonal antipeptide antibodies

Immunogens	Antibody	Isotype	Affinity constant (M^{-1})
CT-TT	CT07	IgG$_2$	0.9×10^{10} (to CT)
CT-TT	CT08	IgG$_1$	3.0×10^{10} (to CT)
KC-TT	KC01	IgG$_1$	1.5×10^{9} (to KC)
PQN-34-TT	KC04	IgG$_1$	3.0×10^{8} (to KC)
PKG-16-TT	CT19	IgG$_1$	6.8×10^{7} (to PKG-16)
PKG-16-TT	CT20	IgG$_1$	6.1×10^{7} (to PKG-16)

myeloma cell line using polyethylene glycol, and hybridoma supernatants were screened for specific antibody production using an enzyme-linked immunoadsorbent assay (ELISA) system (see next section). The antibody-secreting hybridomas were cloned twice by limiting dilution. We obtained large amounts of monoclonal immunoglobulins by using protein-A affinity chromatography of ascitic fluids produced after i.p. inoculation of nude mice with 5×10^5 hybridoma cells [24].

Using this strategy, we generated a large library of monoclonal antipeptide antibodies and then estimated the affinity constant of these antibodies using RIAs. For this purpose, radiolabeling of CT and PYN-22 with ^{125}I was performed using the Iodogen reagent [15, 29]. The PKG-16 synthetic peptide did not include a tyrosine residue and was therefore radiolabeled according to the technique described by Bolton and Hunter [9]. Radiolabeled peptides were incubated with serial dilutions of monoclonal antibody overnight at 4°C with radiolabeled peptides, and the reaction was stopped either by precipitating the unbound labeled peptide by addition of dextran-coated charcoal, in the case of [^{125}I]CT or [^{125}I]PYN-22, or by precipitating antibody-bound labeled peptide using polyethylene glycol, in the case of [^{125}I]PKG16. The affinity constant of monoclonal antibodies was evaluated from RIA-binding data [41]. Table 1 summarizes the immunochemical characteristics of some of the antibodies we obtained. It is noteworthy that the affinity constant of these monoclonal antipeptide antibodies was higher than $10^7/M$, whereas the binding of antibodies to free peptides is usually marked by relatively low affinity, in the 10^4 to $10^7/M$ range [20]. Indeed, four out of our six mAbs display an affinity constant of between 3×10^8 and $3 \times 10^{10}/M$. While it is true that these antibodies were selected from a broad library of antipeptide mAbs, we nonetheless confirm that a monoclonal antipeptide antibody of high affinity can be raised using, as immunogen, synthetic peptides conjugated to a carrier [4].

Immunochemical Mapping of Calcitonin and Related Peptides

In order to determine precisely the antigenic regions recognized by monoclonal antipeptide antibodies, we used a panel of different techniques including ELISA, competitive inhibition ELISA, and competitive RIA.

First, we evaluated the direct binding of mAbs to peptides immobilized on solid-phase support by ELISA, as previously described [6, 29]. Briefly, peptide-coated microtiter plates were incubated with the mAbs, and binding was revealed using peroxidase-conjugated anti-mouse immunoglobulin rabbit anti-serum and O-phenylenediamine as a chromogenic substrate. The reaction could be quantified by measuring optical density at 492 nm. We used this technique as a screening method for hybridomas, as well as to evaluate the binding of mAbs to various peptides. In our hands, it was extremely sensitive and could even detect the binding of low-affinity mAbs which were not reactive in liquid-phase RIA [31, 33]. Results of ELISA enabled us to distinguish between two categories of anti-CT mAbs: one, represented by antibody CT08, bound to CT, PQN-34, PTN-47, and PCN-57; this category of antibody bound to an epitope common to all these peptides. Another category, represented by antibody CT07, bound to CT, but not to peptides with sequences mimicking precursors, and recognized an epitope restricted to mature CT.

These results indicated that CT bore at least two different epitopes. We attempted more precisely to map these epitopes using subpeptides. However, with this technique, we obtained unreproducible results with short-sized peptides (less than 15 amino acids) (P. Motté, P. Ghillani, D. Bellet, unpublished data). In addition, it did not make possible the computation of an affinity constant of the antibody for a given peptide. We therefore designed competitive inhibition ELISA to investigate the reaction of mAbs with short peptide sequences and to locate antigenic determinants. Various competitor peptides were incubated at concentrations ranging from 10^{-4} to 10^{-10} M with the monoclonal antibody of choice prior to the ELISA reaction. In order to rank peptide reactivities with a given antibody, we defined the inhibiting concentration 50% (IC_{50}) as the competitor concentration of peptide yielding 50% inhibition of antibody binding to a peptide-coated plate [30]. Likewise, liquid-phase competitive inhibition assays were designed: binding of an antibody to a ^{125}I-labeled peptide was inhibited by increasing concentrations of unlabeled peptides. Likewise, these reactions were quantified by defining the inhibitory dose 50% (ID_{50}) as the dose of peptide inhibiting 50% binding of the mAb to the labeled synthetic peptide [18]. This panel of techniques enabled us to locate precisely the antigenic site recognized by mAbs (Table 2).

In terms of their specificity toward biosynthetic intermediates of CT biosynthesis, our library of mAbs may be divided into four categories. First, mAbs CT08, KC01, and KC04 recognize antigenic regions shared by procalcitonin and by either CT (CT08) or KC (KC01 and KC04). Second, mAb CT20 recognizes an epitope specifically expressed by CT-Gly; this epitope is not shared by either procalcitonin or the mature hormone. Third, mAb CT19 binds to an epitope present on the CT-Gly peptide; this epitope is partially expressed by mature CT, but is not accessible on procalcitonin. Finally, mAb CT07 is directed to an antigenic determinant present only on the mature hormone, but absent from the prohormone. The location of amino acid sequences recognized by these mAbs is schematized in Fig. 4. MAbs CT07, CT08, KC01, KC04, and CT20 are directed against amino acid sequences shorter than 11 residues; these

Table 2. Location of epitope of mAbs

Antibody	Amino acid region
CT07	CT 26-32 NH_2^a
CT08	CT 11-17
KC01	KC 1-11
KC04	KC 12-21
CT19	CT $(18\text{-}26)^b$ + CT-Gly (26-33)
CT20	CT-Gly (26-33)

[a] Binding of CT07 to its epitope requires the presence of a prolinamide residue at the C-terminus
[b] Amino acids involved in the binding of CT19 to the 18-26 region of CT could not be assigned with precision

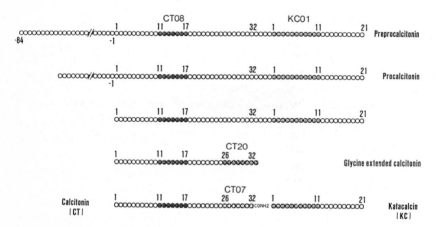

Fig. 4. Schematic representation of antibody-binding regions recognized by monoclonal antipeptide antibodies.

mAbs are probably directed to segmental (continuous) sites usually considered as corresponding to approximately seven residues [5]. In contrast, it is likely that the epitope recognized by CT19 is a topographic (discontinuous) antigenic determinant: this epitope includes residues of the C-terminal octapeptide of CT-Gly, in addition to some residues of the 18-26 region of CT; moreover, we previously described the identification of a distinct topographic site in this region of the procalcitonin molecule [30]. Thus, the presence of peculiar amino acids in this region might create a β-turn folding of procalcitonin and favor the existence of such antigenic determinants [5, 12]. Monoclonal antibodies CT08, KC01, KC04, and CT19 recognize antigenic regions shared by closely related peptides. In contrast, CT07 and CT20 recognize epitopes restricted to either CT or CT-Gly, respectively. It must be emphasized that this restricted specificity is due to the unique recognition of either one amino acid (CT20) or one chemical group (CT07). These results illustrate the selectivity of the immunochemical mapping techniques used in this study.

Design of Two-Site Monoclonal Immunoradiometric Assays

Having produced a library of high-affinity mAbs that recognized distinct epitopes on CT and related peptides, we investigated the possibility of constructing monoclonal immunoradiometric assays specific for mature CT and other intermediates of CT biosynthesis. Such assays have been successfully used in other models and provide both high specificity and high sensitivity [4, 34]. Briefly, "capture" solid-phase supports were prepared by adsorbing mAbs onto polystyrene beads. A serum sample or synthetic peptide diluted in pooled normal human serum and used as standard was incubated with the capture antibody-coated solid-phase support, and molecules bound to the antibody-coated beads were detected using 10^5 cpm of a ^{125}I-radioiodinated second mAb, designated as indicator antibody. Finally, the beads were washed and the bound radioactivity was counted. Nonspecific binding was calculated as the mean counts per minute bound in samples with no synthetic peptide added, and results were expressed as signal-to-noise ratio (S/N). The limit of detection was defined as the lowest dose of synthetic peptide yielding a S/N ratio of 2, corresponding to approximately five standard deviations of the mean to the negative sample.

Two-Site Immunoradiometric Assay for Calcitonin

We hypothesized that a two-site monoclonal immunoradiometric assay (mIRMA) based on the use of an antibody directed to the C-terminus of CT could make possible the specific recognition of mature CT in biological media. Several mAb combinations were tested, and it was observed that the amplitude of the signal generated in such assays was dependent upon the affinities of both the capture and the indicator antibody: the higher the affinities, the lower the dose of CT which could be detected. In order to obtain optimal sensitivity, CT07 and CT08 were selected as capture and indicator antibody, respectively. Using overnight incubation and 200 µl as the sample volume, the limit of detection was 10 pg/ml CT. Using various experimental approaches, we also demonstrated that this assay was indeed specific for mature CT [18, 32, 33]. First, no signal was generated when peptides analogous to CT precursors and lacking the C-terminal carboxamide residue were tested. Second, it was possible specifically to recognize mature CT in the presence of its precursors; indeed, binding of CT to the CT07-CT08 combination was not modified when either PTN-47 or PTG-23 synthetic peptides were added in the incubation medium up to a 10^5-fold molar excess. Moreover, these data were confirmed by studying the immunoreactive profile detected in the serum by the CT07-CT08 assay. Native serum displayed several peaks of immunoreactivity of various molecular weights; however, the immunoreactivity coeluted with monomeric CT after guanidine denaturation and dithiotreitol reduction (Fig. 5). Taken together, these results demonstrate that the CT07-CT08 assay is specific for mature CT even in the presence of other species related to CT. It is noteworthy that this assay does not require either extraction or concentration of the sample to achieve its sensitivity and specificity. Also, as the C-terminal carboxamide is mandatory for biological activity of CT, the CT07-CT08 assay may be used for the measurement of the circulating active hormone. The analytical performances of this assay were excellent (F. Troalen, P. Ghillani, L. Fougeat, C. Bohuon, unpublished data) and are reported in Tables 3 and 4.

In a clinical evaluation of this assay [33], the normal range in healthy subjects was found to be < 10 pg/ml. We have used this assay mainly for screening and controlling medullary carcinoma of the thyroid (MCT), and have found it to be extremely sensitive in detecting small tumors in high-risk families;

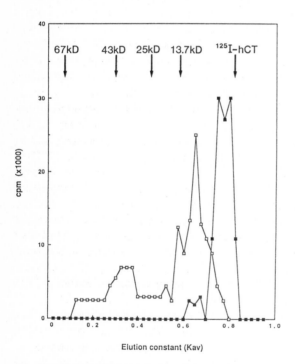

Fig. 5. Immunoreactive profile defined by mIRMAs CT07-CT08 (*solid symbols*) and KC01-CT08 (*open symbols*) in serum of a patient with MCT, after guanidine denaturation, reduction by alkylation, and gel filtration on a Sephadex G-75 column as described by Motté et al. [29]

Table 3. Intraassay coefficient of variation (CV) of the CT07-CT08 mIRMA for CT

Sample concentration (pg/ml)	0	16.3	72	1776
Number of repeats	14	15	15	15
Standard deviation	12.1	16.5	44.2	958
CV (%)	32.7	9.1	4.9	2.5

Table 4. Recovery of added CT to a serum sample containing 60.3 pg/ml CT

Added (pg/ml)	3.35	18	170	890
Recovery (%)	98	91	75	94

indeed, we were able to detect the presence of a 1.3-mm-diameter tumor burden in a 15-year-old male solely on the basis of CT level measurement using the monoclonal CT07-CT08 assay, whereas CT was not detectable using classic RIAs. Useful information has also been obtained from a retrospective study involving 59 patients followed at the Institut Gustave-Roussy for more than 20 years. We found that the postoperative CT level was an excellent indicator of cervical lymph node (CLN) involvement: patients with CLN involvement at the time of surgery had significantly elevated serum CT levels after surgery, and their CT levels were increased by pentagastrin stimulation. We also explored 289 subjects from 74 at-risk families, with each family including at least one subject bearing MTC (J.P. Travagli, P. Gardet, M. Schlumberger, P. Motté, B. Caillou, C. Parmentier, unpublished data). Serum CT levels were measured using both a classic polyclonal RIA (RIA-MatII, Mallinkrodt) and CT07-CT08 mIRMA. Out of 289 subjects, 15 underwent total thyroidectomy with neck dissection. Presurgery basal CT levels were abnormal in only 1/15 patients when using RIA; in contrast, using CT07-CT08 mIRMA, 15/15 patients had abnormal CT levels. Pentagastrin stimulation tests were also performed in these subjects: 11/15 subjects had abnormal results using RIA whereas 15/15 patients had abnormal results using mIRMA. Anatomopathological examination of surgical specimens revealed carcinomatous foci in 13/15 patients; such foci were associated with C-cell hyperplasia in 11/13 subjects. Strikingly, the other two patients had evidence only of bilateral C-cell hyperplasia without tumoral foci. Basal and pentagastrin-stimulated CT levels were found to be in the normal range at 6–95 months after surgery for 15/15 patients using mIRMA. The use of monoclonal antipeptide antibodies for the assay of CT thus provided a reliable basis for the detection and treatment of MTC at a pretumoral stage. Moreover, we are hopeful that the use of detection techniques which are more sensitive than radioisotopes, such as enzyme amplification [36], will enable CT levels to be evaluated under physiological conditions.

Two-Site Immunoradiometric Assay for Calcitonin Precursors

A similar concept was applied to the measurement of CT precursors in serum. Monoclonal antibodies KC01 and CT08 were used to develop an assay that detected CT precursors. KC01 was used as capture antibody and CT08 as radiolabeled indicator; thus, only species which simultaneously bore a KC-associated and CT-associated epitope, i.e., CT precursors, could generate a signal in this assay. Indeed, we showed that only peptides PTN-47 and PCN-57 did so, whereas mature CT, KC, and CT-glycine did not. We also demonstrated that the signal generated by PTN-47 was not significantly modified when either mature CT or CT-glycine was added in the medium up to a 25 000-fold molar excess. The sensitivity of this assay was 100 pg/ml PTN-47 synthetic peptide [18]. In a preliminary clinical evaluation of this assay, we found no detectable procalcitonin in the serum of normal subjects. In contrast, there was constant elevation of procalcitonin in MCT patients. In the latter, procalcitonin and CT were simultaneously present in serum. The immunoreactive profile was studied using this assay, and the pattern confirmed the presence of CT biosynthetic precursors in serum of patients bearing MCT (Fig. 5).

We also found that the procalcitonin level was increased after pentagastrin stimulation; the peak/basal ratio was lower than values obtained in the CT assay. The usefulness of this assay for early detection and monitoring of MCT and its relevance to other CT-secreting tumors is currently under investigation.

Two-Site Immunoradiometric Assay for CT-Glycine

Finally, we investigated the possibility of developing an assay specific for the putative CT-Gly intermediate. For this purpose, CT20 was used as a capture antibody and CT08 as indicator. This combination enabled a dose of 100 pg/ml CT-glycine to be detected in serum. As already observed with the other two mAb-based assays, the presence of CT or procalcitonin in the incubation medium did not significantly alter the binding of CT-glycine to the CT20-CT08 combination.

Early attempts to assay CT-glycine in serum showed an absence of this species in normal serum, but a significant elevation in MCT patients with high serum CT levels. The significance of the presence of CT-glycine is currently under study; however, it strongly suggests that CT-glycine is a biosynthetic intermediate leading to mature CT.

Conclusions

We have produced and characterized a library of mAbs directed against several distinct epitopes of CT and its precursors. Special attention has been paid to the design of immunization procedures, carefully selecting the composition and structure of peptides used as haptens, strictly controlling each step in the synthesis of peptides and their conjugation, and, finally, monitoring the antibody response of the animals. Our strategy has led to the selection of high-affinity monoclonal antipeptide antibodies. The epitope-binding region recognized by each antibody has been precisely determined using a panel of different techniques, including solid-phase and liquid-phase assays. In addition, we have designed new methods for the measurement of CT-related peptides in biological media with distinct specificities for CT precursors, CT-glycine intermediate, and mature CT, respectively. The restricted specificity of these assays has been established by testing the reactivities of different peptides and the assays have been used to define the immunoreactive profile detected in the serum. Finally, we have conducted clinical validation of the CT-specific assay, and are currently evaluating the other two assays.

The use of high-affinity mAbs of predetermined specificity enables immuno-radiometric assays to be developed which have both high sensitivity and defined specificity. This study confirms the advantage of such assays, as previously demonstrated for glycoproteins such as human chorionic gonadotropin [4, 34] and thyroglobulin (M. Schlumberger et al., unpublished data). In our opinion, the CT07-CT08 assay has a definite advantage in that it is specific for mature CT, thus providing a clear-cut difference between the normal and pathological state, compared with RIAs. Of immediate benefit to the patients is, of course, the earlier detection of tumors and even pretumoral foci. In the near future, it is likely that a combination of improved immunoassays and genetic probes will make highly accurate screening of families possible, and will provide physicians and surgeons with safer diagnoses [16]. Finally, we are confident that this approach may eventually be applied to other molecules, including certain hormones and tumor-associated antigens.

Acknowledgments. This work was supported by grants from the Association pour la Recherche sur le Cancer (ARC), and from the Institut Gustave-Roussy, Villejuif (France). P. Motté was the recipient of a Research Fellowship from ARC. The authors wish to thank Dr. G. Alberici for his help in peptide synthesis; Drs B. Caillou, P. Gardet, C. Parmentier, P. Rougier, M. Schlumberger, and J.P. Travagli for their help in clinical studies; and J.L. Bobot, L. Fougeat, and Y. Smith for their technical assistance.

References

1. Alberici G, Freier C, Pallardy M, Motté P (1988) Anti-hapten antibodies. Biofutur 70:57–60
2. Audibert F, Jolivet M, Chedid L, Arnon R, Sela M (1982) Successful immunization with a totally synthetic diphtheria vaccine. Proc Natl Acad Sci USA 79:5042–5046
3. Bellet D, Schlumberger M, Bidart JM, Assicot M, Caillou B, Motté P, Vignal A,

Bohuon C (1983) Production and in vitro utilization of monoclonal antibodies to human thyroglobulin. J Clin Endocrinol Metab 56:530–533

4. Bellet DH, Ozturk M, Bidart JM, Bohuon CJ, Wands JR (1986) Sensitive and specific assay for human chorionic gonadotropin (hCG) based on anti-peptide and anti-hCG monoclonal antibodies: construction and clinical implications. J Clin Endocrinol Metab 63:1319–1327

5. Berzofski JA (1985) Intrinsic and extrinsic factors in protein antigenic structure. Science 229:932–937

6. Bidart JM, Ozturk M, Bellet DH, Jolivet M, Gras-Masse H, Troalen F, Bohuon CJ, Wands JR (1985) Identification of epitopes associated with hCG and the β-hCG carboyl terminus by monoclonal antibodies produced against a synthetic peptide. J Immunol 134:457–464

7. Bikle DD (ed) (1983) Assays for calcium-regulating hormones. Springer, Berlin Heidelberg New York

8. Biozzi G, Asofsky R, Leiberman R, Stiffel G, Mouton D, Benacerraf B (1970) Serum concentrations and allotypes of immunoglobulins in two lines of mice genetically selected for "high" and "low" antibody synthesis. J Exp Med 132:752–764

9. Bolton AE, Hunter WM (1973) The labelling of proteins to high specific radioactivities by conjugation to a ^{125}I-containing acylating agent. Biochem J 133:529–535

10. Bradbury AF, Finnie MD, Smyth DG (1982) Mechanism of C-terminal amide formation by pituitary enzymes. Nature 298:686–689

11. Catherwood BD, Deftos LJ (1984) General principles, problems and interpretation in the radioimmunoassay of calcitonin. Biomed Pharmacother 38:235–241

12. Chou PY, Fasman GD (1978) Prediction of the secondary structure of proteins from their amino acid sequence. Adv Enzymol 47:45–55

13. Del Valle J, Sugano K, Yamada T (1987) Progastrin and its glycine-extended post-translational processing intermediates in human gastrointestinal tissues. Gastroenterology 92:1908–1912

14. Foster GV, Baghdiantz A, Kumar MA, Slack E, Soliman HA, McIntyre I (1964) Thyroid origin of malignancy. Nature 202:1303–1305

15. Fraker PJ, Speck JC (1978) Protein and cell membrane iodination with a sparingly soluble chloramide 1,3,4,6-tetrachloro 3a,6a-diphenylglycoluryl. Biochem Biophys Res Commun 80:849–860

16. Gagel RF, Tashjian AH Jr, Cummings T, Papathanasopoulos N, Kaplan MM, DeLellis RA, Wolfe HJ, Reichlin S (1988) The clinical outcome of prospective screening for multiple endocrine neoplasia type 2A. An 18-year experience. N Engl J Med 318:478–484

17. Gardet P, Parmentier C (1984) Le cancer médullaire de la thyroide. Protocole de détection, de traitement, et de surveillance proposé par le GETC. In: Lemerle J (ed) Actualités carcinologiques. Masson, Paris, pp 69–78

18. Ghillani P, Motté P, Bohuon C, Bellet D (1988) Monoclonal anti-peptide antibodies as tools to dissect closely related gene products: a model using peptides encoded by the calcitonin gene. J Immunol 141:3156–3163

19. Goltzman D, Tischler AS (1978) Characterization of the immunochemical forms of calcitonin released by a medullary thyroid carcinoma in tissue culture. J Clin Invest 61:449–456

20. Gose AC, Karush F (1988) Induction of polyclonal antibody responses to cholera toxin by the synthetic peptide approach. J Immunol 25:223–229

21. Hazard JD, Hawk WA, Crile C Jr (1959) Medullary (solid) carcinoma of the thyroid: a clinicopathologic entity. J Clin Endocrinol Metab 19:152–161

22. Leff SE, Evans RM, Rosenfeld MG (1987) Splice commitment dictates neuron-specific alternative RNA processing in calcitonin/CGRP gene expression. Cell 48:517–524

23. Le Moullec JM, Julienne A, Chenais J, Lasmoles F, Guliana JM, Milhaud G, Moukhtar MS (1984) The complete sequence of human preprocalcitonin. FEBS Lett 167:93–97

24. Manil L, Motté P, Pernas P, Troalen F, Bohuon C, Bellet D (1986) Evaluation of protocols for purification of mouse monoclonal antibodies. Yield and purity in two dimensional gel electrophoresis. J Immunol Methods 90:25–37

25. Mathew CGP, Chin KS, Easton DF, Thorpe K et al. (1987) A linked genetic marker for multiple endocrine neoplasia type 2A on chromosome 10. Nature 328:527–528

26. McIntyre I, Girgis SI, Hillyard CJ (1984) Essential steps in the measurement of normal circulating levels of calcitonin. Biomed Pharmacother 38:230–234

27. Merrifield RB (1986) Solid phase synthesis. Science 232:341–352

28. Moe A, Kaiser BC (1985) Design, synthesis, and activity of peptides with calcitonin-like structure. Biochemistry 24:112–125

29. Motté P, Vauzelle P, Alberici G, Troalen F, Bohuon C, Bellet D (1986) Radio-iodination of human calcitonin using the iodogen reagent. J Immunol Methods 87:223–227

30. Motté P, Alberici G, Ait-Abdellah M, Bellet D (1987a) Monoclonal antibodies distinguish synthetic peptides that differ in one chemical group. J Immunol 138:3332–3338

31. Motté P, Alberici G, Ait-Abdellah M, Bohuon C, Bellet D (1987b) Utilization of synthetic peptides in the study of calcitonin and biosynthetic precursors for calcitonin. Nucl Med Biol 14:289–294

32. Motté P, Ait-Abdellah M, Vauzelle P, Gardet P, Bohuon C, Bellet D (1987c) A two-site immunoradiometric assay for serum calcitonin using monoclonal anti-peptide antibodies. Henry Ford Hosp Med J 35:129–132

33. Motté P, Vauzelle P, Gardet P, Ghillani P, Caillou B, Parmentier C, Bohuon C, Bellet D (1988) Construction and clinical validation of a sensitive and specific assay for serum mature calcitonin using monoclonal anti-peptide antibodies. Clin Chim Acta 174:35–54

34. Ozturk M, Berkowitz R, Goldstein D, Bellet D, Wands JR (1988) Differential production of hCG and free subunits in gestational trophoblastic disease. Am J Obstet Gynecol 158:193–198

35. Pearse AGE (1966) The cytochemistry of the thyroid C-cells and their relationship to calcitonin. Proc R Soc Lond [Biol] 164:478–487

36. Seth R, Motté P, Wimalawansa S, Kehely A, Self CH, Bellet D, Bohuon C, MacIntyre I (1988) A sensitive and specific two-site enzyme-immunoassay for human calcitonin using monoclonal antibodies. J Endocrinol 119:351–357

37. Simpson NE, Kidd KK, Goodfellow PJ, McDermid H et al. (1987) Assignment of multiple endocrine neoplasia type 2A to chromosome 10 by linkage. Nature 328:528–530

38. Sipple JH (1984) MEN 2 syndromes: historical perspectives. Henry Ford Hosp Med J 32:219–221

39. Takahashi H, Wands JR (1988) Development of monoclonal antibodies to hepatitis

B virus. In: Young H, McMillan A (ed) Immunological diagnosis of sexually transmitted diseases. Dekker, New York, pp 451–469

40. Tashjian AH Jr, Howland BG, Melvin KEW, Hill CS (1970) Immunoassay of human calcitonin. Clinical measurement, relation to serum calcium and studies in patients with medullary carcinoma. N Engl J Med 285:1115–1120

41. Van Heyningen VD, Brock JH, Van Heyningen S (1983) A simple method for ranking the affinities of monoclonal antibodies. J Immunol Methods 62:147–157

42. Williams ED (1966) Histogenesis of medullary carcinoma of the thyroid. J Clin Pathol 19:114–118

Subject Index